Breast Disease (Second Series) Test and Syllabus

Edward A. Sickles, M.D.
Section Chairman

Judy M. Destouet, M.D.
G. W. Eklund, M.D.
Stephen A. Feig, M.D.
Valerie P. Jackson, M.D.

 American College of Radiology
Reston, Virginia   1993

Sets Published

Chest Disease	Diagnostic Ultrasound
Bone Disease	Breast Disease
Genitourinary Tract Disease	Bone Disease IV
Gastrointestinal Disease	Pediatric Disease III
Head and Neck Disorders	Chest Disease IV
Pediatric Disease	Neuroradiology
Nuclear Radiology	Gastrointestinal Disease IV
Radiation Pathology and	Nuclear Radiology IV
Radiation Biology	Magnetic Resonance
Chest Disease II	Radiation Bioeffects and
Bone Disease II	Management
Genitourinary Tract Disease II	Genitourinary Tract Disease IV
Gastrointestinal Disease II	Head and Neck Disorders IV
Head and Neck Disorders II	Pediatric Disease IV
Nuclear Radiology II	Breast Disease II
Cardiovascular Disease	
Emergency Radiology	**Sets in Preparation**
Bone Disease III	Musculoskeletal Disease
Gastrointestinal Disease III	Diagnostic Ultrasonography II
Chest Disease III	Chest Disease V
Pediatric Disease II	Neuroradiology II
Nuclear Radiology III	Gastrointestinal Disease V
Head and Neck Disorders III	Emergency Radiology II
Genitourinary Tract Disease III	Nuclear Radiology V

Note: While the American College of Radiology and the editors of this publication have attempted to include the most current and accurate information possible, errors may inadvertently appear. Diagnostic and interventional decisions should be based on the individual circumstances of each case.

SET 36:
Breast Disease (Second Series) Test and Syllabus

Editor in Chief

BARRY A. SIEGEL, M.D., Professor of Radiology and Medicine and Director, Division of Nuclear Medicine, Mallinckrodt Institute of Radiology, Washington University School of Medicine, St. Louis, Missouri

Associate Editor

DAVID H. STEPHENS, M.D., Professor of Radiology, Mayo Medical School; Department of Diagnostic Radiology, Mayo Clinic, Rochester, Minnesota

Section Editor

EDWARD A. SICKLES, M.D., Professor of Radiology and Chief, Breast Imaging Section, Department of Radiology, University of California School of Medicine, San Francisco, California

Co-Authors

JUDY M. DESTOUET, M.D., Chief of Mammography, Drs. Copeland, Hyman, and Shackman, P.A., Baltimore, Maryland

G. W. EKLUND, M.D., Clinical Associate Professor of Radiology, University of Illinois College of Medicine at Peoria, and Medical Director, Susan G. Komen Breast Center, an affiliate of St. Francis Medical Center, Peoria, Illinois

STEPHEN A. FEIG, M.D., Professor of Radiology, Jefferson Medical College, and Director, Breast Imaging Center, Department of Radiology, Thomas Jefferson University Hospital, Philadelphia, Pennsylvania

VALERIE P. JACKSON, M.D., Professor of Radiology, Chief of Breast Imaging, Indiana University of School of Medicine, Indianapolis, Indiana

AMERICAN COLLEGE OF RADIOLOGY
PROFESSIONAL SELF-EVALUATION AND CONTINUING EDUCATION PROGRAM

Publishing Coordinators:	G. Rebecca Haines and Thomas M. Rogers
Administrative Assistant:	Marcy Olney
Production Editor:	Sean M. McKenna
Copy Editors:	Yvonne Strong and John N. Bell
Text Processing:	Fusako T. Nowak
Composition:	Karen Finkle
Index:	EEI, Inc., Alexandria, Va.
Lithography:	Lanman Progressive, Washington, D.C.
Typesetting:	Publication Technology Corp., Fairfax, Va.
Printing:	John D. Lucas Printing, Baltimore, Md.

Library of Congress Cataloging-in-Publication Data

Breast disease (second series) test and syllabus / Edward A. Sickles, section chairman ; Judy M. Destouet ... [et al.].

    p. cm. — (Professional self-evaluation and continuing education program; set 36)

    "Committee on Professional Self-Evaluation and Continuing Education, Commission on Education, American College of Radiology"—Cover.

    Includes bibliographical references and index.

    ISBN 1-55903-037-2 : $200.00. — ISBN 1-55903-000-3 (series)

    1. Breast radiography—Examinations, questions, etc. 2. Breast diseases—radiography—examination questions. I. Sickles, Edward A. II. Destouet, Judy M. III. American College of Radiology. Commission on Education. Committee on Professional Self-Evaluation and Continuing Education. IV. Series.

    [DNLM: W1 PR606 set 36 1993 / WP 18 B828 1993]

RG493.5.R33B74   1993

618.1'90757'076—dc20

DNLM/DLC   93-41764

for Library of Congress   CIP

Additional Contributors

KEVIN W. McENERY, M.D., Instructor of Radiology, Washington University School of Medicine, Mallinckrodt Institute of Radiology, St. Louis, Missouri

TRACY L. ROBERTS, M.D., Assistant Professor of Radiology, Breast Imaging Section, Mallinckrodt Institute of Radiology, Washington University School of Medicine, St. Louis, Missouri

Section Chairman's Preface

This is the second *Breast Disease Test and Syllabus* in the Professional Self-Evaluation and Continuing Education (PSECE) program of the American College of Radiology (ACR). The volume was written and extensively revised over a very short time span, from mid-1992 to mid-1993. As a result, when published at the end of 1993 it will be about as current as is possible for a multi-authored endeavor of such complexity.

The content of the *Breast Disease Test and Syllabus* indeed reflects the state of breast imaging in the mid-1990s. (1) Due to the almost complete disappearance of xeroradiography, all of the mammograms we display are screen-film images. (2) There is full discussion of the current role of ultrasonography, both as an aid to diagnosis and as a guide for lesion localization and percutaneous tissue sampling. (3) Particular emphasis has been placed on interventional procedures, including the use of stereotactic localization devices to facilitate sampling of nonpalpable, mammographically detected lesions. (4) Within the past year, the ACR has published a lexicon of standard terminology for mammography, in an attempt to increase the consistency and clarity of reports. We employ this new terminology throughout the volume, not only to serve as an example of how it can be used, but especially to encourage its usage by all radiologists. (5) The past several years also have brought forth a greatly increased understanding of the factors needed to produce excellent quality mammographic images, including equipment features, exposure techniques, film processing, breast positioning, and quality assurance procedures. These new concepts have been incorporated into several test questions and extensive related discussions, in order to bring the reader up to date with current practice. (6) Throughout the *Breast Disease* syllabus, we have organized the case material and discussions using a problem-oriented approach rather than the disease-oriented format that has been traditional in previous PSECE volumes. This much more closely parallels the experience encountered in clinical breast imaging, in which, for example, one will be presented with a noncalcified circumscribed (well-defined) mass, not a known fibroadenoma or simple benign cyst. The reader should find especially instructive the case on triangulating the location of lesions from their apparent positions on standard craniocaudal and mediolateral oblique views and the case on evaluating mammographic findings seen only on one standard view, since these important subjects have received little attention in prior publications.

As chairman of the committee chosen to write the *Breast Disease Test and Syllabus*, I want to acknowledge the major contributions of my fellow committee members: Drs. Judy M. Destouet, G. W. Eklund, Stephen A. Feig, and Valerie P. Jackson. They played an important role in case selection, sharing of illustrative materials, and in review and constructive criticism of all the test questions and discussions. As a result, they each have been instrumental in producing the entire volume, not just in writing the cases that bear their names as authors.

On behalf of the *Breast Disease* Committee, I also want to thank the Associate Editors of the PSECE program for their help in completing this project. Dr. Anthony V. Proto provided the ideal balance of urging and encouragement in keeping the manuscript production process running smoothly. Dr. David H. Stephens supplied many insightful comments in reviewing all of the test questions and syllabus discussions. However, the bulk of the credit goes to Dr. Barry A. Siegel, Editor in Chief of the PSECE program. His uncanny ability to identify inconsistencies and potentially confusing terminology in test questions and discussions, his absolute mastery of the English language in suggesting concise and precise corrections, and his steadfast insistence on completeness and clinical relevance all combined to hone the rough-edged document produced initially into this highly polished volume. Despite the fact that his name does not appear after any of the individually attributed cases, his contribution to each case was substantial.

Finally, acknowledgements would be incomplete without recognizing the highly competent and cheerful assistance of the ACR publications staff. Rebecca Haines supervises a very efficient and effective operation in book production. Sean M. McKenna and especially Thomas M. Rogers labored hard and long in translating typed manuscripts and photographic prints into highly readable book format and in shuttling the 25 separate manuscripts and page proofs back and forth between authors, editors, and other members of the ACR publications staff.

Edward A. Sickles, M.D.
Section Chairman

Editor's Preface

I am pleased to introduce *Diseases of the Breast (Second Series) Test and Syllabus* to the members of the American College of Radiology (ACR). This volume represents the 36th in the ACR's series of diagnostic radiology syllabi and is published as the College's Professional Self-Evaluation and Continuing Education (PSECE) Program enters its 23rd year. As is outlined more completely in Dr. Edward Sickles' preface, this syllabus is designed to provide our program participants with a problem-oriented guide to many of the most common diagnostic and management dilemmas faced by radiologists who perform breast imaging. Particular emphasis is given to the important role of the radiologist in further characterizing abnormalities detected by screening mammography and in defining what additional diagnostic or therapeutic steps are necessary in individual patients. This volume both complements and updates the information presented in the first breast disease syllabus, published in 1988, and will no doubt be an important added component of the College's broadly based programs committed to ensuring that women have access to breast imaging services of the highest quality.

Dr. Edward A. Sickles and his co-authors—Drs. Judy M. Destouet, G. W. Eklund, Stephen A. Feig and Valerie P. Jackson—have done an outstanding job of crafting this volume, and they have done so in near record time for a self-evaluation package. In large part, this reflects Ed Sickles' clear vision from the outset of the goals for this project, his mastery of a problem-oriented approach to the subject matter, his exceptional leadership of an expert team of breast imaging specialists, and his careful attention to style and editorial detail. Accordingly, working with Ed greatly lessened the editorial burdens borne by me and Dr. David H. Stephens, Associate Editor for this volume, and made our tasks both quite pleasurable and highly instructive. Ed and his co-authors have given freely and selflessly of their time and wisdom in preparing this edition, and all radiologists will be indebted to them for their consummate voluntary efforts.

The publications staff of the American College of Radiology deserve special and continuing thanks for their substantial efforts in support of the PSECE Program. G. Rebecca Haines ably leads a highly professional and competent staff. She and Thomas M. Rogers, who most directly oversees the mechanics of syllabus production, contribute greatly to the success of this program because of their absolute commitment to quality.

That they are empowered to do so is testimony to the vision of the College's leadership in its continuing support of the PSECE Program.

Finally, as editors and authors, those of us who work on behalf of this program must not lose sight of the fact that its success depends completely on the support of all radiologists, both those in practice and those in training, who seek to reap some educational benefit from our efforts. We thank these many radiologists for their collective vote of confidence.

Barry A. Siegel, M.D.
Editor in Chief

Labeling Codes

The American College of Radiology recommends the use of the following standard notations in breast radiography (Reprinted with permission from Hendrick RE, Bassett LW, Dodd GD, et al. Radiologic technologist's manual. Reston, VA: American College of Radiology; 1992:58.) The abbreviations MLO, CC, and XCCL are used throughout this test and syllabus without introduction.

ACR Labeling Codes for Positioning

	Labeling Code	Purpose
Laterality		
Right	R[a]	
Left	L[a]	
Projection / Position		
Mediolateral oblique	MLO	Standard view
Craniocaudal	CC	Standard view
90° Lateral		
Mediolateral	ML	Localize, define
Lateromedial	LM	Localize, define
Spot compression		Define
Magnification	M[a]	Define
Exaggerated craniocaudal	XCCL	Localize
Cleavage	CV	Localize
Axillary tail	AT	Localize, define
Tangential	TAN	Localize, define
Roll	RL (rolled lateral)[b]	Localize, define
	RM (rolled medial)[b]	Localize, define
Caudocranial	FB (from below)	Define
Lateromedial oblique	LMO	Define
Superolateral to inferomedial oblique	SIO	Define
Implant displaced	ID	Augmented breast

    [a]Used as a prefix before the projection. For example, RMMLO means "Right Magnification Mediolateral Oblique."

    [b]Used as a suffix after the projection. For example, LCCRL means "Left Craniocaudal Upper Breast Tissue Rolled Laterally."

Breast Disease (Second Series) Test

For you to derive the maximum benefit from this program, you should complete the following test, and send your answer sheet to the ACR for scoring, before you proceed to the syllabus.

If for any reason you refer to the syllabus material, or any other references, in answering the questions, please be sure to so indicate when answering Question 118, the first demographic question. Your score will then not be used in developing the norm tables.

NOTE: You must return your answer sheet for scoring, whether or not you use reference materials, in order to claim the 20 hours of Category I credit.

Category I credit is valid for this publication from January 1994 through January 1997. Category I credit review will be conducted in January 1997 and every three years thereafter.

CASE 1: Questions 1 through 5

This 64-year-old asymptomatic woman had mammographic screening after a normal breast physical examination. You are shown the MLO view of the right breast (Figure 1-1) and a photographic enlargement of the upper portion of this image (Figure 1-2). The finding illustrated in these mammograms was not seen on the CC view (not shown).

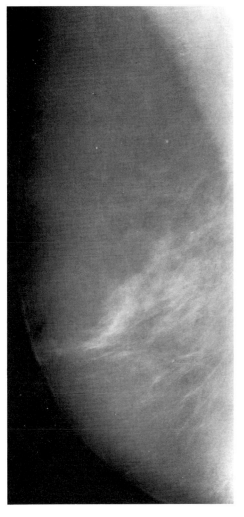

Figure 1-1

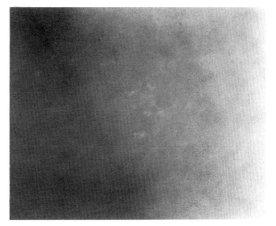

Figure 1-2

CASE 1 (Cont'd)

1. Which *one* of the following is the LEAST likely explanation for the finding?

    (A) Deodorant artifact
    (B) Dust artifact
    (C) Sclerosing adenosis
    (D) Atypical hyperplasia
    (E) Ductal carcinoma *in situ*

2. The patient was recalled for additional mammographic imaging. Which *one* of the following is the BEST sequence for obtaining additional images?

    (A) XCCL view, cleavage view, MLO view
    (B) Cleavage view, XCCL view, MLO view
    (C) XCCL view, MLO view, cleavage view
    (D) Cleavage view, MLO view, no XCCL view
    (E) XCCL view, MLO view, no cleavage view

3. The finding was seen only on the repeat MLO view. A 90° lateral view was then obtained. You are shown the entire image (Figure 1-3) and a photographic enlargement of the upper portion of the image (Figure 1-4). Which *one* of the following BEST describes the location of the mammographic finding?

    (A) Upper outer breast, between 10 o'clock and 11 o'clock
    (B) Upper outer breast, between 1 o'clock and 2 o'clock
    (C) Upper central breast, at 12 o'clock
    (D) Upper inner breast, between 10 o'clock and 11 o'clock
    (E) Upper inner breast, between 1 o'clock and 2 o'clock

4. The next step should be:

    (A) cleavage view with the X-ray tube angled 5° away from the MLO projection
    (B) XCCL view with the X-ray tube angled 5° toward the MLO projection
    (C) CC view with no breast compression
    (D) CC view
    (E) craniocaudal projection lumpogram of the upper central breast

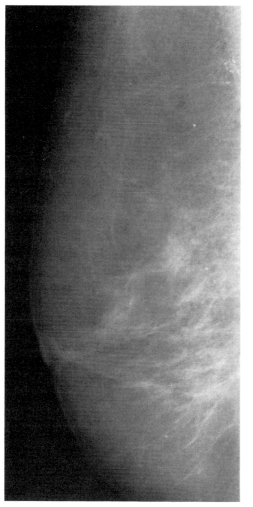

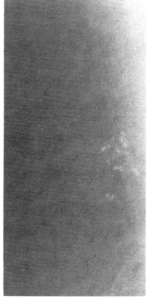

Figure 1-3   **Figure 1-4**

5. The additional view chosen in the previous question again showed the mammographic finding, but neither this view nor spot-compression magnification views portrayed it any more clearly than in Figures 1-2 and 1-4. The next step should be:

   (A) routine mammographic screening in 1 year
   (B) follow-up mammography in 6 months
   (C) breast ultrasonography
   (D) breast CT scan
   (E) preoperative needle localization

CASE 2: Questions 6 through 10

This 58-year-old asymptomatic woman underwent mammographic screening after a normal breast physical examination. You are shown the CC (Figure 2-1) and MLO (Figure 2-2) views of the left breast from that examination, as well as a photographic enlargement of a portion of the CC view (Figure 2-3).

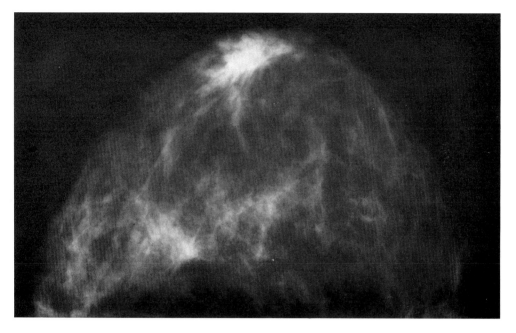

Figure 2-1

6. Which *one* of the following is the LEAST likely explanation for the mammographic findings?

   (A) Carcinoma, upper outer quadrant
   (B) Carcinoma, lower outer quadrant
   (C) Cyst
   (D) Postsurgical scar tissue
   (E) Summation shadow

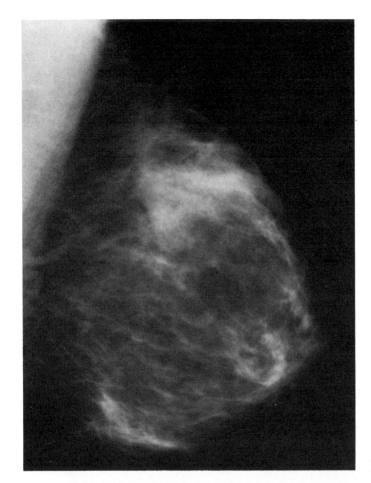

Figure 2-2

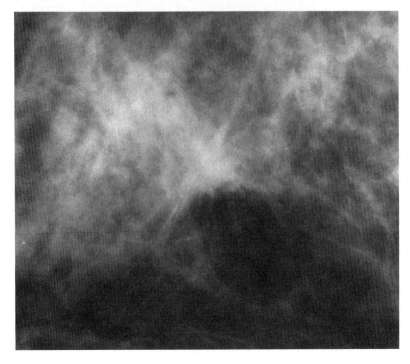

Figure 2-3

7. In the diagnosis of the lesion in the test patient, which *one* of the following should be the next step?

    (A) Routine mammographic screening in 1 year
    (B) Follow-up mammography in 6 months
    (C) Ultrasonography
    (D) Additional mammographic imaging
    (E) Needle localization

QUESTIONS 8 THROUGH 10: MARK YOUR ANSWER SHEET TRUE (T) OR FALSE (F) FOR EACH OF THE RESPONSE CHOICES.

8. Concerning ultrasonography of a nonpalpable, well-defined, 1-cm mass,

    (A) nonvisualization nearly always necessitates biopsy
    (B) identification of a solid, irregular, hypoechoic mass nearly always necessitates biopsy
    (C) Doppler imaging reliably discriminates benign from malignant masses
    (D) it generally should not be performed until the lesion is identified on at least two mammographic projections

9. Additional mammographic images likely to help differentiate a mass seen on only one standard projection from a summation shadow include:

    (A) 90° lateral view
    (B) view with 5 to 10° tube angulation from the view demonstrating the finding
    (C) tangential view
    (D) "roll" view
    (E) spot-compression view
    (F) magnification view

CASE 2 (Cont'd)

10. Concerning preoperative needle localization of a density seen on only one standard mammographic projection,

   (A) biopsy is the preferred management option when the density appears irregular and spiculated
   (B) a 90° lateral mammogram should be deferred until the day of surgery to minimize inconvenience to the patient
   (C) localization by a conventional technique cannot be performed until the mammographic density is clearly identified on an additional mammographic view
   (D) even without additional mammographic views, stereotactic localization will permit placement of a needle within the density in nearly all cases

CASE 3: Questions 11 through 14

This asymptomatic 50-year-old woman, who had a normal physical examination 2 weeks earlier, underwent baseline mammographic screening. You are shown 50° MLO (A) and CC (B) views of both breasts (Figure 3-1).

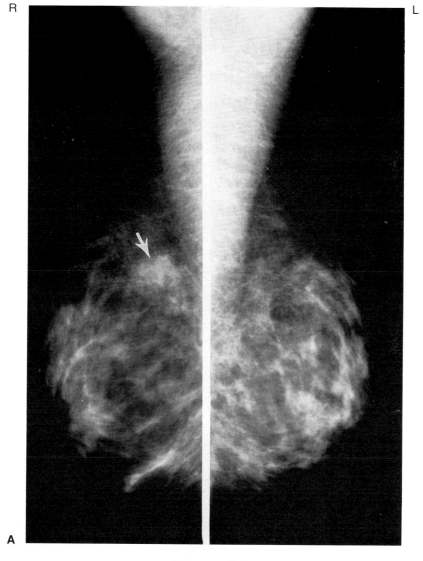

Figure 3-1

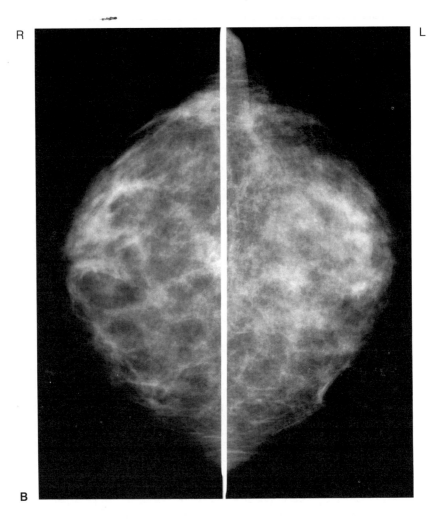

R   L

B

QUESTIONS 11 THROUGH 14: MARK YOUR ANSWER SHEET TRUE (T) OR FALSE (F) FOR EACH OF THE RESPONSE CHOICES.

11.   Plausible reasons why a poorly marginated density (arrow) is seen in the right breast only on the MLO view include the following:

    (A) it is located too far laterally to be seen on a CC image
    (B) it is located too far medially to be seen on a CC image
    (C) it is located too high in the superior portion of the breast to be seen on a CC image
    (D) it represents a summation shadow
    (E) it is masked by overlapping parenchymal elements

12. Concerning the axillary tail of the breast,

(A) it occasionally exists as an isolated density

(B) it is less frequently the site of breast cancer than is the lower medial quadrant of the breast

(C) it is less frequently the site of benign masses than is the lower medial quadrant of the breast

(D) much of this tissue can be pulled into the field of a standard CC image

13. Concerning the anticipated location of mammographically identified lesions,

(A) an upper medial lesion and a lower lateral lesion can superimpose on an MLO view

(B) a medial lesion will project in a more cephalic position with respect to the nipple on the MLO view than on the 90° lateral view

(C) a small right-breast carcinoma just under the skin, causing slight skin thickening and retraction on the inferior skin margin of an MLO image, is more likely to be located at the 4 o'clock position than at the 6 o'clock position

(D) a lesion that is 4 cm directly behind the nipple will project directly behind the nipple on both the 90° lateral and MLO views

(E) a lesion located at the 9 o'clock position in the left breast, 3 cm from the nipple, will be more sharply defined on a 90° lateromedial view than on an MLO view

14. Concerning "blind areas" associated with routine mammographic views,

(A) the upper posterior breast is usually excluded from view on the CC image

(B) medial breast tissue is usually excluded from view on the MLO image

(C) glandular tissue wrapping around the upper lateral margin of the pectoral muscle is usually excluded from view on the MLO image

(D) routine positioning at 45° virtually eliminates blind areas on the MLO image

(E) a lesion at the 6 o'clock position, 1 cm anterior to the pectoral muscle and 2 cm above the inframammary fold, will most probably be excluded from view on the CC image if the inframammary fold is elevated before the breast is positioned on the film holder

CASE 4: Questions 15 through 17

You are shown MLO (A) and CC (B) mammograms of both breasts of a 54-year-old woman (Figure 4-1). (The fingerprint artifact superimposed on the upper aspect of the right breast on the MLO view should be disregarded.)

R   L

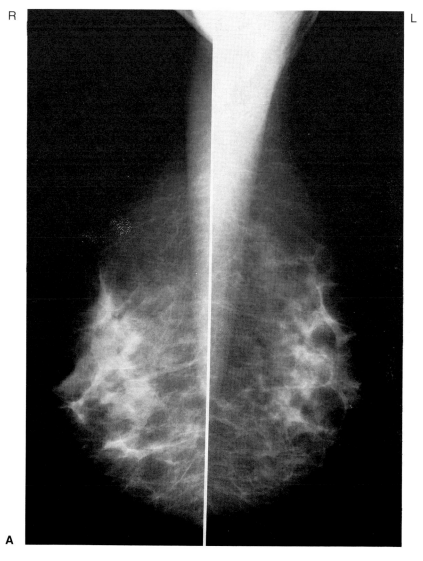

A

Figure 4-1

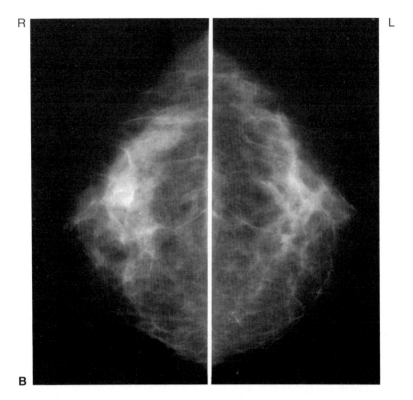

15. Which *one* of the following BEST describes the technical quality of the test images?

    (A) Underexposed with low contrast
    (B) Inadequate compression
    (C) Not enough pectoral muscle included
    (D) Motion unsharpness (blurring)
    (E) Excellent images

CASE 4 (Cont'd)

QUESTIONS 16 AND 17: MARK YOUR ANSWER SHEET TRUE (T) OR FALSE (F) FOR EACH OF THE RESPONSE CHOICES.

16. Given unacceptable motion unsharpness on a mammogram taken with the parameters of 25 kVp, +1 density setting, 320 mAs, and 5-cm compression, corrective measures that would decrease the effects of motion include:

    (A) decreasing the density setting
    (B) decreasing the kVp
    (C) use of a manual technique of 27 kVp and 250 mAs
    (D) increasing compression
    (E) moving the photocell from under dense glandular tissue to under fatty tissue

17. Concerning the phototimer in a mammographic unit,

    (A) it is located between the breast and the film
    (B) it senses the amount of radiation entering the breast
    (C) its primary function is to adjust the mA to achieve a specific film density for the selected kVp
    (D) it regulates the amount of radiation reaching the screen
    (E) its accuracy must be assessed every 6 months to meet American College of Radiology accreditation standards

CASE 5: Questions 18 through 21

You are shown a CC view of the right breast of an 82-year-old woman (Figure 5-1), which was obtained with the following technical factors: 26 kVp, 2-cm compression, 0 density setting, resulting in 28 mAs.

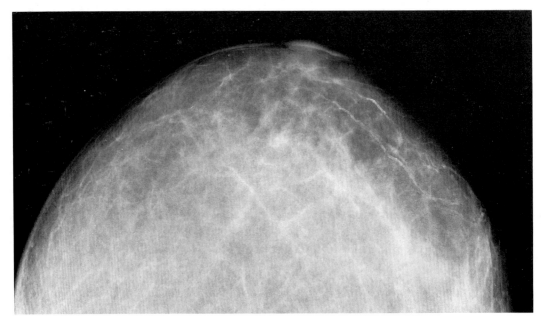

Figure 5-1

QUESTIONS 18 THROUGH 21: MARK YOUR ANSWER SHEET TRUE (T) OR FALSE (F) FOR EACH OF THE RESPONSE CHOICES.

18. Adjustments in technique that would result in an improved image include:

   (A) reducing the kVp to 23
   (B) increasing compression
   (C) changing to a manual technique of 26 kVp with 80 mAs
   (D) increasing density setting to +1

CASE 5 (Cont'd)

19. An increase in kVp with a fixed mAs would increase the:

    (A) radiation dose
    (B) exposure time
    (C) scatter radiation
    (D) image contrast
    (E) optical density of the image

20. An increase in mAs with a fixed kVp would increase the:

    (A) radiation dose
    (B) exposure time
    (C) scatter radiation
    (D) image contrast
    (E) optical density of the image

21. An increase in image contrast would be expected with the use of:

    (A) a grid
    (B) increased compression
    (C) an increase in the density setting
    (D) extended development time
    (E) a smaller focal spot

You are shown a phototimed left CC mammogram of a 57-year-old woman (Figure 6-1).

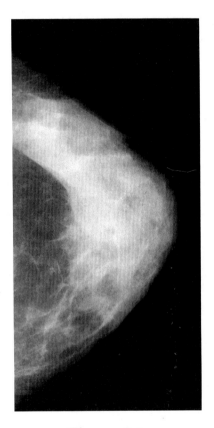

Figure 6-1

22. Which *one* of the following is the BEST explanation for the appearance of the test image?

    (A) mAs "cutoff" (tube limit exceeded)
    (B) Incompletely developed film
    (C) High kVp (>28)
    (D) Improper placement of the photocell
    (E) Parenchyma too dense for phototiming

QUESTIONS 23 THROUGH 25: MARK YOUR ANSWER SHEET TRUE (T) OR FALSE (F) FOR EACH OF THE RESPONSE CHOICES.

23. Circumstances usually requiring the use of a manual technique, as opposed to phototiming, include:

(A) imaging dermal calcifications in tangent to the skin
(B) taking a standard MLO view of an augmented breast
(C) ductography
(D) a small breast with a 3-cm fibroadenoma
(E) a large fibrofatty breast with a 3-cm lipoma

24. Concerning single-emulsion film,

(A) it has as much silver as does double-emulsion film
(B) it requires a longer development time to achieve the same optical density obtained with double-emulsion film
(C) extended developer processing prolongs the life of the X-ray tube
(D) artifacts and scratches are more commonly seen than with double-emulsion film
(E) it should be developed at 33.3°C (92°F)

25. Concerning the tube limit or mAs "cutoff" when phototiming,

(A) the Food and Drug Administration requires that mammographic units terminate exposure at 400 mAs
(B) if mAs cutoff has occurred and the film was overexposed, lowering the kVp would result in a lighter film
(C) if mAs cutoff has occurred and the film was underexposed, increasing the density by one step would result in a darker film
(D) if mAs cutoff has occurred and the film was underexposed, increasing the kVp would result in a darker film

You are shown MLO (Figure 7-1), CC (Figure 7-2), and spot-compression magnification (Figure 7-3) views of the left breast from a baseline screening mammogram of a 59-year-old woman.

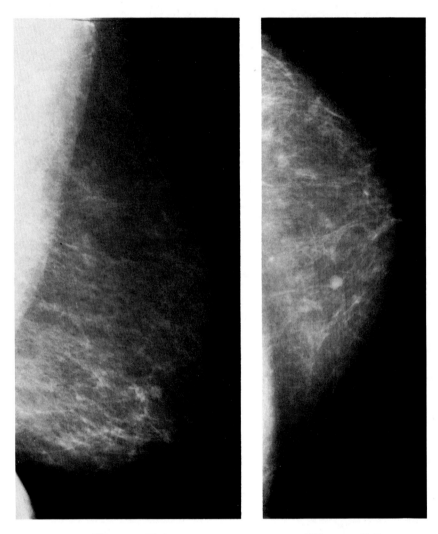

Figure 7-1   Figure 7-2

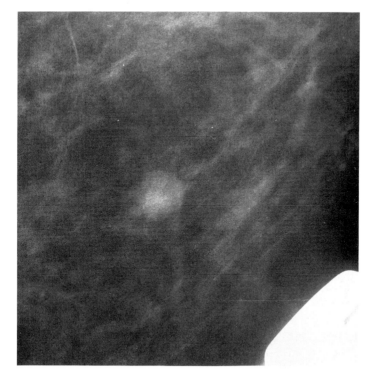

Figure 7-3

26. Which *one* of the following is the MOST appropriate next step?

    (A) Clinical correlation
    (B) Follow-up mammography in 3 months
    (C) Follow-up mammography in 6 months
    (D) Routine mammographic screening in 1 year
    (E) Surgical biopsy

27. The probability of carcinoma in a nonpalpable, completely smooth, noncalcified solid mass less than 1 cm in diameter is:

    (A) 2%
    (B) 5%
    (C) 10%
    (D) 20%
    (E) 30%

28. Follow-up mammography in 6 months is MOST appropriate for which *one* of the following lesions?

    (A) 1-cm cyst
    (B) 7-mm completely smooth, noncalcified mass
    (C) 3-cm smooth noncalcified mass
    (D) 1.3-cm ill-defined noncalcified mass
    (E) 1.5-cm smooth noncalcified mass with mixed fat and soft tissue density

This 43-year-old woman presented with pain in the left breast. You are shown a spot-compression magnification CC view of the left breast (Figure 8-1). She has had no prior mammograms.

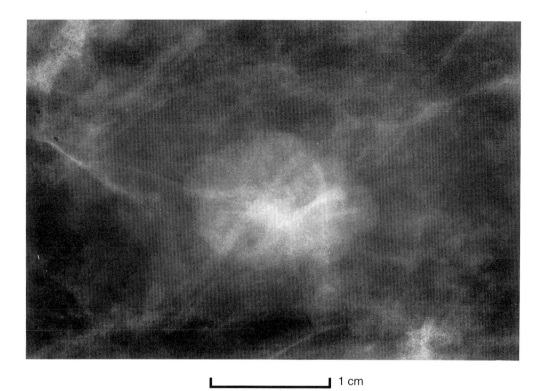

⊢————————⊣ 1 cm

Figure 8-1

29. Which *one* of the following is the MOST likely diagnosis?

(A) Phyllodes tumor
(B) Fibroadenoma
(C) Invasive ductal carcinoma
(D) Ductal carcinoma *in situ*
(E) Complex cyst

30. Which *one* of the following is the LEAST appropriate next step?

(A) Routine screening mammography in 1 year
(B) Follow-up mammography in 6 months
(C) Ultrasonography
(D) Fine-needle aspiration biopsy
(E) Surgical biopsy

QUESTIONS 31 THROUGH 33: MARK YOUR ANSWER SHEET TRUE (T) OR FALSE (F) FOR EACH OF THE RESPONSE CHOICES.

31. Concerning phyllodes tumor,

(A) it usually presents as a large, rapidly enlarging mass
(B) 5 to 10% of these tumors are malignant
(C) its peak incidence occurs between the ages of 60 and 70 years
(D) the mammographic appearance is similar to that of a large fibroadenoma
(E) on ultrasonography, small fluid-filled spaces are occasionally seen within the tumor

32. Concerning fibroadenomas,

(A) they are multiple in approximately 15% of patients
(B) they usually occur in women between the ages of 35 and 45 years
(C) they usually develop coarse calcification after involution
(D) they are associated with an increased risk for breast cancer
(E) the frequency of carcinoma in fibroadenomas is approximately 5%

CASE 8 (Cont'd)

33. Concerning circumscribed carcinoma,

    (A) invasive ductal carcinoma accounts for 20% of cases
    (B) magnification mammography often shows one or more indistinct borders
    (C) it can be reliably differentiated from a benign circumscribed mass by ultrasonography
    (D) papillary carcinoma typically appears as a circumscribed mass
    (E) cyst aspiration cytology is the most accurate way to diagnose intracystic carcinoma

This 52-year-old asymptomatic woman was referred for her first mammographic screening after a recent normal breast physical examination. A 1-cm noncalcified mass in the upper outer quadrant of the left breast was seen. You are shown the portion of the MLO view that includes the mass (Figure 9-1).

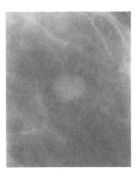

Figure 9-1

34. Which *one* of the following is the LEAST likely diagnosis?

   (A) Cyst
   (B) Fibroadenoma
   (C) Hamartoma
   (D) Carcinoma
   (E) Raised skin lesion

For each numbered nonpalpable lesion listed below (Questions 35 through 39), select the *one* lettered sequence of ultrasonography (US) and spot-compression magnification mammography (SM) (A, B, C, D, or E) that is MOST appropriate in conducting the imaging work-up. Each lettered work-up sequence may be used once, more than once, or not at all.

35. 1.2-cm fairly well defined upper outer right breast mass
36. 1-cm ovoid well-defined retroareolar left breast mass containing eight discrete calcifications
37. 1.6-cm spiculated upper outer left breast mass associated with focal skin thickening and retraction
38. 0.6-cm spiculated upper inner right breast mass
39. 1.3-cm fairly well defined round density identified in the outer aspect of the left breast only on the craniocaudal view

(A) US first, SM second
(B) SM first, US second
(C) US, no SM
(D) SM, no US
(E) Neither US nor SM first

QUESTIONS 40 AND 41: MARK YOUR ANSWER SHEET TRUE (T) OR FALSE (F) FOR EACH OF THE RESPONSE CHOICES.

40. Spot-compression magnification mammography would prompt biopsy of a 1-cm fairly well defined mass seen on a standard mammogram by demonstrating:

(A) the margins to be more well defined
(B) the borders to be microlobulated
(C) the contour to be more irregular
(D) a few spiculations at the border
(E) multiple tiny calcifications within the mass

41. Types of carcinoma that are usually seen as fairly well defined masses at mammography include:

   (A) lobular carcinoma *in situ*
   (B) comedocarcinoma
   (C) colloid carcinoma
   (D) medullary carcinoma
   (E) invasive ductal carcinoma

CASE 10: Questions 42 through 49

This 38-year-old woman has a palpable mass in the upper outer right breast. You are shown MLO (A) and CC (B) mammograms (Figure 10-1).

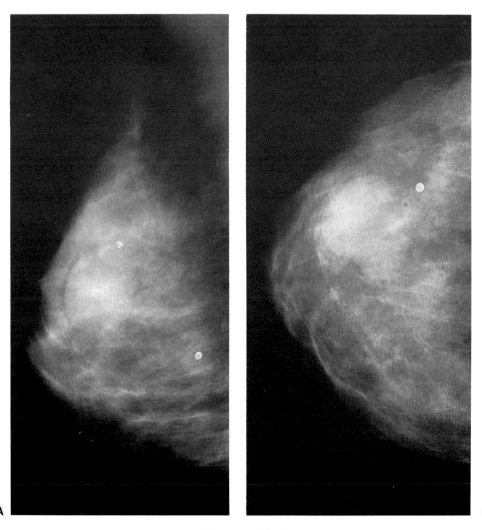

A　　　　　　　　　　　　　　　　　　　　　　**B**

Figure 10-1

42. Which *one* of the following is the MOST likely diagnosis?

(A) Cyst
(B) Medullary carcinoma
(C) Papilloma
(D) Intracystic carcinoma
(E) Hamartoma

QUESTIONS 43 AND 44: MARK YOUR ANSWER SHEET TRUE (T) OR FALSE (F) FOR EACH OF THE RESPONSE CHOICES.

43. Reliable methods for distinguishing a cyst from a sharply circumscribed solid mass include:

(A) ultrasonography
(B) needle aspiration
(C) magnification mammography
(D) pneumocystography
(E) physical examination
(F) MRI

44. Findings that preclude ultrasonographic diagnosis of a simple benign cyst include:

(A) low-level internal echoes
(B) compressibility
(C) slightly irregular walls
(D) acoustic enhancement behind the lesion
(E) acoustic attenuation behind the lesion
(F) edge refraction

CASE 10 (Cont'd)

For each numbered breast disorder listed below (Questions 45 through 48), select the *one* lettered sonographic finding (A, B, C, D, or E) that is MOST closely associated with it. Each lettered sonographic finding may be used once, more than once, or not at all.

45. Invasive ductal carcinoma
46. Hemorrhagic cyst
47. Intracystic papillary carcinoma
48. Hamartoma

(A) Heterogeneous solid smooth mass
(B) Smooth hypoechoic mass with low-level internal echoes
(C) Complex mass with solid projection into the anechoic area of the lesion
(D) Hyperechoic solid mass with lateral shadows
(E) Irregular hypoechoic mass with posterior attenuation

49. Which *one* of the following is the MOST important meaning of the halo sign?

(A) The mass is benign
(B) The mass is malignant
(C) The border of the mass is smooth
(D) The mass is a cyst
(E) A partial halo sign is highly suggestive of an intracystic carcinoma

CASE 11: Questions 50 through 54

This 61-year-old woman has a palpable mass in the right breast. You are shown right MLO (Figure 11-1), left MLO (Figure 11-2), right CC (Figure 11-3), and left CC (Figure 11-4) baseline mammograms.

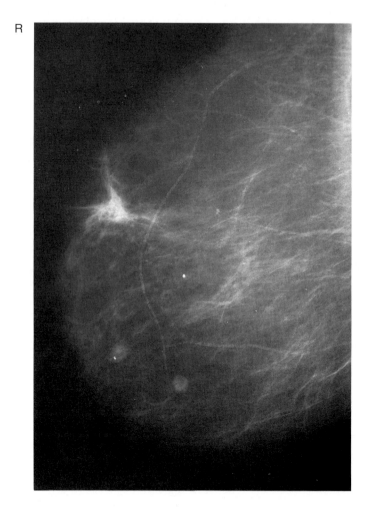

Figure 11-1

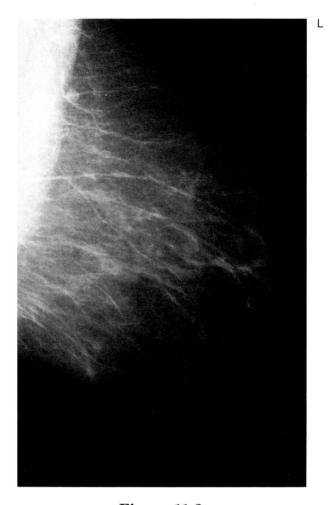

L

Figure 11-2

50. Which *one* of the following is the MOST likely diagnosis for the 1-cm smooth mass, containing a single coarse calcification, in the lower outer right breast?

(A) Medullary carcinoma
(B) Cyst
(C) Hamartoma
(D) Involuting fibroadenoma
(E) Lymph node

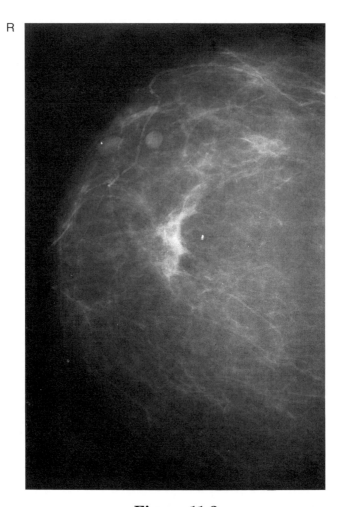

Figure 11-3

51. The single MOST important abnormality is:

  (A) the 1-cm smooth mass, containing a single coarse calci-
      fication, in the lower outer right breast

  (B) the 8-mm smooth noncalcified nodule in the lower outer
      right breast

  (C) the ill-defined 3-cm asymmetric density with internal
      lucency in the upper central right breast

  (D) the 2-mm calcification in the central right breast, 7 cm
      deep to the nipple

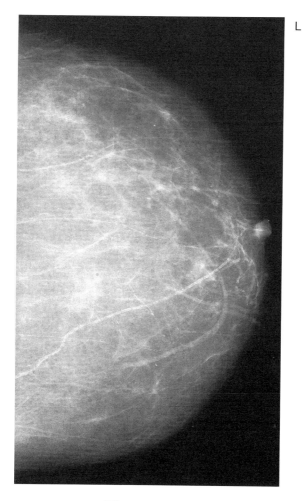

L

Figure 11-4

52. The NEXT step should be:

    (A) routine screening mammography in 1 year
    (B) follow-up mammography in 6 months
    (C) ultrasonography
    (D) biopsy

QUESTIONS 53 AND 54: MARK YOUR ANSWER SHEET TRUE
(T) OR FALSE (F) FOR EACH OF THE RESPONSE CHOICES.

53. Concerning spiculated lesions,

   (A) they most probably represent invasive lobular carci-
        noma
   (B) radial scar cannot be reliably differentiated from carci-
        noma by mammography
   (C) radial scar cannot be reliably differentiated from carci-
        noma by physical examination
   (D) postsurgical scar can be identical in appearance to
        breast carcinoma on mammography
   (E) ultrasonography reliably differentiates between asym-
        metric glandular tissue and breast carcinoma

54. Concerning medullary carcinoma of the breast,

   (A) it is the most common type of circumscribed carcinoma
        of the breast
   (B) calcifications are a common mammographic feature
   (C) internal necrosis is frequently found histologically
   (D) posterior shadowing on sonograms is common

This 55-year-old woman has a palpable mass at 3 o'clock in the outer left breast. You are shown CC (A) and 90° lateral (B) views from her mammography examination (Figure 12-1).

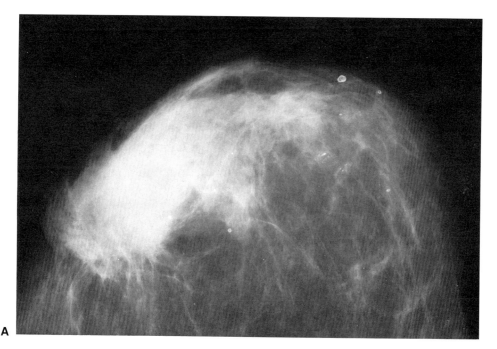

A

Figure 12-1

55. Which *one* of the following is the MOST likely diagnosis?

    (A) Galactocele
    (B) Hamartoma
    (C) Hematoma
    (D) Fat necrosis
    (E) Sarcoma

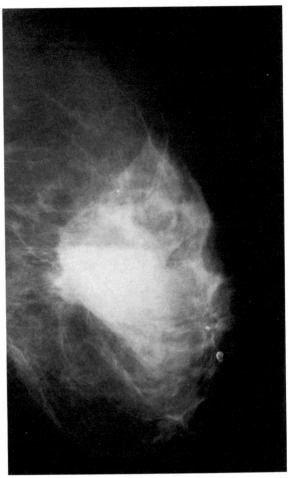

B

QUESTIONS 56 THROUGH 58: MARK YOUR ANSWER SHEET TRUE (T) OR FALSE (F) FOR EACH OF THE RESPONSE CHOICES.

56. Hamartomas of the breast:

    (A) have malignant potential
    (B) are characteristically firm on palpation
    (C) often result in asymmetric breast size
    (D) contain lobular and ductal epithelium
    (E) are occasionally anechoic on ultrasonography

57. Concerning fat necrosis,

    (A) calcifications are linear and branching
    (B) history of a surgical biopsy is usually present
    (C) oil cysts are a mammographic manifestation
    (D) biopsy is usually necessary for confirmation of diagnosis
    (E) parenchymal distortion is occasionally an associated finding

58. Concerning patients undergoing breast conservation therapy,

    (A) mammographic changes stabilize within 1 year
    (B) any new calcifications should be biopsied
    (C) most recurrent carcinomas develop 2 years or more after lumpectomy
    (D) 70% of recurrent carcinomas are detected only by mammography
    (E) a postlumpectomy mammography examination helps exclude residual tumor

This 62-year-old asymptomatic woman underwent mammographic screening. She is on estrogen replacement therapy and has a negative family history for breast cancer. You are shown MLO (Figure 13-1) and CC (Figure 13-2) views of the right breast. You are also shown her MLO and CC right-breast mammograms from 2 years earlier (Figures 13-3 and 13-4, respectively).

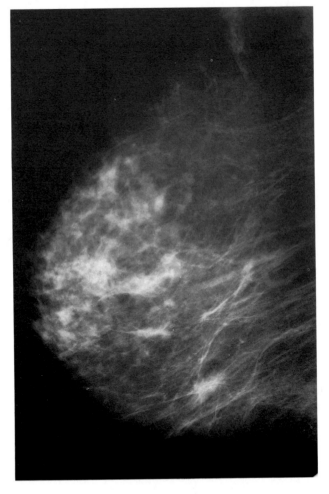

Figure 13-1

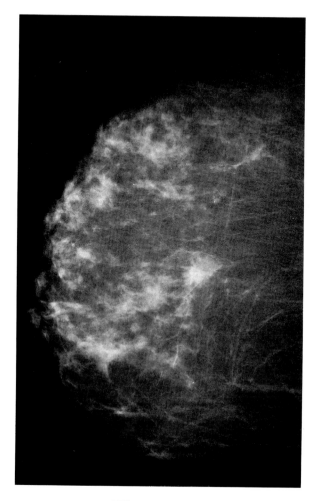

Figure 13-2

59. Which *one* of the following BEST characterizes the mammographic findings?

   (A) Probably benign disease, unchanged
   (B) Probably benign disease, changed
   (C) Suspicious for malignant disease, unchanged
   (D) Suspicious for malignant disease, changed

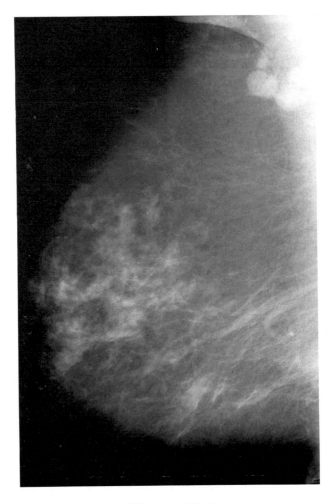

Figure 13-3

60. An abnormality requiring further evaluation appears in which *one* of the following locations?

   (A) Upper outer quadrant
   (B) Upper inner quadrant
   (C) Lower outer quadrant
   (D) Lower inner quadrant
   (E) Subareolar region

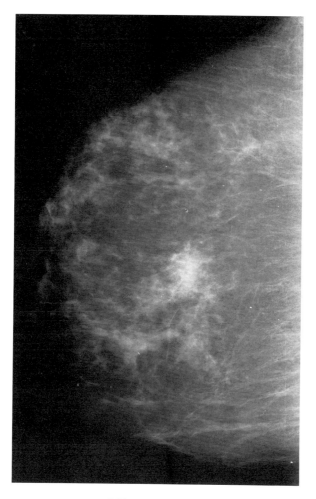

Figure 13-4

QUESTIONS 61 THROUGH 63: MARK YOUR ANSWER SHEET TRUE (T) OR FALSE (F) FOR EACH OF THE RESPONSE CHOICES.

61. Appropriate further imaging evaluation of the test patient includes:

   (A) 90° lateral view
   (B) spot-compression magnification view
   (C) "nipple-in-profile" view
   (D) ultrasonography

62. Concerning a developing density,

   (A) a new density in a premenopausal woman is almost always an indication for biopsy
   (B) a new density in a postmenopausal woman is almost always an indication for biopsy
   (C) a new 1-cm smooth, noncalcified, nonpalpable mass should be evaluated by ultrasonography
   (D) the most frequent cause is trauma to the breast

63. Concerning the effects of estrogen replacement therapy,

   (A) a diffuse increase in fibroglandular density develops in most patients
   (B) breast cysts develop in most patients
   (C) diffuse skin thickening usually develops
   (D) the relative risk of breast cancer is increased approximately threefold

This 41-year-old woman underwent mammography after a 1-cm firm mobile mass was palpated in her upper outer left breast. You are shown the CC (A) and 90° lateral (B) views (Figure 14-1).

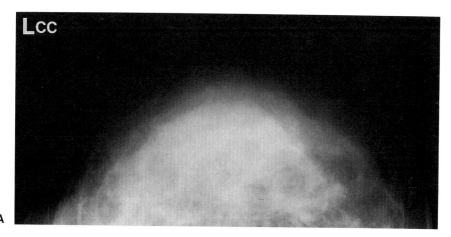

Figure 14-1

64. Which *one* of the following BEST describes the mammographic findings with respect to the palpable mass?

   (A) No useful information
   (B) Cystic or solid benign mass
   (C) Probably benign mass
   (D   Mass, suspicious for malignancy
   (E) Mass, highly suspicious for malignancy

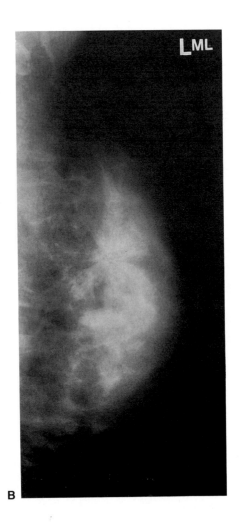

QUESTIONS 65 THROUGH 67: MARK YOUR ANSWER SHEET TRUE (T) OR FALSE (F) FOR EACH OF THE RESPONSE CHOICES.

65. Further imaging evaluation of the test patient should include:

   (A) review of the CC view to confirm proper placement of the "CC" marker
   (B) shallow oblique (from CC) view
   (C) spot-compression magnification views of the mammographic abnormality
   (D) CC and 90° lateral views with a metallic marker placed over the palpable mass
   (E) spot-compression tangential view of the palpable mass

66. Use of a metallic marker for evaluation of a palpable mass:

   (A) requires the mammography technologist to place the marker over the single point on the breast at which the mass is most readily palpable
   (B) often intereferes with mammographic interpretation
   (C) indicates whether the palpable mass is included in the mammographic image
   (D) indicates whether the palpable mass and a mammographically identified mass are one and the same

67. Appropriate reasons for obtaining a spot-compression tangential view for evaluation of a palpable mass include:

   (A) determining whether the mass is within the skin
   (B) determining whether there is associated skin thickening
   (C) better defining the features of the margins of the mass
   (D) demonstrating a mass not seen on routine views

CASE 15: Questions 68 through 72

This 44-year-old asymptomatic woman with a normal breast physical examination underwent mammographic screening, which revealed an isolated cluster of tiny calcifications. You are shown photographic enlargements from the CC (A) and MLO (B) views (Figure 15-1).

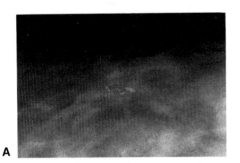 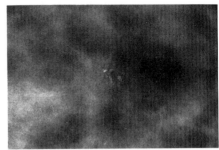

A   B

Figure 15-1

68. Which *one* of the following is the BEST interpretation of the test images?

 (A) Sedimented calcium in tiny benign cysts
 (B) Benign skin calcifications
 (C) Incompletely evaluated calcifications
 (D) Probably benign calcifications
 (E) Calcifications suspicious for malignancy

69. Which *one* of the following is the MOST appropriate next step?

 (A) Routine mammographic screening in 1 year
 (B) Follow-up mammography in 6 months
 (C) Tangential views
 (D) Spot-compression magnification views
 (E) Preoperative needle localization

QUESTIONS 70 THROUGH 72: MARK YOUR ANSWER SHEET TRUE (T) OR FALSE (F) FOR EACH OF THE RESPONSE CHOICES.

70. When undertaking further imaging evaluation of an isolated cluster of tiny calcifications, useful information is likely to be provided by:

    (A) tangential projection mammography
    (B) 90° lateral projection mammography
    (C) spot-compression mammography
    (D) magnification mammography
    (E) shallow oblique (from any standard) projection mammography

71. Concerning magnification in mammography,

    (A) it is best performed by combining conventional mammographic imaging with the use of a powerful magnifying lens
    (B) images demonstrate both increased spatial resolution and reduced system noise
    (C) the nominal size of the X-ray focal spot should be ≤0.3 mm
    (D) the simultaneous use of spot-compression and magnification techniques usually provides more mammographic information than the use of either technique alone
    (E) the use of an oscillating grid usually improves the mammographic image

72. Potential explanations for blurring of a magnification mammogram by comparison with a standard image include use of a:

    (A) faster screen-film combination
    (B) longer X-ray exposure
    (C) higher kVp
    (D) 0.1-mm focal spot
    (E) 2x magnification tray

A 57-year-old asymptomatic woman underwent her first screening mammography examination. You are shown CC (A) and MLO (B) views of the right breast (Figure 16-1) demonstrating an isolated cluster of calcifications (arrows), which was further evaluated on a spot-compression magnification MLO view (Figure 16-2).

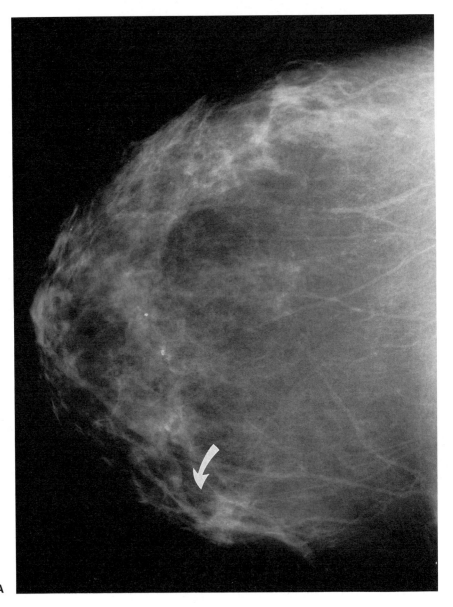

A

Figure 16-1

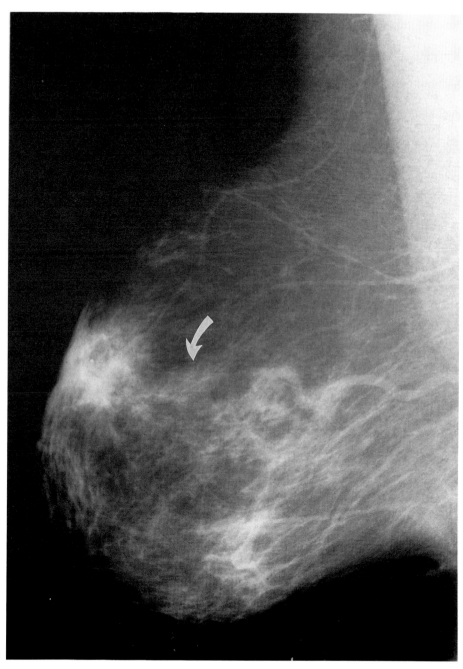

B

1 cm

Figure 16-2

73. The NEXT step should be:

    (A) follow-up mammography in 6 months
    (B) tangential view
    (C) 90° lateral view
    (D) needle localization

74. In a patient with nonspecific calcifications, a change to a
    more specific mammographic appearance over 6 months is
    MOST likely with:

    (A) fat necrosis
    (B) sebaceous gland calcification
    (C) sclerosing adenosis
    (D) milk of calcium in cysts
    (E) arteriosclerosis

75. Magnification views are LEAST helpful in evaluating which *one* of the following types of calcifications?

    (A) Arteriosclerotic
    (B) Secretory
    (C) Sebaceous gland
    (D) Milk of calcium
    (E) Sclerosing adenosis

QUESTION 76: MARK YOUR ANSWER SHEET TRUE (T) OR FALSE (F) FOR EACH OF THE RESPONSE CHOICES.

76. Dermal calcifications are associated with:

    (A) keloids
    (B) raised nevi
    (C) tattoos
    (D) trichinosis
    (E) burns

You are shown a spot-compression magnification view obtained following the first screening mammography examination of a 50-year-old asymptomatic woman (Figure 17-1).

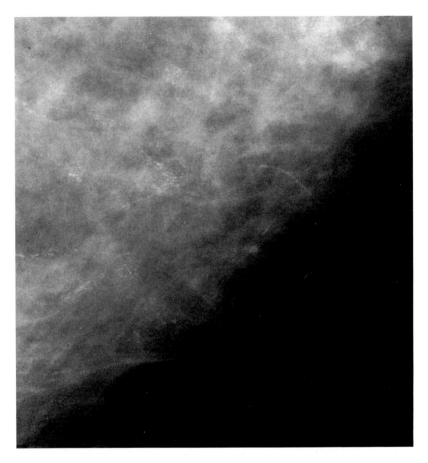

Figure 17-1

77. The NEXT step should be:

   (A) excisional biopsy
   (B) fine-needle aspiration biopsy
   (C) follow-up mammography in 3 months
   (D) follow-up mammography in 6 months
   (E) follow-up mammography in 1 year

QUESTION 78: MARK YOUR ANSWER SHEET TRUE (T) OR FALSE (F) FOR EACH OF THE RESPONSE CHOICES.

78. Calcifications are found predominantly within ducts in:

   (A) ductal hyperplasia
   (B) secretory disease (plasma cell mastitis)
   (C) comedocarcinoma
   (D) Paget's disease of the nipple
   (E) sclerosing adenosis

79. Which *one* of the following types of calcifications is LEAST likely to be associated with carcinoma?

   (A) Linearly distributed
   (B) Branching
   (C) Casting
   (D) Solid round or oval
   (E) Ringlike

80. In the absence of calcifications elsewhere in the breast, biopsy of a solitary cluster of indeterminate microcalcifications should be considered if their number equals or exceeds:

   (A) $2/cm^2$
   (B) $5/cm^2$
   (C) $10/cm^2$
   (D) $15/cm^2$
   (E) $20/cm^2$

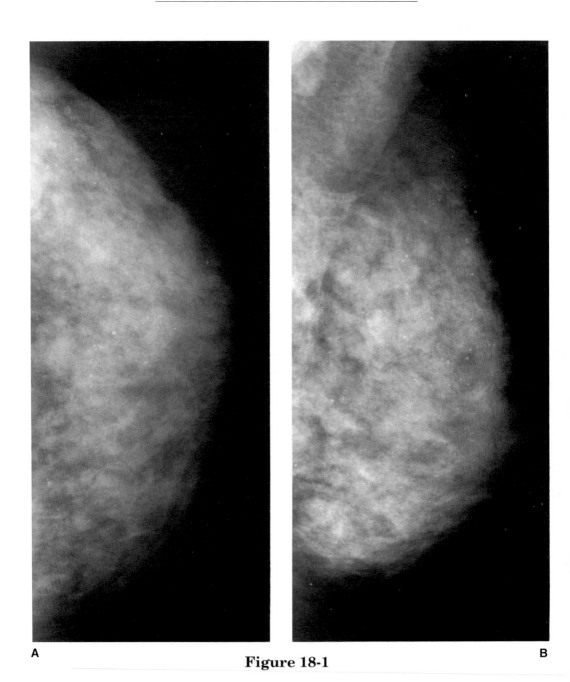

A

B

Figure 18-1

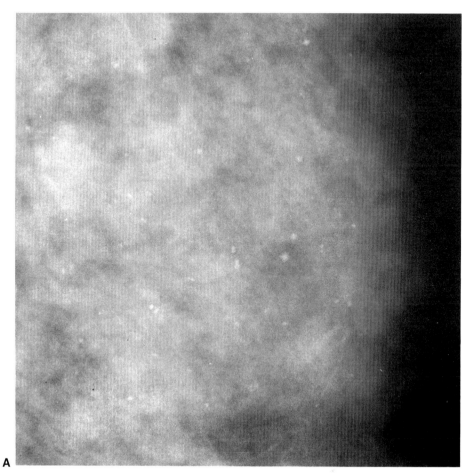

A

Figure 18-2

You are shown CC (A) and MLO (B) views of the left breast from the mammography examination of a 60-year-old asymptomatic woman who underwent right mastectomy 4 years ago (Figure 18-1). Corresponding spot-compression magnification views are also shown (Figure 18-2).

81. Which *one* of the following is the MOST likely cause of the calcifications?

    (A) Atypical hyperplasia
    (B) Sclerosing adenosis
    (C) Ductal carcinoma *in situ* (comedo)
    (D) Ductal carcinoma *in situ* (micropapillary)
    (E) Lobular neoplasia

MLO

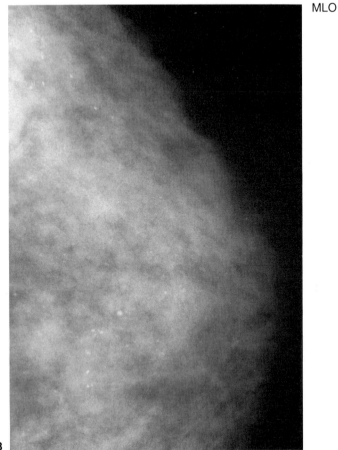

B

QUESTIONS 82 THROUGH 84: MARK YOUR ANSWER SHEET TRUE (T) OR FALSE (F) FOR EACH OF THE RESPONSE CHOICES.

82. Calcifications in adenosis:

    (A) occur primarily in acini
    (B) are most often in the upper-outer quadrant
    (C) often have hollow centers
    (D) are often rod-shaped
    (E) are usually scattered in distribution

83. Concerning ductal carcinoma *in situ*,

    (A) it is synonymous with comedocarcinoma
    (B) multicentricity describes tumors that involve more than one quadrant
    (C) it is often multicentric
    (D) an extensive intraductal component reduces the effectiveness of radiation therapy
    (E) it is a precursor of invasive disease

84. Concerning lobular carcinoma *in situ*,

    (A) it has a poorer prognosis than lobular neoplasia
    (B) it occurs primarily in ducts
    (C) it is less aggressive than ductal carcinoma *in situ*
    (D) the mammographic findings are specific
    (E) it usually progresses to invasive disease

You are shown photographic enlargements of CC (A) and 90° mediolateral (B) spot-compression magnification views obtained following the first mammographic screening examination of a 50-year-old asymptomatic woman (Figure 19-1).

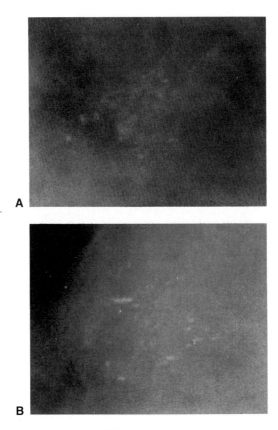

Figure 19-1

85. Which *one* of the following is the MOST likely diagnosis?

    (A) Fat necrosis
    (B) Microcystic hyperplasia
    (C) Ductal carcinoma *in situ*
    (D) Lobular neoplasia
    (E) Ductal ectasia

QUESTION 86: MARK YOUR ANSWER SHEET TRUE (T) OR
FALSE (F) FOR EACH OF THE RESPONSE CHOICES.

86.   Characteristics of calcifications in microcysts as seen on a
      lateral view include:

      (A)   crescent shape
      (B)   semilunar shape
      (C)   horizontal orientation
      (D)   upper margins better defined than lower margins
      (E)   appearance similar to that on the CC view

87.   In a solitary cluster of microcalcifications, the characteristic
      MOST suspicious for malignancy is:

      (A)   variation in density
      (B)   variation in size
      (C)   oval shape
      (D)   number of calcifications more than 10
      (E)   dot-dash appearance

QUESTION 88: MARK YOUR ANSWER SHEET TRUE (T) OR
FALSE (F) FOR EACH OF THE RESPONSE CHOICES.

88.   Characteristics of secretory calcifications include:

      (A)   location in the duct wall
      (B)   polarity toward the nipple
      (C)   smoothly tapered shape
      (D)   hollow, cylindrical shape
      (E)   unilaterality

You are shown CC (A and B) and MLO (C and D) views of both
breasts from the first screening examination of a 40-year-old
asymptomatic woman with no breast cancer risk factors (Figure
20-1). Spot-compression magnification CC (A) and MLO (B) views
of the left breast obtained following this screening examination
are also shown (Figure 20-2).

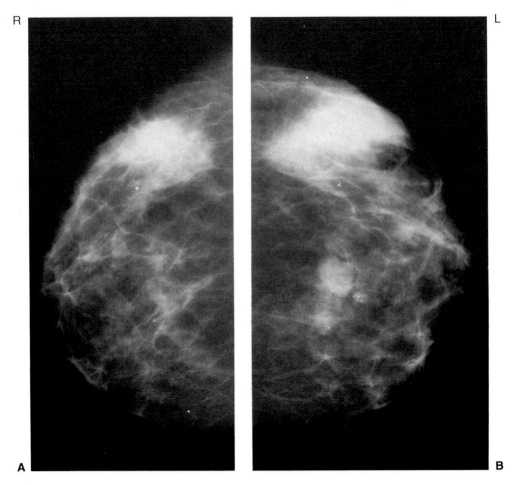

R   L

A   B

Figure 20-1

R

L

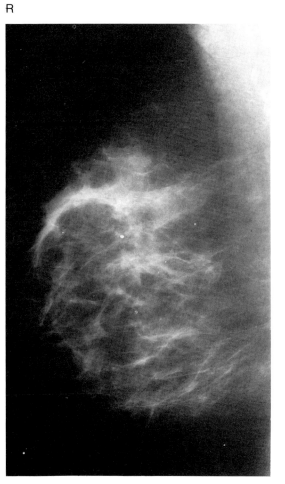

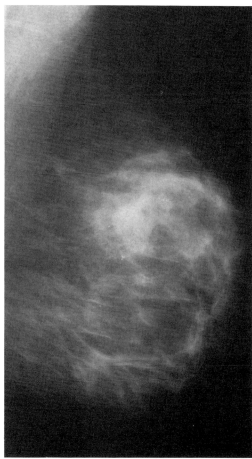

C

D

89. The NEXT step should be:

    (A) ultrasonography
    (B) biopsy
    (C) follow-up mammography in 6 months
    (D) follow-up mammography in 1 year
    (E) follow-up mammography in 2 years

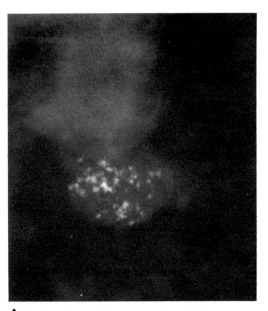 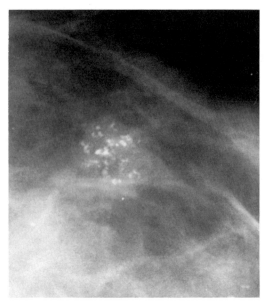

A   B

Figure 20-2

QUESTIONS 90 THROUGH 92: MARK YOUR ANSWER SHEET TRUE (T) OR FALSE (F) FOR EACH OF THE RESPONSE CHOICES.

90. Distributions of fine calcifications in a circumscribed mass indicating that it is benign include:

    (A) predominantly central
    (B) eccentric
    (C) diffuse
    (D) predominantly marginal
    (E) ringlike peripheral

91. Distributions of coarse calcifications in a circumscribed mass indicating the need for biopsy include:

    (A) predominantly central
    (B) eccentric
    (C) diffuse
    (D) predominantly marginal

92. Types of calcifications in a circumscribed mass indicating that it is benign include:

    (A) irregular shape, ringlike distribution
    (B) thick, curvilinear, peripheral distribution
    (C) thin, curvilinear distribution
    (D) plaquelike
    (E) popcornlike

You are shown standard MLO (A) and CC (B) mammograms of augmented breasts (Figure 21-1).

R   L

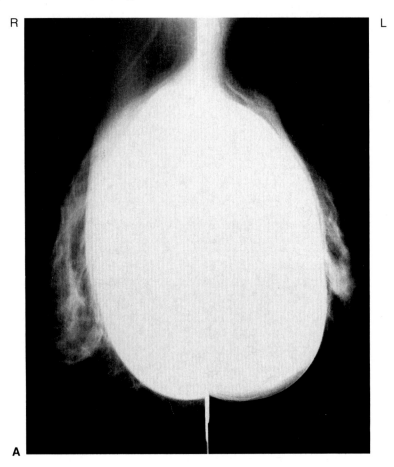

A

Figure 21-1

QUESTION 93: MARK YOUR ANSWER SHEET TRUE (T) OR FALSE (F) FOR EACH OF THE RESPONSE CHOICES.

93. The mammograms demonstrate:

   (A) double-lumen implants
   (B) subpectoral implants
   (C) leakage of silicone
   (D) capsular contracture
   (E) capsular calcification

R

L

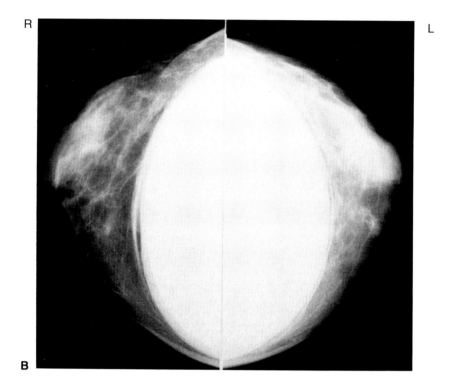

B

94. The NEXT step should be:

   (A) ultrasonography
   (B) modified compression mammography
   (C) axillary mammographic view
   (D) CT scan
   (E) MRI

QUESTIONS 95 THROUGH 97: MARK YOUR ANSWER SHEET TRUE (T) OR FALSE (F) FOR EACH OF THE RESPONSE CHOICES.

95. Concerning mammography of the augmented breast,

(A) detection of lesions is easier in patients with saline-filled implants than in those with silicone-filled implants

(B) phototiming should not be used for implant-displaced views

(C) by including implant-displaced views, the augmented breast is imaged as completely as the breast without an implant

(D) it is essential to use a high-kVp technique

96. Concerning encapsulation of an implant,

(A) it is the result of fibrosis developing around the implant wall

(B) it occurs more often in patients with subglandular implants than in those with subpectoral implants

(C) it is suggested by the shape of the implant on mammography

(D) mammography is the most reliable method for its detection

(E) calcium deposition occurs on the surface of the implant wall

(F) firm encapsulation is a contraindication to mammography

97. Concerning implant rupture or leakage,

(A) a soft, palpable bulge in the side of an implant is most likely a pocket of free silicone

(B) peri-implant calcification is an important mammographic sign of silicone leakage

(C) dense lymph nodes with loss of fatty hila suggest lymphatic sequestration of silicone

(D) a closed capsulotomy occasionally results from compression during mammography

(E) saline-filled implants are less prone to decompression than are silicone-filled implants

CASE 22: Questions 98 through 101

A new circumscribed, 8-mm bilobed mass (arrows) was found on MLO (A) and CC (B) mammograms (Figure 22-1) in this 44-year-old woman. The lesion was not palpable. Ultrasonography (not shown) demonstrated a hypoechoic mass with low-level internal echoes.

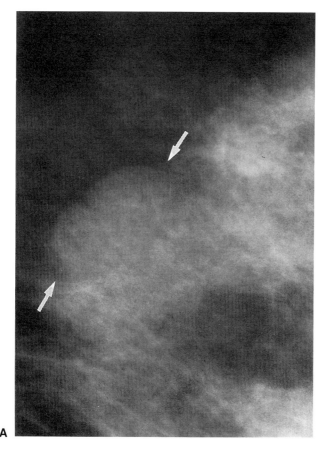

A

Figure 22-1

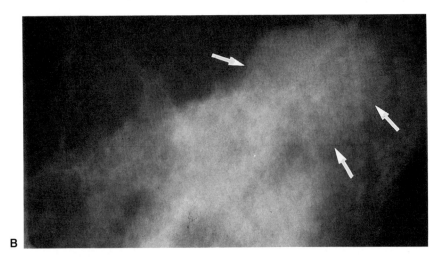

B

QUESTIONS 98 THROUGH 101: MARK YOUR ANSWER SHEET TRUE (T) OR FALSE (F) FOR EACH OF THE RESPONSE CHOICES.

98. A reasonable next step would be:

   (A) sonographic fine-needle aspiration
   (B) stereotactic fine-needle aspiration
   (C) freehand needle localization
   (D) grid coordinate needle placement
   (E) follow-up mammography in 6 months
   (F) follow-up ultrasonography in 6 months

99. Concerning aspiration of cystic lesions,

   (A) it is indicated if a mural nodule is seen on ultrasonography
   (B) bloody aspirates should be sent for cytologic testing
   (C) postaspiration mammography is essential
   (D) multiloculated cysts should be aspirated
   (E) an associated cancer is usually adjacent to a cyst rather than within the wall

100. Intracystic papillary lesions:

    (A) are usually found in women under age 50
    (B) when malignant, are usually *in situ*
    (C) usually present with bloody nipple discharge
    (D) usually appear as circumscribed masses
    (E) usually contain microcalcifications

101. Concerning sonographically guided aspiration of breast masses,

    (A) it requires the use of a needle-guide attachment
    (B) visualization of the needle tip requires the use of a burnished needle
    (C) the use of a sector transducer rather than a linear-array transducer is preferred
    (D) it should not be attempted for lesions ≤1 cm in diameter

This 43-year-old woman was referred for needle localization of a nonpalpable lesion in the left breast. You are shown MLO (A) and CC (B) mammograms of both breasts (Figure 23-1).

R   L

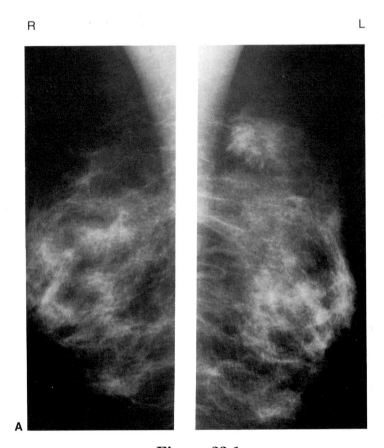

A

Figure 23-1

102. The NEXT step should be:

    (A) needle localization
    (B) ultrasonography
    (C) spot-compression mammogram
    (D) tangential mammogram
    (E) follow-up mammography in 6 months

CASE 23 (Cont'd)

R

L

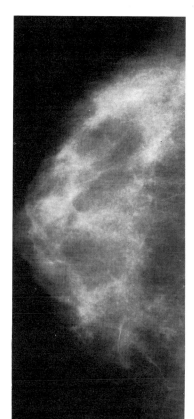
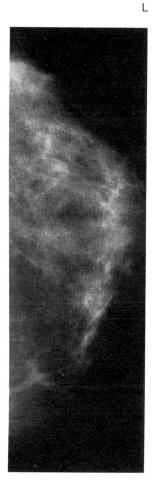

B

QUESTIONS 103 THROUGH 105: MARK YOUR ANSWER
SHEET TRUE (T) OR FALSE (F) FOR EACH OF THE
RESPONSE CHOICES.

103. Reasonable explanations for asymmetric density seen on a
mammogram include:

    (A) invasive lobular carcinoma
    (B) exogenous estrogen therapy
    (C) mastitis
    (D) prior surgery
    (E) congestive heart failure

104. Concerning acute mastitis,

    (A) calcifications are frequently present
    (B) fluid collections identifiable by sonography are present in most patients
    (C) purulent discharge from the nipple is a frequent presenting complaint
    (D) an associated abscess is usually subareolar
    (E) no organism is cultured on aspirates in more than 50% of cases

105. Concerning invasive lobular carcinoma,

    (A) presenting physical findings are subtle or nonspecific in most patients
    (B) presenting mammographic findings are subtle or nonspecific in most patients
    (C) it constitutes 30% of invasive breast carcinoma
    (D) it often contains round, punctate calcifications
    (E) it is often more conspicuous on the CC view than on the MLO view

This 84-year-old woman was referred for needle localization of microcalcifications associated with an area of increased density in the right breast. You are shown CC (A) and 90° lateral (B) mammograms (Figure 24-1) and a photographic enlargement of the 90° lateral view (Figure 24-2). The microcalcifications and density are indicated by arrows. This lesion was not present on mammograms taken 14 months previously.

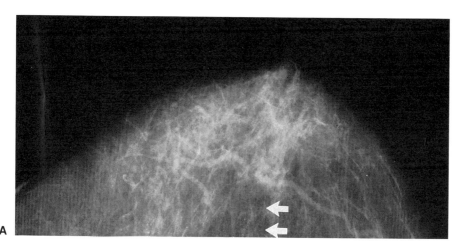

A

Figure 24-1

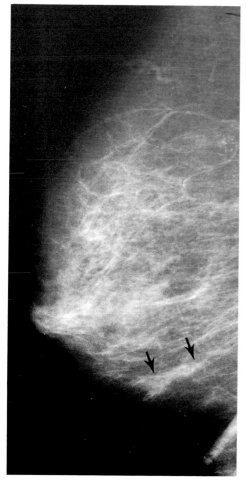

B

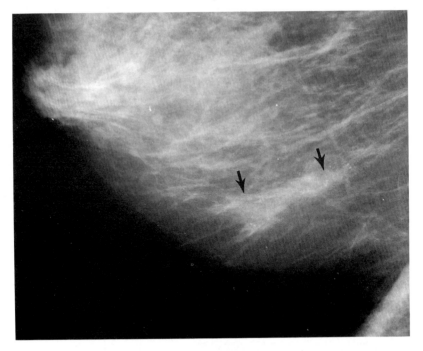

Figure 24-2

106. Which *one* of the following would be the BEST approach to localize this lesion?

    (A) Mediolateral
    (B) Superior (CC)
    (C) Lateromedial
    (D) Inferior (caudocranial)
    (E) Periareolar

CASE 24 (Cont'd)

QUESTIONS 107 AND 108: MARK YOUR ANSWER SHEET TRUE (T) OR FALSE (F) FOR EACH OF THE RESPONSE CHOICES.

107. Concerning specimen radiography,

   (A) it confirms excision of the lesion
   (B) it is not necessary for a lesion palpated in the specimen
   (C) it is essential only for assessment of lesions containing calcifications
   (D) a magnification technique should be used routinely
   (E) it facilitates detection of tumor extending to the margin of resection
   (F) radiographs of tissue blocks should be performed if resected calcifications are not seen on histologic sections

108. Concerning microcalcifications seen on specimen radiographs,

   (A) they nearly always correspond to the location of histologically demonstrated carcinoma
   (B) if distant from the resected mass, they generally indicate intraductal extension of tumor
   (C) those composed of calcium oxalate are better seen histologically with polarized light than on hematoxylin-and-eosin-stained sections
   (D) they are a common manifestation of lobular neoplasia (lobular carcinoma *in situ*)

This 70-year-old woman underwent mammographic screening. You are shown CC (A) and MLO (B) views (Figure 25-1). A 6-mm density (arrows) not present 1 year ago was detected on the CC view. You are also shown CC (A) and 90° lateral (B) spot-compression magnification views (Figure 25-2). Spiculated margins are seen clearly on the CC view but are barely visible on the 90° lateral view (arrows). The patient is a poor operative risk.

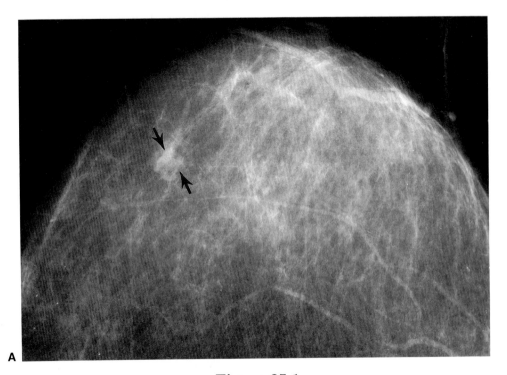

Figure 25-1

109. The NEXT step should be:

   (A) follow-up mammography in 6 months
   (B) sonographically guided fine-needle aspiration cytology or core biopsy
   (C) stereotactic fine-needle aspiration or core biopsy
   (D) grid coordinate needle localization

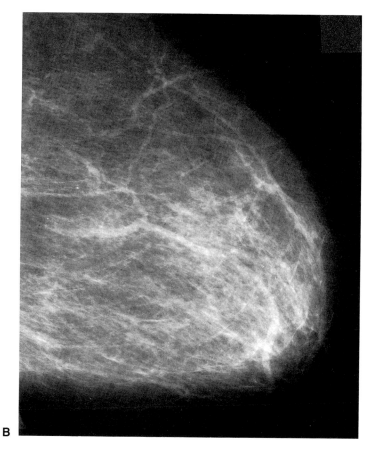

B

Figure 25-1 (Continued)

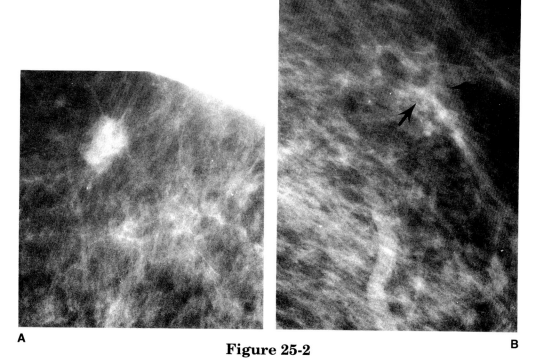

A

Figure 25-2

B

QUESTIONS 110 THROUGH 112: MARK YOUR ANSWER SHEET TRUE (T) OR FALSE (F) FOR EACH OF THE RESPONSE CHOICES.

110. Concerning stereotactic procedures,

    (A) they require expensive, specialized equipment
    (B) they are highly operator dependent
    (C) they require a cooperative patient
    (D) they permit more precise wire localization

111. Stereotactically guided procedures are preferable to the use of a grid coordinate system for:

    (A) biopsy of loosely grouped calcifications
    (B) biopsy of a mass smaller than 1 cm
    (C) biopsy of a deep lesion in a large breast
    (D) aspiration of a cyst smaller than 1 cm

112. Concerning stereotactic devices,

    (A) prone systems facilitate procedures in less cooperative patients
    (B) prone systems facilitate sampling of lesions adjacent to the chest wall
    (C) upright systems are designed to obtain cytological samples only
    (D) each upright system works only with the mammography unit(s) of that manufacturer
    (E) upright systems cost less than prone systems

CASE 25 (Cont'd)

For each numbered statement listed below (Questions 113 to 117), indicate whether it is MORE closely associated with core biopsy (A) or fine-needle aspiration cytology (B), equally associated with both (C), or associated with neither (D). Each lettered option may be used once, more than once, or not at all.

113. The pathologist needs special training for interpretation of the specimen
114. Invasive carcinoma is reliably differentiated from *in situ* carcinoma
115. Sclerosing duct hyperplasia (radial scar) is reliably diagnosed
116. Only one specimen is required for diagnosis
117. Fibroadenoma is reliably diagnosed

    (A)   Core biopsy
    (B)   Fine-needle aspiration cytology
    (C)   Both
    (D)   Neither

DEMOGRAPHIC DATA QUESTIONS

Please answer all of the questions below. The data you provide will be used to supply information that will allow you to compare your performance on the examination with that of others at similar levels of training and with similar backgrounds, and for purposes of planning continuing education projects. Please answer each question as accurately and as objectively as possible. Please mark the *one* BEST response for each question. Recall, of course, that we do *not* want individual names. Our analyses will reflect only categories and groups; everything will remain completely anonymous and no attempt will be made to identify any specific individual.

118. The ACR will be evaluating the questions in this examination to determine their degree of difficulty and to determine the success of the examination as an instrument of self-evaluation and continuing education. To assist the ACR, please indicate in which of the following ways you took this examination.

    (A) Used reference materials or read the syllabus portion of this book to assist in answering some portion of the examination
    (B) Did not use reference materials and did not read the syllabus portion of this book while taking the examination

119. How much residency and fellowship training in Diagnostic Radiology have you completed?

    (A) None
    (B) Less than 1 year
    (C) 1 year
    (D) 2 years
    (E) 3 years
    (F) 4 or more years

120. When did you finish your residency training in Radiology?

    (A) More than 10 years ago
    (B) 5 to 10 years ago
    (C) 1 to 5 years ago
    (D) Less than 1 year ago
    (E) Not yet completed
    (F) Radiology is not my specialty

121. Have you been certified by the American Board of Radiology in Diagnostic Radiology?

    (A) Yes
    (B) No

122. Have you completed fellowship training in Breast Imaging?

    (A) Yes
    (B) No

123. Which one of the categories listed below BEST describes the setting of your practice in the immediate past 3 years? (For residents and fellows, in which one did you or will you spend the major portion of your residency or fellowship?)

    (A) Community or general hospital—less than 200 beds
    (B) Community or general hospital—200 to 499 beds
    (C) Community or general hospital—500 or more beds
    (D) University-affiliated hospital
    (E) Office practice

124. In which one of the following general areas of Radiology do you consider yourself MOST expert?

    (A) Breast Imaging
    (B) Chest radiology
    (C) Musculoskeletal radiology
    (D) Gastrointestinal radiology
    (E) Genitourinary radiology
    (F) Head and neck radiology
    (G) Neuroradiology
    (H) Pediatric radiology
    (I) Cardiovascular radiology
    (J) Other

125. In which one of the following radiologic modalities do you consider yourself MOST expert?

    (A) General angiography
    (B) Interventional radiology
    (C) Magnetic resonance imaging
    (D) Nuclear radiology
    (E) Ultrasonography
    (F) Computed tomography
    (G) Radiation therapy
    (H) Other

Breast Disease
(Second Series)

Table of Contents

The Table of Contents is placed in this unusual location so that the reader will not be distracted by the answers before completeing the test. A detailed index of the areas considered in this syllabus is provided (beginning on p. 357) for further reference.

Breast Disease
(Second Series)
Syllabus

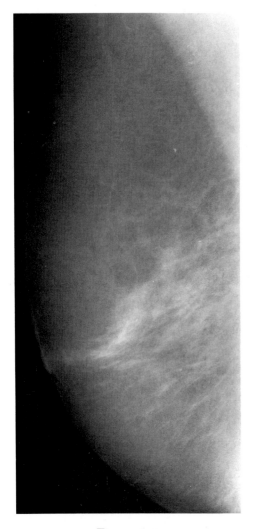

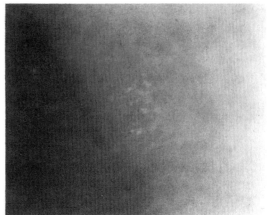

Figure 1-1   *Figure 1-2*

Figures 1-1 and 1-2. This 64-year-old asymptomatic woman had mammographic screening after a normal breast physical examination. You are shown the MLO view of the right breast (Figure 1-1) and a photographic enlargement of the upper portion of this image (Figure 1-2). The finding illustrated in these mammograms was not seen on the CC view (not shown).

Case 1: Triangulating the Location of a Lesion by Using the Oblique View

Question 1

Which *one* of the following is the LEAST likely explanation for the finding?

    (A) Deodorant artifact
    (B) Dust artifact
    (C) Sclerosing adenosis
    (D) Atypical hyperplasia
    (E) Ductal carcinoma *in situ*

In its entirety, this case addresses the process of triangulating the location of a mammographic lesion by using the MLO view. Figures 1-1 through 1-4 indicate the location of the test patient's lesion on MLO and 90° lateral views. However, the 90° lateral view becomes part of the imaging workup only later (see Question 3), so consideration of its findings will be deferred for now.

The MLO mammogram shown in Figure 1-1 demonstrates a grouping of 15 to 20 small calcifications in the uppermost portion of the image, projected over the pectoral muscle shadow. There is no suggestion of an associated mass. Figure 1-2 is a photographic enlargement of the area of interest and provides a view equivalent to that obtained by using a 2x magnifying lens. It shows the multiple calcific particles to be variable in size, nonuniform in density, and indistinct in shape.

The fact that the calcifications were not seen on the CC mammogram (not shown) adds no useful information to narrow the differential diagnosis, because a lesion that appears to be so close to the chest wall and so distant from the nipple is unlikely to be included on a standard CC view. Even with optimal patient positioning, including elevation of the inframammary fold, the far lateral mammary tissues are routinely cut off the CC view; occasionally, the very uppermost part of the breast is also

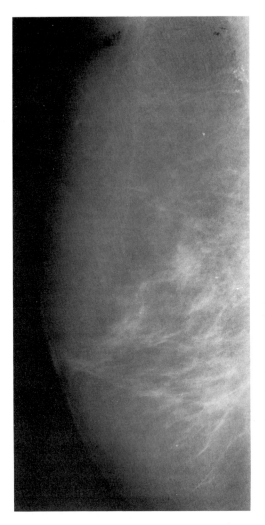

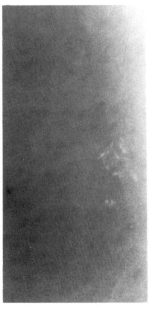

Figure 1-3 (see page 9)   *Figure 1-4 (see page 9)*

excluded. Thus, possible explanations for the mammographic finding in the test patient must include the full spectrum of lesions that simulate or actually represent clustered microcalcifications.

One possible cause is deodorant artifact (Option (A)). The zinc- or aluminum-containing preservatives in many deodorants produce mammographic shadows that are similar in density and size to true breast microcalcifications. Most commonly, this finding projects over the axillary tail region of the breast or over the axilla itself, sites that are entirely consistent with the location of the radiodense particles seen on the MLO view in Figure 1-1. However, deodorant artifact usually occupies a larger area and involves many more individual particles than are observed in this image. Furthermore, when deodorant particles are extensive in distribution, some of them will by chance be imaged tangentially and will therefore demonstrate their true dermal location. Unfortunately, these mammographic features often cannot be used when only a few calcific particles are present, as in the test patient, since it is unlikely that any particles will be projected tangentially. Therefore, the mammographic information provided in Figures 1-1 and 1-2 is insufficient to either establish or exclude the possibility of deodorant artifact.

The calcific particles seen in the test image are even more likely to represent true intramammary calcifications. A wide variety of histologic abnormalities, both benign and malignant, present as clustered microcalcifications. Sclerosing adenosis (Option (C)) is very common among the benign lesions. It involves proliferation of the intralobular ducts, accompanied by an overgrowth of the other components of the lobule. Dense hyalinization produces the "sclerosing" component of this entity. There does not appear to be any increased predisposition for malignancy. Most often, the microcalcifications seen in patients with sclerosing adenosis are widely distributed throughout both breasts, but biopsy of an isolated cluster of calcifications not infrequently discloses this diagnosis.

Atypical hyperplasia (Option (D)), whether ductal, lobular, or mixed, also presents mammographically as an isolated cluster of microcalcifications. The calcific particles are usually neither characteristically benign nor malignant but, rather, appear to be indeterminate in nature; this is totally consistent with the calcifications seen in the test image. Both bland and atypical hyperplasias of the breast are benign proliferative lesions. However, when a substantial degree of cellular atypia accompanies the hyperplastic changes, the lesion carries a significant risk for subsequent breast carcinoma, approximately 5 times that of normal breast tissue. The risk is even higher, more than 10 times normal, if atypical hyperplasia is found in a woman who has a strong family history of breast cancer.

Ductal carcinoma *in situ* (DCIS) (Option (E)) is a histologically malignant lesion, usually detected at mammographic screening by virtue of the clustered microcalcifications with which it typically presents. The large-cell (or comedo) type of DCIS often displays characteristic fine calcific particles, many of which are linear or branching in shape. The small-cell types of DCIS, called cribriform and micropapillary, more commonly display even smaller calcific particles, which are so tiny that their individual shapes cannot be resolved. Despite these differences, all DCIS lesions can produce a mammographic appearance identical to that seen in the test image.

Finally, dust artifact occasionally simulates breast calcification, but in most cases the true nature of this condition can be suspected on the basis of its mammographic features, even when it occurs in a clustered distribution. Characteristically, particles of dust appear more dense and much more sharply defined than those of intramammary calcification. Dust particles appear to be "too" dense because, by being trapped between the film and the intensifying screen, they permit no light at all from the screen to blacken the film; they appear "too" sharply defined since there can be absolutely no geometric unsharpness when the dust is in direct contact with the recording system. The calcific particles seen in the test image are variable in density and indistinct in shape, and therefore they are very unlikely to represent dust artifact **(Option (B) is correct).** This statement is valid even though, like the calcifications shown in Figures 1-1 and 1-2, virtually all examples of clustered dust artifact are found on only one of the two views that make up the standard mammographic examination.

Question 2

The patient was recalled for additional mammographic imaging. Which *one* of the following is the BEST sequence for obtaining additional images?

   (A) XCCL view, cleavage view, MLO view
   (B) Cleavage view, XCCL view, MLO view
   (C) XCCL view, MLO view, cleavage view
   (D) Cleavage view, MLO view, no XCCL view
   (E) XCCL view, MLO view, no cleavage view

The art of problem-solving mammography involves choosing the various additional projections that are most likely to answer specific unresolved imaging questions and planning the sequence of views that is likely to produce the correct answer most convincingly, with as few exposures as possible.

The test case concerns a very common problem, i.e., the lesion seen on only one standard mammographic projection. The solution to this problem depends to a great extent on the nature of the mammographic finding. For an apparent mass, the most likely explanation is superimposition of normal areas of fibroglandular tissue; therefore, the initial workup is usually planned to establish or exclude the possibility of summation shadow (see Case 2). For apparently clustered microcalcifications (the situation in the test case), it is very unlikely that the finding represents superimposition of isolated calcific particles; therefore, the radiologist normally assumes that a cluster is truly present and begins the workup by distinguishing between the two causes of why the cluster was not seen on one projection.

The first cause of nonvisualization of clustered microcalcifications is poor mammographic technique. A variety of deficiencies can produce this problem, especially if the calcifications are subtle in presentation. The most common deficiencies are underexposure, motion unsharpness, and geometric unsharpness. These are usually readily apparent to the experienced observer; in fact they were not present in the test images (CC view not shown).

The other cause of nonvisualization is that the lesion is so far from the nipple that it has been excluded from the field of view. Assuming that the breast has been positioned properly during exposure, the best way to evaluate whether calcifications have been cut off a given image is to measure the straight-line distance from the nipple to the lesion on the view where the lesion is seen and then to trace an arc of this measured length, centered at the nipple, on the view where the lesion is not seen. If the arc extends beyond the back edge of this radiograph (as it did on the CC view of the test patient), or even if the arc comes within 1 cm of the edge of the film, it is likely that the calcifications were excluded from the view.

In this situation, the next step in evaluation is to obtain a radiograph that includes deeper breast tissues. The MLO view usually images more tissue close to the chest wall than does the CC view. Therefore, the common scenario (true in the test case as well) is that clustered calcifications are seen on the MLO view alone and that a modified CC view is needed. By repeating a CC view with the patient turned either laterally or medially, deeper tissues on one side of the breast can be included, at the expense of including less tissue on the other side. One might argue that the initial exaggerated CC view should always be designed to include more lateral breast tissue, not only because the outermost portion of the breast is often cut off the standard CC view, but also because many more clusters of calcifications are seen laterally rather than medially. However, there is a more sensible approach to deciding the direction in which to exaggerate the CC view, one that is tailored to the specifics of the case being evaluated. This approach uses the location of the calcifications as actually seen on the MLO view to indicate whether they should be found either laterally or medially on the CC view. As illustrated in Figures 1-5 and 1-6, far-lateral breast lesions usually project somewhere in the upper half of the breast on the MLO view, whereas far-medial lesions are ordinarily seen in the lower half of the MLO image. Therefore, in the test patient, the fact that clustered calcifications are seen very near the top of the MLO image indicates that they are probably located in the lateral aspect of the breast and that they are almost certainly not located far medially. Consequently, the next step in mammographic imaging should

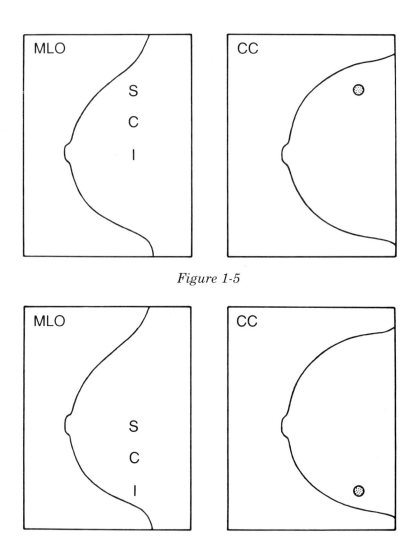

Figure 1-5

Figure 1-6

Figures 1-5 and 1-6.   Drawings of standard MLO and CC projection mammograms illustrate the range of locations of lesions on the MLO view for known locations on the CC view (S = superior; C = central; I = inferior location as found on the 90° lateral view [not shown]). Figure 1-5 demonstrates that far-lateral lesions are seen somewhere in the upper half of an MLO projection mammogram. Figure 1-6, drawn for far-medial lesions, indicates that they project in the lower half of the breast on an MLO view. (Reprinted with permission from Sickles [10].)

be to obtain an exaggerated CC view directed laterally (the so-called XCCL view). Furthermore, there would appear to be no value in attempting an exaggerated CC image directed medially (usually taken as a cleavage view [see Question 4]), either as the first step (Options (B) and (D)) or as a subsequent step (Options (A) and (C)) in evaluation.

If an XCCL view still fails to include the calcifications, the chance that these particles actually represent deodorant artifact would increase in probability to the point that it would be useful to repeat the MLO view on which they were initially seen after the patient washes off any residual deodorant from her breast and axilla. Intramammary calcifications would still be visualized, but deodorant artifact would not.

Thus, in planning the sequence of additional images to obtain for the test patient, the first radiograph should be an XCCL view and should be followed (if necessary) by a repeat MLO view after skin washing **(Option (E) is correct).** There would be no need for a cleavage view, since it would be virtually impossible for calcifications projected so high up on the MLO view to be located very far medially on the CC view.

Question 3

The finding was seen only on the repeat MLO view. A 90° lateral view was then obtained. You are shown the entire image (Figure 1-3 [see page 4]) and a photographic enlargement of the upper portion of the image (Figure 1-4 [see page 4]). Which *one* of the following BEST describes the location of the mammographic finding?

    (A) Upper outer breast, between 10 o'clock and 11 o'clock
    (B) Upper outer breast, between 1 o'clock and 2 o'clock
    (C) Upper central breast, at 12 o'clock
    (D) Upper inner breast, between 10 o'clock and 11 o'clock
    (E) Upper inner breast, between 1 o'clock and 2 o'clock

Visualization of the clustered microcalcifications on the repeat MLO view, taken after skin washing, excludes the possibility of deodorant artifact (and dust artifact as well, although this was never a strong consideration), thus effectively establishing the diagnosis of intramammary calcifications. However, the location of the calcifications remains undetermined because they are still seen only on the MLO projection.

This situation prompted the next step in the workup, i.e., obtaining a 90° lateral projection mammogram (Figure 1-3 [see page 4]). The calcifications are seen once again, still located in the uppermost portion of the image, now projected over the anterior edge of the pectoral muscle shadow. The photographic enlargement of this mammogram (Figure 1-4 [see page 4]) demonstrates that although the calcific particles are portrayed somewhat more clearly than on the initial MLO view, their individual shapes remain indistinct.

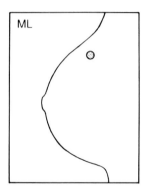 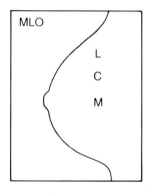 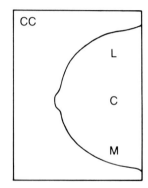

Figure 1-7

Figures 1-7 through 1-9. Drawings of standard 90° lateral (ML), MLO, and CC projection mammograms illustrate how to determine the expected location of a lesion on the CC view when its location is known on both the 90° lateral and the MLO views. Use the drawings by choosing among the three possible locations of the lesion on the MLO view and then finding the corresponding location on the CC view. L = lateral; C = central; M = medial. Figure 1-7 should be used for lesions seen in the upper aspect of the breast on the 90° lateral view. Figures 1-8 and 1-9 should be used for lesions seen in the central and lower aspects of the breast on the 90° lateral view, respectively. (Reprinted with permission from Sickles [10].)

The 90° lateral view also provides useful information about the three-dimensional location of the clustered microcalcifications; this is obtained by triangulation, using the MLO and lateral views. Among the simplest visual aids available to learn how to make triangulation estimates are the line drawings presented in Figure 1-7. As explained in the figure legend, one may use these drawings by identifying the known locations of the abnormality on lateral and MLO view drawings and then consulting the CC view drawing to obtain the expected location of the lesion on this projection, which is orthogonal to the lateral projection. Thus, the abnormality in the test patient, which is located in the uppermost aspect of the breast on both the lateral and MLO views, would be found in the far outer region of the breast on the CC view. This establishes the site of the lesion to be in the middle of the upper outer quadrant of the breast, in effect excluding locations in the upper central and upper inner quadrants (Options (C), (D), and (E)).

The midportion of the upper outer quadrant of the left breast corresponds to a clock face position of between 1 o'clock and 2 o'clock (Option (B)). However, referring back to the initial description of the test images, the clustered calcifications were in the right breast, within which the cor-

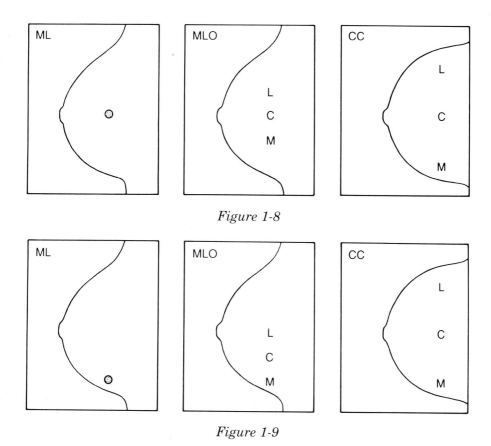

Figure 1-8

Figure 1-9

responding upper outer quadrant location is found between 10 o'clock and 11 o'clock **(Option (A) is correct).**

This apparently trivial exercise in determining clock face position actually has considerable significance in the daily practice of mammography. First, when assigning the clock face position of a known-quadrant lesion, one must be very careful to note the breast in which the lesion is located, since the combination of quadrant and clock face descriptors for lesions in the right and left breasts are different for all positions except 6 o'clock and 12 o'clock (e.g., the upper outer quadrant of the right breast is found between 9 o'clock and 12 o'clock whereas the same quadrant of the left breast is located between 12 o'clock and 3 o'clock). Second, by describing all breast lesions according to the side, quadrant, and clock face position, the radiologist provides a very helpful internal consistency check to use when signing or otherwise verifying transcribed mammography reports, a task that is ordinarily performed without access to the pertinent films. Right-left confusion occurs only rarely but can have disastrous consequences. Such an internal consistency check will permit the radiologist to know that there has been an error in either dictation or transcription if the report describes an impossible combination of descriptors (e.g., upper outer quadrant of the right breast at the 2 o'clock position).

For those interested in using the previously described line drawings for triangulation of all lesions initially identified on MLO and 90° lateral views, Figures 1-8 and 1-9 are supplied to complement those in Figure 1-7, by providing information on lesion location for abnormalities situated elsewhere than in the upper aspect of the breast on the 90° lateral view.

Question 4

The next step should be:

    (A) cleavage view with the X-ray tube angled 5° away from the MLO projection
    (B) XCCL view with the X-ray tube angled 5° toward the MLO projection
    (C) CC view with no breast compression
    (D) caudocranial view
    (E) CC projection lumpogram of the upper central breast

The next step in the problem-solving mammography workup involves obtaining an additional mammogram in whichever modified CC projection is most likely to include the clustered calcifications, which have yet to be seen on an orthogonal view. Of course, the choice of which view to obtain will be governed by the result of the triangulation procedure described previously.

Had one (erroneously) concluded that the lesion was located in the upper inner quadrant of the breast, it would have been proper to modify the standard CC view to include the most medial breast tissues close to the sternum. The cleavage view is a modified CC view that includes the medial portions of both breasts, often somewhat more of the ipsilateral breast than of the contralateral breast. It is probably the most effective view if one wishes to include medial breast tissue by using a craniocaudally directed X-ray beam. There is no reason to take a cleavage view with the X-ray tube angled 5° away from the MLO projection (Option (A)); vertical beam orientation is preferable.

Had one (erroneously) concluded that the lesion was located in the upper breast at the 12 o'clock position, it would have been proper to modify the standard CC view by encouraging inclusion of the uppermost central breast tissues. A lesion in this part of the breast is very difficult to image on the CC view because as compression is applied inferiorly, the lesion is likely to slip back toward the chest wall, behind the back of the

compression paddle. Simply repeating a CC projection exposure with
maximum elevation of the inframammary fold might solve the problem
without need for further maneuvers, since the compression paddle might
have to travel inferiorly to a much lesser extent in achieving taut breast
compression, thereby maintaining the lesion within the field of view.
However, this approach does not work in every case, and alternative
methods might be chosen. One approach would be to repeat the CC view
with no compression (Option (C)). However, this would probably fail to
display the calcifications, even if they were included in the image, owing
to a combination of motion unsharpness (compression usually restrains
breast motion), geometric unsharpness (the area of interest would not be
compressed inferiorly, closer to the film), and underexposure (the breast
would not be flattened to uniform thickness). A potentially more successful approach would be to obtain a caudocranial view (Option (D)), which
is taken by placing the film holder at the uppermost part of the breast
and applying compression from below. A final, equally successful method
would be to obtain a CC projection lumpogram of the upper central
breast (Option (E)), in effect compressing only the uppermost central
breast tissues within which the suspect lesion was located.

However, triangulation actually showed the calcifications to be
located high up and far lateral within the upper outer quadrant of the
breast. The most successful modification of the CC view in this circumstance is an XCCL view with the X-ray tube angled 5° toward the MLO
projection **(Option (B) is correct).** The purpose of the slight tube angulation is to allow the compression paddle to clear the humeral head as it
travels inferiorly. This avoids the need to move the shoulder out of the
way, a maneuver that may cause the outermost portion of the breast to
become dislodged from the field of view.

Question 5

The additional view chosen in the previous question again showed the mammographic finding, but neither this view nor spot-compression magnification views portrayed it any more clearly than in Figures 1-2 and 1-4. The next step should be:

(A) routine mammographic screening in 1 year
(B) follow-up mammography in 6 months
(C) breast ultrasonography
(D) breast CT scan
(E) preoperative needle localization

Figure 1-10 shows the successful slightly angled XCCL view of the
test patient, which indeed includes the clustered microcalcifications at

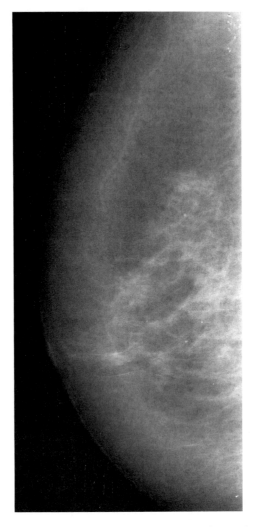

Figure 1-10. Same patient as in Figures 1-1 through 1-4. The same breast as seen in the test figures was imaged by using an XCCL view with the X-ray tube angled 5° toward the MLO projection. The cluster of tiny calcifications is now included in this variant of the CC view, located very far laterally in the axillary tail region of the breast.

the far lateral aspect of the breast. The calcific particles still appear indistinct in shape on this view, as they did on additional spot-compression magnification views (not shown). It is very doubtful that breast ultrasonography (Option (C)) or a breast CT scan (Option (D)) would contribute meaningful information to characterize the lesion better; the resolution of these procedures is far inferior to that of mammography, and therefore the calcifications probably would not be seen at all.

Before making a final mammographic diagnosis, it is the practice of many experienced radiologists to perform internal consistency checks of lesion location and depth, by using the several views on which an abnormality is visible, to confirm that the finding seen on each view is indeed the same lesion. Unlike the workup carried out with the test patient, most mammographic abnormalities are identified first on MLO and CC views, with subsequent triangulation being performed to locate the lesion on a 90° lateral view. The line drawings presented in Figures 1-11 through 1-13 are used for this purpose, with the internal consistency check of lesion location usually carried out starting with the CC and MLO views and then continuing to the 90° lateral view. Figures 1-14 through 1-16 illustrate the method used for this procedure, as well as for the consistency check of lesion depth.

It is now appropriate to make a mammographic diagnosis and to recommend appropriate subsequent management. The clustered microcalcifications in the test patient are variable in size and density and indistinct in shape. This combination of mammographic features indicates a likelihood of malignancy of approximately 20 to 25%. With such a relatively high probability of carcinoma, it would be inappropriate to recommend either routine mammographic screening in 1 year (Option (A)) or follow-up mammography in 6 months (Option (B)). Rather, the calcifications should be interpreted as being suspicious for malignancy, accompanied by a recommendation that biopsy be considered, perhaps with the aid of preoperative needle localization if a mass is not readily palpable even in retrospect **(Option (E) is correct).**

Edward A. Sickles, M.D.

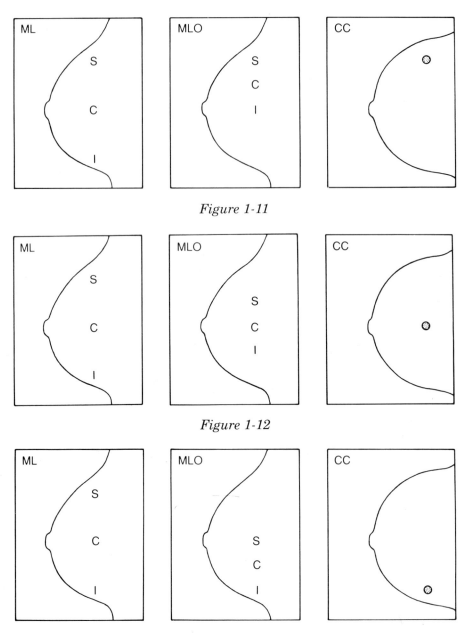

Figure 1-11

Figure 1-12

Figure 1-13

Figures 1-11 through 1-13. Drawings of standard 90° ML, MLO, and CC projection mammograms illustrate how to determine the expected location of a lesion on the 90° lateral view when its location is known on both the MLO and CC views. Use the drawings by choosing among the three possible locations of the lesion on the MLO view and then finding the corresponding location on the 90° lateral view. S = superior; C = central; I = inferior. In each set of illustrations, note that a straight line drawn between the location of an abnormality on the CC and MLO views can be extended to its expected location on the 90° lateral view. Figures 1-11, 1-12, and 1-13 should be used for lesions seen in the lateral, central, and medial aspects of the breast on the CC view, respectively. (Reprinted with permission from Sickles [10].)

16

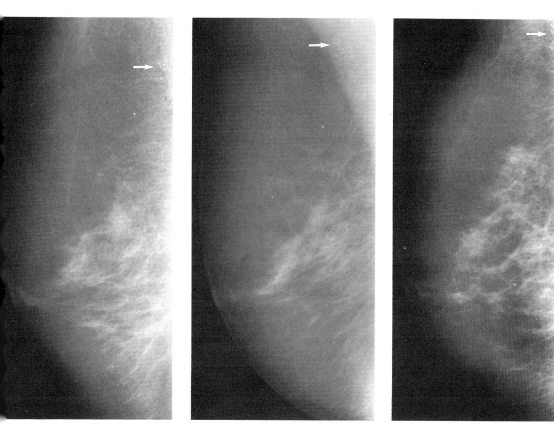

Figure 1-14   *Figure 1-15*   *Figure 1-16*

Figures 1-14 through 1-16 (Same as Figure 1-3, Figure 1-1, and Figure 1-10, respectively).   Internal consistency checks of lesion location and depth. You are again shown the whole-breast mammograms that demonstrate the clustered calcifications (arrow) on the 90° lateral (Figure 1-14), MLO (Figure 1-15), and XCCL (Figure 1-16) projections. These images are displayed in similar orientation to the line drawings shown in Figures 1-11 through 1-13, with the MLO view in between the other two, the breast facing in the same direction, the projection marker in the same corner of the radiograph, and the nipple at the same vertical level on all three radiographs. The internal consistency check for lesion location is confirmed by drawing an imaginary line between the lesion as seen on the CC and MLO views and then noting that a direct extension of this line further to the left predicts the actual location of the lesion on the 90° lateral view. The consistency check for lesion depth is validated by comparing the straight-line distance from the nipple to the lesion on each view.

SUGGESTED READINGS

CALCIFICATIONS SEEN ON ONLY ONE STANDARD MAMMOGRAPHIC PROJECTION

1. Homer MJ. Mammographic interpretation: a practical approach. New York: McGraw-Hill; 1991:34–47
2. Ikeda DM. Mammographic analysis of breast calcifications. In: Sickles EA, Kopans DB (eds), Syllabus for the categorical course on breast imaging. Reston, VA: American College of Radiology; 1990:47–55
3. Kopans DB. Breast imaging. Philadelphia: JB Lippincott; 1989:86–96
4. Lanyi M. Diagnosis and differential diagnosis of breast calcifications. Berlin: Springer-Verlag; 1986
5. Sickles EA. Breast calcifications: mammographic evaluation. Radiology 1986; 160:289–293

TRIANGULATING THE LOCATION OF A LESION BY USING THE OBLIQUE VIEW

6. Eklund GW. Problem-solving mammography. In: Sickles EA, Kopans DB (eds), Syllabus for the categorical course on breast imaging. Reston, VA: American College of Radiology; 1990:69–75
7. Eklund GW, Cardenosa G. The art of mammographic positioning. Radiol Clin North Am 1992; 30:21–53
8. Kopans DB. Breast imaging. Philadelphia: JB Lippincott; 1989:43–59
9. Kopans DB, Waitzkin ED, Linetsky L, et al. Localization of breast lesions identified on only one mammographic view. AJR 1987; 149:39–41
10. Sickles EA. Practical solutions to common mammographic problems: tailoring the examination. AJR 1988; 151:31–39
11. Sickles EA. Tailoring the mammogram: problem solving and special views. In: Thrall JH (ed), Current practice of radiology. St. Louis: BC Decker; 1993:393–402
12. Swann CA, Kopans DB, McCarthy KA, White G, Hall DA. Localization of occult breast lesions: practical solutions to problems of triangulation. Radiology 1987; 163:577–579

Notes

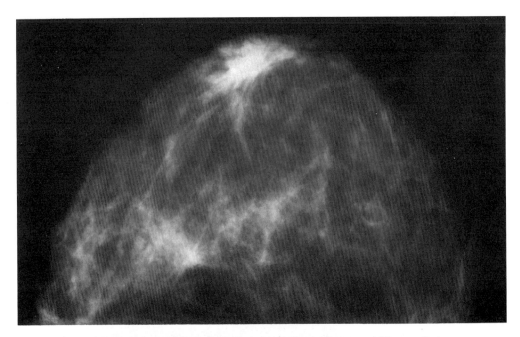

Figure 2-1

Figures 2-1 through 2-3. This 58-year-old asymptomatic woman underwent mammographic screening after a normal breast physical examination. You are shown the CC (Figure 2-1) and MLO (Figure 2-2) views of the left breast from that examination, as well as a photographic enlargement of a portion of the CC view (Figure 2-3).

Figure 2-2

20

Case 2: Lesion Seen on Only One Standard Mammographic Projection

Question 6

Which *one* of the following is the LEAST likely explanation for the mammographic findings?

(A) Carcinoma, upper outer quadrant
(B) Carcinoma, lower outer quadrant
(C) Cyst
(D) Postsurgical scar tissue
(E) Summation shadow

The CC views shown in Figures 2-1 and 2-3 demonstrate a poorly defined, irregular area of fibroglandular density in the lateral aspect of the breast, with some suggestion of the presence of spiculation (arrows, Figure 2-4). However, these observations cannot be confirmed with certainty on the MLO projection (Figure 2-2). It is true that on this view, in the inferior aspect of the breast, there is a poorly defined area of fibroglandular density similar in size to and at approximately the same depth from the nipple as the lesion seen on the CC view (open arrow, Figure 2-5). On the other hand, equidistant from the nipple there is also a considerably larger area of fibroglandular density in the upper aspect of the breast, within which the finding on the CC view could easily be obscured (arrows, Figure 2-5). Moreover, it is possible that there is no abnormality at all but, rather, that the finding on the CC view represents superimposition of innocuous areas of benign fibroglandular tissue.

Therefore, from the mammographic information available from the two standard projection images, there are two potential locations for an ill-defined breast lesion in this case: one in the upper outer quadrant and the other in the lower outer quadrant. Alternatively, the "lesion" may simply be a summation shadow (Option (E)). In addition, assuming that

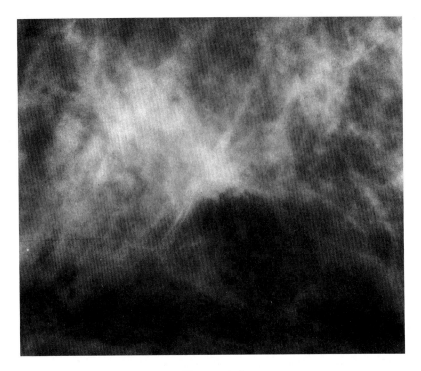

Figure 2-3

a breast mass is truly present, its irregular and perhaps spiculated borders require the differential diagnosis to include such abnormalities as carcinoma (Options (A) and (B)), postsurgical and post-inflammatory scar tissue (Option (D)), radial scar, and abscess. A cyst, on the other hand, is a very unlikely diagnosis because in the great majority of cases such a lesion demonstrates round or oval contours with well-defined smooth borders **(Option (C) is correct).** Although a thick-walled cyst occasionally shows irregular margins because of an abundant chronic inflammatory reaction, spiculation is rarely if ever seen. Furthermore, although it is not unusual for some or even most of the borders of a simple cyst to be obscured by nearby fibroglandular tissue, when the borders of a cyst are adjacent to fat they should not appear as irregular and ill defined as those seen in the test images.

Question 7

In the diagnosis of the lesion in the test patient, which *one* of the following should be the next step?

    (A) Routine mammographic screening in 1 year
    (B) Follow-up mammography in 6 months
    (C) Ultrasonography
    (D) Additional mammographic imaging
    (E) Needle localization

The major diagnostic distinction to be made in the test patient is whether the finding seen on only one standard mammographic view represents a true breast mass or a summation shadow. In this commonly encountered situation, there is sometimes enough information already available on the CC and MLO images to establish a diagnosis of summation shadow. This requires (1) assurance that the second standard view includes a sufficient amount of breast tissue close to the chest wall so that the mammographic finding could not have been cut off, and (2) absence of any area or areas of surrounding isodense fibroglandular tissue on the second standard view that could obscure the finding. The easiest way to carry out these two assessments is to measure the straight-line distance from the nipple to the suspect finding on the first standard view and then use this length in making appropriate measurements on the second view.

As discussed above, in the test patient there are indeed areas on the MLO view that may correspond to the finding on the CC view, so that a confident diagnosis of summation shadow cannot be made from the two standard views alone. Carcinoma remains a major diagnostic possibility, and therefore the next step in management should not be either routine mammographic screening in 1 year (Option (A)) or follow-up mammography in 6 months (Option (B)). Similarly, the diagnosis of summation shadow cannot be excluded from an evaluation of the two standard views, and so it would be inappropriate to recommend needle localization (Option (E)) as the next step in the diagnostic work-up.

Ultrasonography (Option (C)) might prove helpful in this patient if it were to demonstrate either a cystic or a solid mass. However, several factors militate against this as an acceptable next step in the imaging strategy for the test patient. (1) Cyst is a very unlikely possibility, as discussed above. (2) For a solid mass, ultrasonography is effective primarily when the three-dimensional location of the lesion is already known (see the discussion of Question 8). (3) Lack of visualization cannot reliably exclude the possibility that the mammographic finding is a true breast mass because many such lesions are not imaged by ultrasonography if

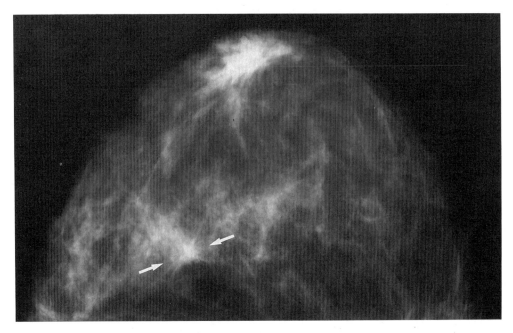

Figure 2-4

Figures 2-4 and 2-5 (Same as Figures 2-1 and 2-2, respectively). Lesion seen on only one standard mammographic projection. Figure 2-4 is the CC view of the test patient, showing a poorly defined, irregular, and possibly spiculated area of fibroglandular density in the lateral aspect of the breast (arrows). Figure 2-5 is the corresponding MLO view, on which the existence of a mass cannot be confirmed, even though there is a mammographic finding in the inferior aspect of the breast that is similar in size and approximately the same depth from the nipple (open arrow). This is because there is also a considerably larger area of fibroglandular density in the upper aspect of the breast (arrows), within which the finding on the CC view could be obscured. Furthermore, it is possible that the finding on the CC view simply represents a summation shadow.

they are small, solid, close to the chest wall, and surrounded by fatty tissue. (4) Even if a mass were found on ultrasonography, additional correlative mammographic imaging would still be required to ensure that the mammographic and ultrasonographic findings represented one and the same lesion.

The proper next step in the diagnostic work-up of the test patient is additional mammographic imaging **(Option (D) is correct).** In almost all cases, such an approach will rapidly and reliably differentiate between a true breast mass and a summation shadow. The various mammographic projections and techniques used for this purpose are

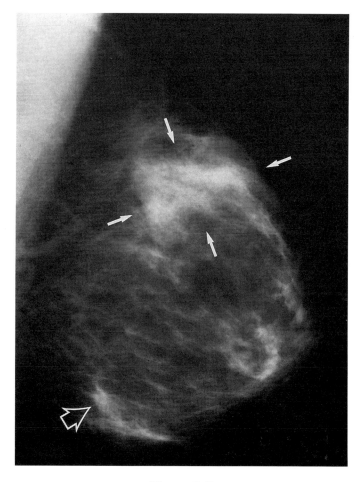

Figure 2-5

described at length in the discussion of Question 9. Findings that prove to represent summation shadows will be interpreted as normal, with a recommendation for subsequent mammographic screening in 1 year. Findings that prove to be true masses may then be evaluated by ultrasonography and spot-compression magnification mammography. Subsequent management will depend on the results of these additional examinations.

Question 8

Concerning ultrasonography of a nonpalpable, well-defined, 1-cm mass,

- (A) nonvisualization nearly always necessitates biopsy
- (B) identification of a solid, irregular, hypoechoic mass nearly always necessitates biopsy
- (C) Doppler imaging reliably discriminates benign from malignant masses
- (D) it generally should not be performed until the lesion is identified on at least two mammographic projections

The principal role of ultrasonography in the evaluation of a mammographically detected well-defined mass is to establish or exclude the diagnosis of simple benign cyst, thereby averting any further work-up for a mass that is purely cystic. If strict ultrasonographic criteria are followed, uncomplicated cysts can be identified with virtually 100% accuracy. This subject is covered more fully in the discussion of Case 10.

Ultrasonographic visualization of solid masses can be much more challenging because, unlike simple cysts, which are anechoic, solid lesions often return low-amplitude echoes, which are very similar to those produced by normal fatty breast tissue. The current practice of using hand-held transducers further confounds detection of some nonpalpable solid masses because it is tedious and time-consuming and because complete coverage of large volumes of breast tissue is very difficult. Therefore, most radiologists defer the use of ultrasonography until a lesion is identified on at least two mammographic projections **(Option (D) is true).** This approach limits the extent of manual scanning to the region defined by mammographic localization and ensures that ultrasonography is used to evaluate only true masses, not summation shadows. Thus, when ultrasonography fails to visualize a mass, the radiologist can conclude not only that the lesion is noncystic (i.e., that it is solid) but also that it is a real and important finding requiring further evaluation. However, biopsy is not needed for many solid masses that are not visualized by ultrasonography **(Option (A) is false).** Rather, masses that have mammographically well-defined margins, especially as seen on spot-compression magnification mammograms, are usually interpreted as "probably benign," with the recommendation for periodic mammographic surveillance.

On the other hand, sonographic findings may indicate a need for biopsy of a mass. When ultrasonography demonstrates that a hypoechoic mass does have irregular margins, particularly if there is decreased through transmission of sound (shadowing), cancer should be suggested. Thus, biopsy nearly always will be recommended under these circumstances despite a "probably benign" mammographic appearance (**Option (B) is true**).

There has been recent interest in the possible clinical utility of the blood flow information provided by Doppler ultrasonographic techniques. This was sparked by a preliminary report that described different flow signals for benign and malignant breast masses. However, more extensive experience has subsequently indicated that Doppler imaging does not reliably differentiate benign from malignant masses (**Option (C) is false**). As a result, these techniques are not widely used in the evaluation of breast lesions, although there has been some recent interest in color Doppler imaging.

Question 9

Additional mammographic images likely to help differentiate a mass seen on only one standard projection from a summation shadow include:

(A) 90° lateral view
(B) view with 5 to 10° tube angulation from the view demonstrating the finding
(C) tangential view
(D) "roll" view
(E) spot-compression view
(F) magnification view

The mammographic work-up of a finding seen on only one standard projection can involve a wide variety of additional views. The specific choice of imaging approach will depend primarily on the depth and location of the suspect finding.

Initially, the radiologist must decide whether the finding was not seen on one view because it was so close to the chest wall that it was cut off the image. If so, the next step in the work-up should be an additional view designed to include deeper breast tissues, at the most likely site of the lesion. For example, an ovoid masslike density seen close to the chest wall on an MLO view might have been cut off the standard CC view because it was located very far laterally in the axillary tail region (if the lesion projects into the upper aspect of the breast on the MLO view) or very far medially near the sternum (if the lesion projects into the lower breast). Exaggerated CC views have been devised to include tissues located around the convexity of the chest wall, either laterally or medially.

On the other hand, if the radiologist concludes that the lesion is sufficiently close to the nipple that it could not have been cut off the second view, the next step in evaluation should be an attempt to distinguish between a true breast mass and a summation shadow. Numerous additional mammographic projections can be used for this purpose, all of which operate on the premise that on a different projection, the superimposition inherent in the production of a summation shadow will no longer be present, whereas a true mass will remain visible.

One such approach is to obtain a 90° lateral view **(Option (A) is true),** which is taken at so different an angle of obliquity from the standard MLO or CC view that repeat visualization of a summation shadow would be virtually impossible. However, such a great change in the obliquity of exposure is not required to prevent duplication of fibroglandular tissue superimposition; all that is needed is a 5 to 10° tube angulation from the view that demonstrated the mammographic finding **(Option (B) is true).** This imaging approach involves only a very slight change in tube angulation, and so it has the additional advantage of causing only a small shift in the location of a true breast mass, thereby considerably limiting the size of the area in which one must search for the suspect finding. Another method of producing a 5 to 10° change in the obliquity of exposure is the use of a "roll" view **(Option (D) is true).** This is done by applying a gentle amount of torque to the breast, as illustrated in Figure 2-6, so that previously overlapping fibroglandular structures are no longer superimposed.

Still other imaging techniques are also successful in differentiating between a true breast mass and a summation shadow. The use of spot compression spreads apart overlying islands of breast tissue more effectively than whole-breast compression, thereby eliminating most summation shadows without resorting to any change in obliquity of exposure **(Option (E) is true).** Magnification mammography not only produces images that depict true masses with greater clarity but also reduces the likelihood of summation shadows because it uses a more divergent (hence differently angled) x-ray beam than conventional exposures **(Option (F) is true).**

The purpose of the tangential view is to project superficially located breast structures as close as possible to the skin. This technique is most useful in establishing the intradermal location of clustered skin calcifications, which are always benign (see the discussion of Case 16). The technique often requires some change in the obliquity of exposure compared with standard mammographic projections, and so it may fortuitously eliminate a summation shadow. However, the tangential view is not designed for, nor is it well suited to, the differentiation between a true breast mass and a summation shadow, since it is difficult to position the breast so that a nonpalpable finding is projected tangentially, especially if the finding simply represents superimposed tissues. As a result, tangential views are not used in the work-up of the lesion seen on only one standard projection **(Option (C) is false).**

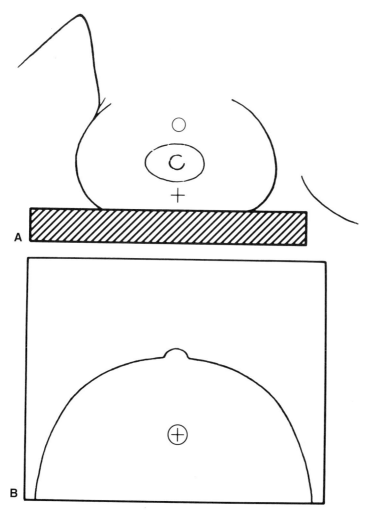

Figure 2-6. Varying the obliquity of mammographic projection by changing the orientation of the breast, using the "rolled" view. (A) This breast has an area of benign fibroglandular tissue at the 12 o'clock position (O) and another at the 6 o'clock position (+). (B) These two areas may superimpose on a standard CC mammogram to create a summation shadow with masslike features. (C) The upper aspect of the breast has been "rolled" laterally, so that the two areas of benign fibroglandular tissue no longer project over each other on straight CC projection. (D) A repeat CC mammogram shows that the summation shadow has disappeared. (Reprinted with permission from Sickles [6].)

Among the various additional mammographic views that can successfully distinguish between a true breast mass and a summation shadow, no one view is inherently superior. Therefore, the choice of

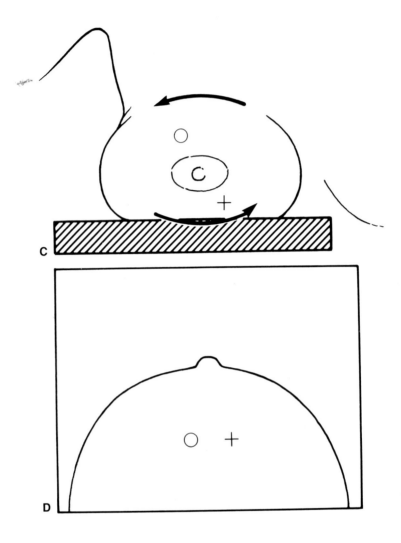

which to use is based primarily on personal preference. To evaluate the finding in the CC view of the test patient (Figure 2-7), an imaging technique that combined the features of several mammographic views into a single additional shallow, oblique, spot-compression magnification exposure was used (Figure 2-8). The disappearance of the suspect finding on this extra view permits the confident mammographic diagnosis of summation shadow. The rationale behind the strategy of combination-view imaging is that the several component techniques operate by different mechanisms: shallow oblique positioning by producing a slight change in obliquity of exposure, spot compression by spreading apart superimposed islands of fibroglandular tissue, and magnification by providing for increased image clarity and detail. Thus, the imaging advantages of the

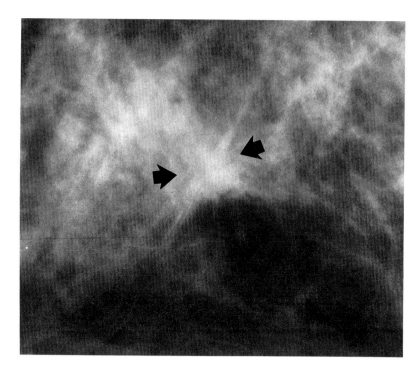

Figure 2-7 (Same as Figure 2-3). Summation shadow. Figure 2-7 is a photographic enlargement of a portion of the CC view of the test patient, showing a poorly defined, irregular area of fibroglandular density (arrows) that appears to have somewhat spiculated margins. This finding could not be confirmed with certainty on the MLO view.

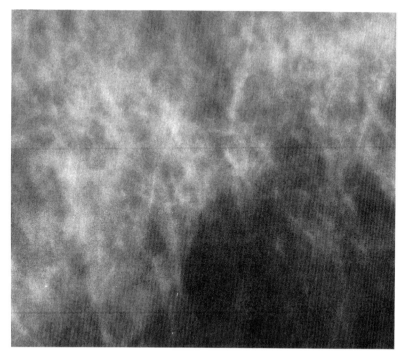

Figure 2-8. Same patient as in Figures 2-1 through 2-5 and in Figure 2-7. On this shallow oblique, spot-compression magnification view of the area of interest, the suspect finding is no longer seen. When a mammographic finding seen on only one standard projection cannot be identified on an additional fine-detail view taken with a very slight change in the obliquity of exposure, this provides convincing evidence that the finding was a summation shadow rather than a true abnormality.

31

combined techniques are additive, and the overall result is more mammographic information in a single exposure than would be available from an exposure involving any one technique alone.

Question 10

Concerning preoperative needle localization of a density seen on only one standard mammographic projection,

(A) biopsy is the preferred management option when the density appears irregular and spiculated
(B) a 90° lateral mammogram should be deferred until the day of surgery to minimize inconvenience to the patient
(C) localization by a conventional technique cannot be performed until the mammographic density is clearly identified on an additional mammographic view
(D) even without additional mammographic views, stereotactic localization will permit placement of a needle within the density in nearly all cases

The primary purpose of preoperative needle localization is to guide the surgeon to the region of a nonpalpable lesion and hence ensure its removal by excisional biopsy. However, it is premature to recommend needle localization for a lesion seen on only one standard mammographic projection, even if it appears to have an irregular contour and spiculated borders **(Option (A) is false)**. Several reasons support this conclusion. (1) The spiculated mammographic lesion seen on only one view may actually represent a summation shadow (Figures 2-7 and 2-8), for which needle localization is impossible since there is no true lesion to localize. (2) Until an abnormality is seen on more than one projection, the radiologist cannot describe the three-dimensional location of the lesion. This description permits repeat physical examination directed at the site of the lesion, which should be done before deciding whether needle localization is really necessary; up to 25% of initially nonpalpable abnormalities indeed are palpated in retrospect, thereby averting needle localization. (3) Conventional needle localization techniques require that the target lesion be clearly visualized on two different mammographic views, preferably orthogonal projections, to provide verification in all three dimensions that the needle has been placed in close proximity to the lesion **(Option (C) is true)**.

The goal of demonstrating a suspect mammographic abnormality on orthogonal projections usually prompts the radiologist to obtain a 90° lateral view. If the lesion is already visible on standard CC and MLO views and if the patient has already left the premises, this may be deferred until the day of surgery to minimize inconvenience to the patient. However, for the lesion initially seen on only one standard projection, the 90° lateral view should be obtained before the day of surgery, at the same time that the patient returns for additional imaging to differentiate between a summation shadow and a true breast mass **(Option (B) is false)**. It is inappropriate to do this work-up as part of the needle localization procedure, because surgery will have to be cancelled at the last minute if the finding proves to be a summation shadow, causing unnecessary stress to the radiologist, the surgeon, and especially the patient. Furthermore, costly radiologic and surgical resources are wasted in the process.

Stereotactic devices have been adapted for mammographic use to permit placement of a needle within a nonpalpable lesion in the great majority of cases, so that tissue can be obtained percutaneously for cytologic or histologic evaluation or both. These systems do not use orthogonal views, but it is still necessary to see the target lesion clearly on 30° stereoscopic views for localization to be precise. For the lesion seen initially on only one view, stereotactically guided tissue sampling should not be attempted until the diagnosis of summation shadow has been excluded, in order to avert the morbidity of needle placement for a nonexistent lesion **(Option (D) is false)**.

Edward A. Sickles, M.D.

SUGGESTED READINGS

LESION SEEN ON ONLY ONE STANDARD MAMMOGRAPHIC PROJECTION

1. Berkowitz JE, Gatewood OM, Gayler BW. Equivocal mammographic findings: evaluation with spot compression. Radiology 1989; 171:369–371
2. Eklund GW. Problem-solving mammography. In: Sickles EA, Kopans DB (eds), Syllabus for the categorical course on breast imaging. Reston, VA: American College of Radiology; 1990:69–75
3. Eklund GW, Cardenosa G. The art of mammographic positioning. Radiol Clin North Am 1992; 30:21–53
4. Kopans DB. Breast imaging. Philadelphia: JB Lippincott; 1989:43–59
5. Logan WW, Janus J. Use of special mammographic views to maximize radiographic information. Radiol Clin North Am 1987; 25:953–959
6. Sickles EA. Practical solutions to common mammographic problems: tailoring the examination. AJR 1988; 151:31–39
7. Sickles EA. Combining spot-compression and other special views to maximize mammographic information (letter). Radiology 1989; 173:571
8. Sickles EA. Tailoring the mammogram: problem solving and special views. In: Thrall JH (ed), Current practice of radiology. St. Louis: BC Decker; 1993:393–402

9. Adler DD, Carson PL, Rubin JM, Quinn-Reid D. Doppler ultrasound color flow imaging in the study of breast cancer: preliminary findings. Ultrasound Med Biol 1990; 16:553–559

10. Bassett LW, Kimme-Smith C. Breast sonography. AJR 1991; 156:449–455

11. Bassett LW, Kimme-Smith C, Sutherland LK, Gold RH, Sarti D, King W III. Automated and hand-held breast US: effect on patient management. Radiology 1987; 165:103–108

12. Cosgrove DO, Kedar RP, Bamber JC, et al. Breast diseases: color Doppler US in differential diagnosis. Radiology 1993; 189:99–104

13. Dock W, Grabenwöger F, Metz V, Eibenberger K, Farres MT. Tumor vascularization: assessment with duplex sonography. Radiology 1991; 181:241–244

14. Feig SA. Breast masses. Mammographic and sonographic evaluation. Radiol Clin North Am 1992; 30:67–92

15. Hilton SV, Leopold GR, Olson LK, Willson SA. Real-time breast sonography: application in 300 consecutive patients. AJR 1986; 147:479–486

16. Jackson VP. Breast neoplasms: duplex sonographic imaging as an adjunct in diagnosis (letter). Radiology 1989; 170:578

17. Jackson VP. The role of US in breast imaging. Radiology 1990; 177:305–311

18. Jellins J, Kossoff G, Reeve TS. Detection and classification of liquid-filled masses in the breast by gray scale echography. Radiology 1977; 125:205–212

19. Jokich PM, Monticciolo DL, Adler YT. Breast ultrasonography. Radiol Clin North Am 1992; 30:993–1009

20. Kopans DB. Breast imaging. Philadelphia: JB Lippincott; 1989:227–247

21. McNicholas MMJ, Mercer PM, Miller JC, McDermott EWM, O'Higgins NJ, MacErlean DP. Color Doppler sonography in the evaluation of palpable breast masses. AJR 1993; 161:765–771

22. Mendelson EB. Breast sonography. In: Sickles EA, Kopans DB (eds), Syllabus for the categorical course on breast imaging. Reston, VA: American College of Radiology; 1990:31–45

23. Rubin E, Miller VE, Berland LL, Han SY, Koehler RE, Stanley RJ. Hand-held real-time breast sonography. AJR 1985; 144:623–627

24. Schoenberger SG, Sutherland CM, Robinson AE. Breast neoplasms: duplex sonographic imaging as an adjunct in diagnosis. Radiology 1988; 168:665–668

25. Sickles EA, Filly RA, Callen PW. Benign breast lesions: ultrasound detection and diagnosis. Radiology 1984; 151:467–470

NEEDLE LOCALIZATION

26. Bolmgren J, Jacobson B, Nordenström B. Stereotaxic instrument for needle biopsy of the mamma. AJR 1977; 129:121–125

27. Dowlatshahi K, Gent HJ, Schmidt R, Jokich PM, Bibbo M, Sprenger E. Nonpalpable breast tumors: diagnosis with stereotaxic localization and fine-needle aspiration. Radiology 1989; 170:427–433

28. Fajardo LL, Davis JR, Wiens JL, Trego DC. Mammography-guided stereotactic fine-needle aspiration cytology of nonpalpable breast lesions: pro-

spective comparison with surgical biopsy results. AJR 1990; 155:977–981

29. Homer MJ, Smith TJ, Safaii H. Prebiopsy needle localization. Methods, problems, and expected results. Radiol Clin North Am 1992; 30:139–153

30. Kopans DB. Breast imaging. Philadelphia: JB Lippincott; 1989:320–341

31. Kopans DB, Waitzkin ED, Linetsky L, et al. Localization of breast lesions identified on only one mammographic view. AJR 1987; 149:39–41

32. Löfgren M, Andersson I, Lindholm K. Stereotactic fine-needle aspiration for cytologic diagnosis of nonpalpable breast lesions. AJR 1990; 154:1191–1195

33. Parker SH, Lovin JD, Jobe WE, et al. Stereotactic breast biopsy with a biopsy gun. Radiology 1990; 176:741–747

34. Swann CA, Kopans DB, McCarthy KA, White G, Hall DA. Localization of occult breast lesions: practical solutions to problems of triangulation. Radiology 1987; 163:577–579

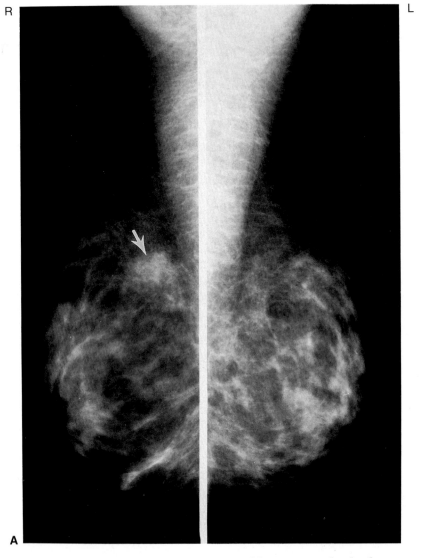

R   L

A

Figure 3-1. This asymptomatic 50-year-old woman, who had a normal physical examination 2 weeks earlier, underwent baseline mammographic screening. You are shown 50° MLO (A) and CC (B) views of both breasts.

Case 3:   Mammographic Positioning

Question 11

Plausible reasons why a poorly marginated density (arrow) is seen in the right breast only on the MLO view include the following:

(A) it is located too far laterally to be seen on a CC image
(B) it is located too far medially to be seen on a CC image
(C) it is located too high in the superior portion of the breast to be seen on a CC image
(D) it represents a summation shadow
(E) it is masked by overlapping parenchymal elements

The breast is a teardrop-shaped gland with a narrow extension toward the axilla. In approximately 11% of women this axillary extension, known as the tail of Spence, is quite prominent, wrapping around and occasionally behind the lateral margin of the pectoralis muscle. A prominent tail of Spence is recognized on the MLO view as fibroglandular tissue superimposed on the upper pectoral muscle. Since the poorly marginated density indicated by the arrow in Figure 3-1A is seen at approximately the same site, it certainly could be within the tail of Spence. Such a laterally located structure will generally be excluded from view on a properly positioned CC image **(Option (A) is true).** The CC view, as correctly performed in the test patient, should include posterior medial breast tissue to the sternal margin so as not to exclude medial breast lesions from the image **(Option (B) is false).**

Traditional teaching of mammographic positioning for the CC view has called for positioning the film holder at the level of the inframammary fold (IMF) when the breast is unsupported, implying that this neutral IMF position is a fixed and immobile landmark. However, the IMF is actually very mobile and can be elevated from 1 to 7 cm, depending on the size of the breast, natural skin elasticity, and the degree of breast ptosis. The CC images (Figure 3-1B) were obtained without attention to breast mobility in that the IMF was not elevated. If the IMF is not elevated when the patient is positioned for the CC view, upper posterior

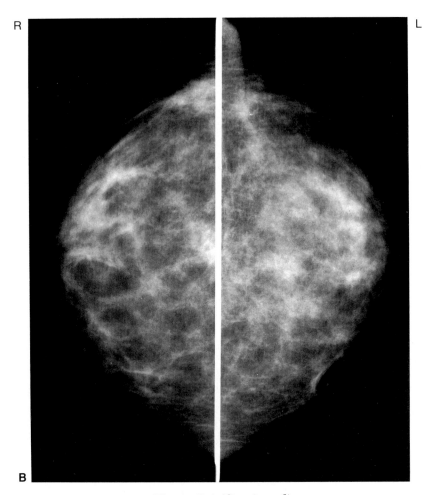

R   L

B

Figure 3-1 (Continued)

breast tissue may be excluded from view (Figure 3-2A) **(Option (C) is true).** If the IMF is elevated and the film holder is then positioned at the level of the elevated IMF, the compression paddle has less distance to travel across the upper breast to achieve the same degree of compression, thus permitting inclusion of more upper posterior breast tissue in the field of view (Figure 3-2B and C). Figure 3-3 shows the CC images of the test patient obtained with elevation of the IMF.

The only definitive conclusion about location within the breast that can be drawn for a finding seen only on the MLO view is that the finding (if real) lies somewhere along an oblique plane, parallel to that of the X-ray beam, traversing the breast from medial to lateral (Figure 3-4).

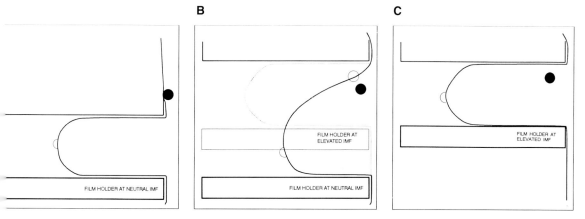

Figure 3-2. (A) Positioning for the CC view with the film holder support-
ing the breast at the neutral level of the inframammary fold (IMF). A
nodule located high and posterior in the breast will be forced out from
under the compression paddle as the paddle is moved down toward the
film holder. (B) Effect of elevating the inframammary fold (IMF) during
positioning for the CC view. This shows the location of the nodule seen in
panel A, before compression is applied. By first elevating the IMF, the
compression paddle has less distance to move down over upper posterior
breast tissue to achieve proper compression, thus permitting the high
posterior lesion to remain within the field of view. (C) Positioning for the
CC view after elevation of the inframammary fold (IMF). This shows the
final position of the nodule seen in panel A; it is maintained in the field of
view when the IMF is properly elevated before compression is applied.

Every mammographic density represents a summation of all tissue densities from the point of beam entry to the point of beam exit. Superimposition of parenchymal elements can either mask significant lesions or
create the false impression of masses (Figure 3-5) **(Options (D) and (E)
are true).**

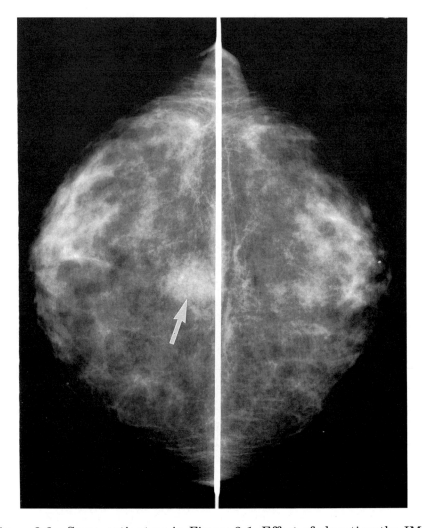

Figure 3-3. Same patient as in Figure 3-1. Effect of elevating the IMF during positioning for the CC view. These CC images were taken after elevation of the IMF. The density initially seen only on the MLO view is now also included (arrow), showing that elevation of the IMF has allowed the density to remain in the field of view on the CC projection. Substantially more breast tissue is usually seen when the CC view is taken with the IMF elevated.

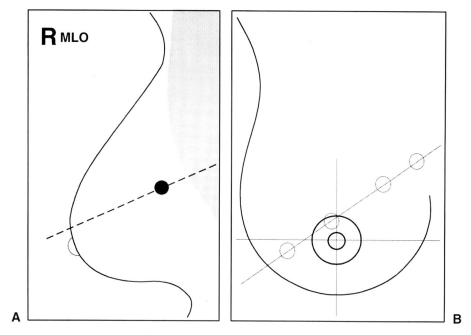

Figure 3-4. Localization of a lesion seen on the MLO view. (A) MLO view of the right breast with a posterior nodule projecting just above the nipple. (B) On the basis of this image alone, one can conclude only that the lesion lies somewhere along the line drawn at the appropriate degree of obliquity through the breast. The lesion could lie at any of the circled locations and still present the image shown in panel A.

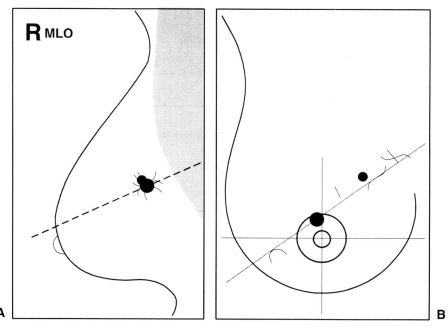

Figure 3-5. Effect of superimposition on any given mammographic image. (A) The "lesion" appears quite real in this single MLO projection. Recall that everything seen at any one location on a single mammographic image represents a superimposition of all structural elements within the breast between the point of entry and point of exit of the X-ray beam. (B) Several benign-appearing structures lying along the plane of the X-ray beam. When superimposed, these structures form a composite that may take on a much more sinister appearance.

Question 12

Concerning the axillary tail of the breast,

    (A) it occasionally exists as an isolated density
    (B) it is less frequently the site of breast cancer than is the lower medial quadrant of the breast
    (C) it is less frequently the site of benign masses than is the lower medial quadrant of the breast
    (D) much of this tissue can be pulled into the field of a standard CC image

In some women with a prominent axillary "tail," the fibroglandular tissue can be seen mammographically as a separate or free island of tissue **(Option (A) is true).** When prominent and dense, this island of tissue can be mistaken for a mass. History becomes important in the diagnostic evaluation, because this tissue responds in similar fashion to the rest of the gland, becoming tender in the premenstrual period and enlarging during pregnancy. When associated with an accessory nipple, this tissue has presented as a lactating "accessory breast" in the postpartum period. To visualize the entire axillary tail properly during mammography, careful attention to positioning, perhaps including an XCCL view, is required.

Most of the glandular tissue of the breast is in the upper outer quadrant, which may explain why over half of all breast cancers and benign masses occur in this region. Similarly, more than 10% of breast cancers and benign masses occur in the axillary tail, whereas fewer than 10% of cancers and benign masses are found in the lower medial quadrant **(Options (B) and (C) are false).**

The XCCL view is designed to visualize lateral breast tissue that may extend lateral to or behind the lateral margin of the pectoral muscle. This view is performed with the patient rotated to bring the anterior axillary line into contact with the anterior edge of the film holder. The gantry is routinely angled 5° toward the MLO projection to allow the compression paddle to clear the humeral head. A useful maneuver to minimize the amount of lateral tissue excluded from the standard CC view is performed just before the compression paddle is engaged; the technologist pulls as much lateral breast onto the film as possible, being careful not to exclude any of the medial tissue (Figure 3-6) **(Option (D) is true).** XCCL views are indicated only when it is apparent that breast tissue is "cut off" or excluded from the lateral aspect of the standard CC image. Properly performed, the CC view is an image of all but the far-lateral portion of the breast.

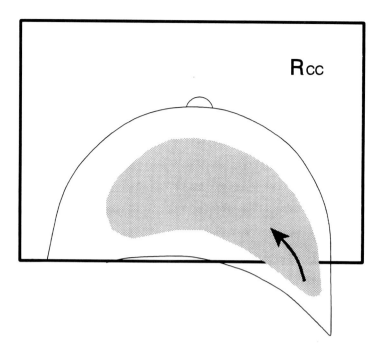

Figure 3-6. Including the axillary tail of the breast on the CC view. This diagram shows the portion of the breast that is usually excluded from the image on a standard CC view. The need for an additional XCCL view to include this area can often be eliminated by pulling lateral breast tissue onto the film (arrow) just before the compression paddle is engaged. It is important that no medial breast tissue be excluded in the process.

Question 13

Concerning the anticipated location of mammographically identified lesions,

    (A) an upper medial lesion and a lower lateral lesion can superimpose on an MLO view

    (B) a medial lesion will project in a more cephalic position with respect to the nipple on the MLO view than on the 90° lateral view

    (C) a small right-breast carcinoma just under the skin, causing slight skin thickening and retraction on the inferior skin margin of an MLO image, is more likely to be located at the 4 o'clock position than at the 6 o'clock position

    (D) a lesion that is 4 cm directly behind the nipple will project directly behind the nipple on both the 90° lateral and MLO views

    (E) a lesion located at the 9 o'clock position in the left breast, 3 cm from the nipple, will be more sharply defined on a 90° lateromedial view than on an MLO view

If we imagine an X-ray beam dividing the right breast through the MLO plane of the nipple (Figure 3-7), we can see that a portion of upper

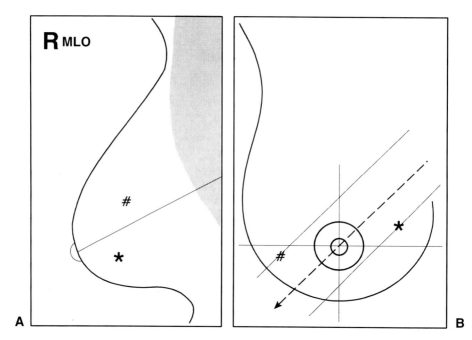

Figure 3-7. Localization of lesions seen on MLO view. (A) MLO view with two lesions. One lesion (#) projects above the nipple, while the other lesion (✳) projects below the nipple. (B) Frontal view of the breast. The first lesion (#) is actually in the lower outer quadrant but is still on the oblique line drawn through a plane projecting above the nipple. The second lesion (✳) is in the upper inner quadrant, although it projects below the nipple in the oblique plane.

medial breast will be included in the lower half of the image, as seen on an MLO projection image. In the MLO view, the point of entry of the X-ray beam is at a more cephalic location than the point of exit and so upper medial lesions and lower lateral lesions can superimpose (Figure 3-5) **(Option (A) is true).** Likewise, a lateral lesion can project in the upper half of the breast, whereas a medial lesion in the same horizontal plane projects in the lower half of the breast (Figure 3-7).

A 90° lateral X-ray beam through the nipple plane will show an upper medial lesion in its true axial plane above the nipple, in a higher position relative to the nipple than when seen in the MLO projection (compare Figure 3-8 with Figure 3-7) **(Option (B) is false).**

Another useful concept in estimating the axial-plane location of a lesion seen on the MLO image is that on this view, lesions projecting in the lower breast, near the skin margin, will probably be located in the medial aspect of the breast. The most inferior or caudal skin margin seen

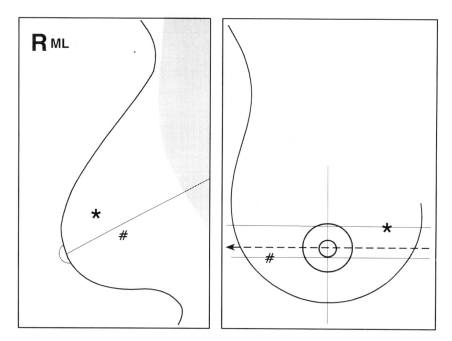

Figure 3-8. Localization of lesions seen on a true lateral view. This figure shows the same two lesions (# ánd ✳) seen in Figure 3-9 as they would be seen in a horizontal-beam true 90° lateral image.

on an MLO image is the skin of the lower medial quadrant of the breast (Figure 3-9). It is this margin that is tangential to the X-ray beam on the MLO view **(Option (C) is true)**.

Yet another useful concept in estimating the axial-plane location of a lesion seen on the MLO image is that most lesions projecting in the upper posterior breast are located laterally in the upper outer quadrant (Figure 3-10). The axillary tail of the breast is the most cephalic-appearing tissue on the MLO view, usually superimposed on the pectoral muscle (Figure 3-10). A properly performed MLO view should include virtually all of the axillary tail.

Lesions located directly posterior to the nipple, in the sagittal and horizontal planes of the nipple, will project at the same location with respect to the nipple on both the MLO and 90° lateral views (Figure 3-11) **(Option (D) is true)**.

The closer a lesion can be positioned against the film, the sharper its features will be seen. The marginal characteristics of a lesion in the upper central breast are optimally visualized and more sharply defined on a caudocranial projection, which will position the lesion closer to the film than they would be on a CC view. Similarly, a medial lesion would be

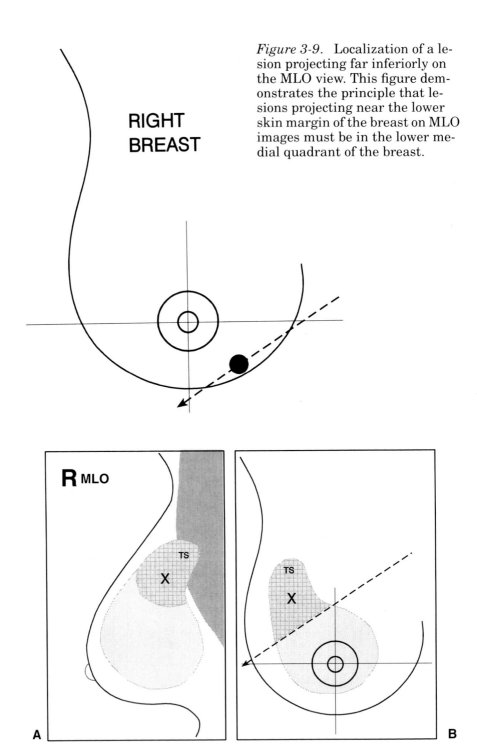

RIGHT BREAST

Figure 3-9. Localization of a lesion projecting far inferiorly on the MLO view. This figure demonstrates the principle that lesions projecting near the lower skin margin of the breast on MLO images must be in the lower medial quadrant of the breast.

R MLO

TS
X

TS
X

A

B

Figure 3-10. Localization of findings projecting far superiorly on the MLO view. The glandular tissue indicated by the darker shading and marked with "X" is the axillary portion of the breast. "TS" indicates the tail of Spence, an extension of the axillary portion of the breast into the axillary area, which occurs in about 11% of women. These illustrations demonstrate the principle that upper posterior tissue, as seen on the MLO view (A), is usually located in the axillary portion of the breast (B).

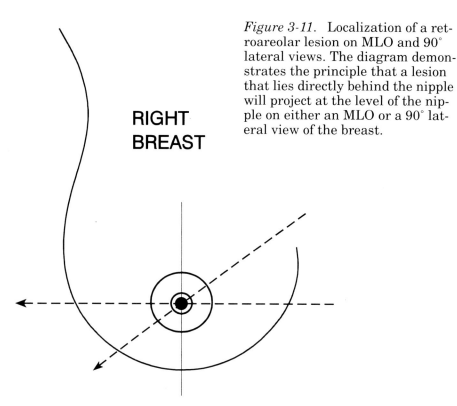

Figure 3-11. Localization of a retroareolar lesion on MLO and 90° lateral views. The diagram demonstrates the principle that a lesion that lies directly behind the nipple will project at the level of the nipple on either an MLO or a 90° lateral view of the breast.

RIGHT BREAST

closer to the film and more sharply defined on a lateromedial image than on a mediolateral image **(Option (E) is true).**

Question 14

Concerning "blind areas" associated with routine mammographic views,

    (A) the upper posterior breast is usually excluded from view on the CC image

    (B) medial breast tissue is usually excluded from view on the MLO image

    (C) glandular tissue wrapping around the upper lateral margin of the pectoral muscle is usually excluded from view on the MLO image

    (D) routine positioning at 45° virtually eliminates blind areas on the MLO image

    (E) a lesion at the 6 o'clock position, 1 cm anterior to the pectoral muscle and 2 cm above the inframammary fold, will most probably be excluded from view on the CC image if the inframammary fold is elevated before the breast is positioned on the film holder

If the film holder is positioned at the level of the neutral IMF, the compression paddle must move across upper posterior breast tissue as compression is applied, resulting in exclusion of upper posterior tissue from view on the CC image (Figure 3-2A). By first elevating the IMF and then positioning the film holder at the elevated position of the fold, the compression paddle has less distance to travel to achieve the same degree of compression (Figure 3-2B and C). This routine maneuver usually leaves upper posterior tissue within the field of view **(Option (A) is false)**.

The upper and medial margins of the breast are relatively immobile; therefore, we must move the breast toward these margins to avoid excluding upper or medial tissue on our images. In standard positioning for the MLO view, the lateral margin of the breast is moved medially, allowing the compression paddle to remain nearer the sternum and maintaining most of the medial tissue within the field of view **(Option (B) is false)**.

In performing the MLO view, lateral breast tissue, including the portion that wraps around the lateral margin of the pectoral muscle, is moved medially and anteriorly, bringing it into the field of view **(Option (C) is false)**. The pectoral muscle itself and the breast tissue lateral to or behind its lateral margin will be superimposed on the MLO image.

The advantages of the MLO view over the 90° lateral view are (1) the ability to pull the breast further off the chest wall, visualizing more breast tissue, and (2) the ability to achieve better compression. The breast is a skin appendage, and, as can be demonstrated with skin in other parts of the body, more skin can be lifted parallel than can be lifted perpendicular to the orientation of underlying muscle fibers. The pectoralis major muscle is obliquely oriented on the chest; therefore, the MLO view is preferred to the 90° lateral view. Pectoral muscles vary in their oblique orientation according to patient habitus, so the optimal degree of obliquity will not be the same for every patient but will vary, from approximately 30° to 60°. Although 45° obliquity is ideal for many patients, it is not optimal for some **(Option (D) is false)**.

To prevent lower posterior breast lesions from being excluded on the CC image, the entire breast must be elevated along with the IMF. The technologist must avoid pulling the skin and IMF away from the chest wall as the IMF is elevated, because otherwise the IMF might be brought up anterior to and in front of a lower posterior lesion, thus excluding it from view. Rather, the IMF should be lifted cephalad along the anterior pectoral fascia, keeping all breast tissue above it. If elevation of the IMF is properly performed, posterior breast tissue should not "drop" behind the film holder **(Option (E) is false)**.

G. W. Eklund, M.D.

SUGGESTED READINGS

1. Bassett LW, Gold RH. Breast radiography using the oblique projection. Radiology 1983; 149:585–587
2. Eklund GW, Cardenosa G. The art of mammographic positioning. Radiol Clin North Am 1992; 30:21–53
3. Kopans DB. Breast imaging. Philadelphia: JB Lippincott; 1989:43–58
4. Logan WW, Janus J. Use of special mammographic views to maximize radiographic information. Radiol Clin North Am 1987; 25:953–959
5. Sickles EA. Practical solutions to common mammographic problems: tailoring the examination. AJR 1988; 151:31–39
6. Swann CA, Kopans DB, McCarthy KA, White G, Hall DA. Localization of occult breast lesions: practical solutions to problems of triangulation. Radiology 1987; 163:557–559
7. Tabar L, Dean PB. Optimum mammographic technique: the annotated cookbook approach. Admin Radiol 1989:54–56

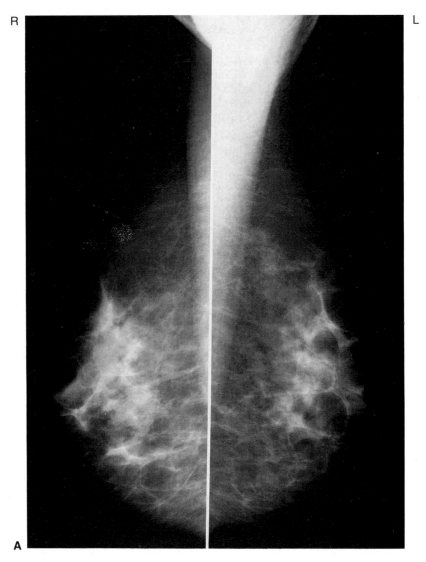

R   L

A

Figure 4-1. You are shown MLO (A) and CC (B) mammograms of both breasts of a 54-year-old woman. (The fingerprint artifact superimposed on the upper aspect of the right breast on the MLO view should be disregarded.)

Case 4: Mammographic Technique and Image Quality: Overview

Question 15

Which *one* of the following BEST describes the technical quality of the test images?

(A) Underexposed with low contrast
(B) Inadequate compression
(C) Not enough pectoral muscle included
(D) Motion unsharpness (blurring)
(E) Excellent images

Optimal mammographic image quality requires proper positioning to ensure visualization of all breast tissue, as well as high contrast and high resolution. Over- or underexposure can result in failure to visualize lesions. Inadequate compression can result in underpenetration of dense glandular elements (underexposure), masking of lesions as a result of superimposed stromal elements, or blurring due to motion. Subtle degrees of motion can render tiny calcifications invisible. The mammographer should look carefully for blurring caused by motion. The lower posterior portion of the breast is most often fatty with fine trabecular markings (Figure 4-2). With the use of a magnifying lens, blurring can best be appreciated by the unsharpness or "fuzziness" of the fine linear structures in this area (Figure 4-3).

The dense parenchymal areas in the test images (Figure 4-1) are well penetrated, and fatty portions are not overexposed; therefore, the film exposure is adequate (Option (A)). Fine trabecular markings remain sharp and distinct, indicating both good compression and lack of motion unsharpness (Options (B) and (D)). The pectoral muscle shadows should be seen down to the level of the nipple on most properly performed MLO views. However, simply showing pectoral muscle down to the level of the nipple does not ensure proper positioning. Note that the anterior margin of the pectoral muscle is projected almost parallel to the back of the images in Figure 4-1A, and then compare the amount and orientation of

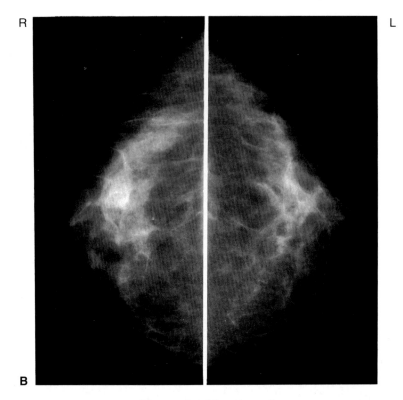

R   L

B

Figure 4-1 (Continued)

the pectoral muscle on these images with those in Figure 4-4, which are images of the test patient taken after the test images. Considerably more pectoral muscle, as well as deeper breast tissue, is seen on the second set of images. Therefore, the primary deficiency in the test images is suboptimal inclusion of pectoral muscles on the MLO view **(Option (C) is correct).** Accordingly, these images cannot be considered excellent in quality (Option (E)).

Failure to move the pectoral muscle and lateral aspect of the breast medially before compression is the most common cause of this deficiency. The lateral and inferior margins of the breast are the mobile margins (Figure 4-5). The lateral margin of the pectoral muscle is unattached to the chest wall (Figure 4-6). Conventional practice directs us to position the mobile breast margins against a stationary film holder; it is therefore necessary to take advantage of breast mobility before placing the breast against the film holder. By first moving the lateral breast and pectoral muscle medially, the compression paddle has less distance to travel across the medial breast to achieve full compression. The net result is

R

L

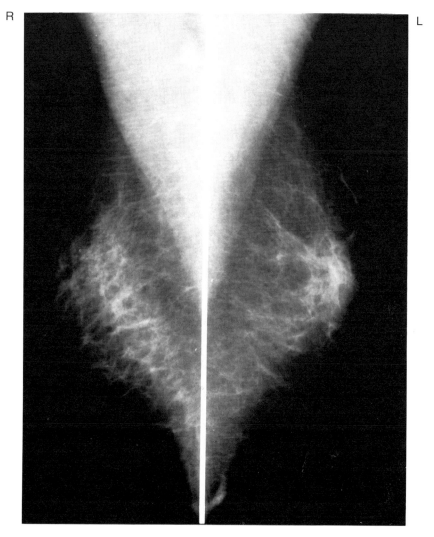

Figure 4-2

Figures 4-2 and 4-3. MLO images with motion unsharpness (blurring). This finding is usually best seen in the lower posterior part of the MLO image. This area is normally fatty with fine trabecular markings (Figure 4-2), which become blurred with motion. Use of a magnifying lens when searching this area for blurring is helpful. This is simulated by photographic enlargements of the lower posterior tissue (Figure 4-3). Note that the trabecular markings on the right side are "fuzzy," suggesting motion unsharpness.

that more medial tissue is seen on the MLO view. Suboptimal inclusion of pectoral muscle on the MLO image should alert the mammographer to the probability of excluded medial breast tissue. Likewise, when posi-

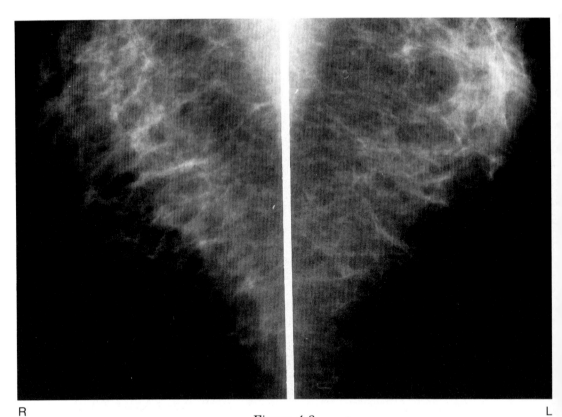

R

L

Figure 4-3

tioning for the CC image, elevation of the inframammary fold before positioning the breast on the film holder reduces the distance that the compression paddle must descend over the upper posterior breast and so reduces the amount of upper posterior tissue excluded from view.

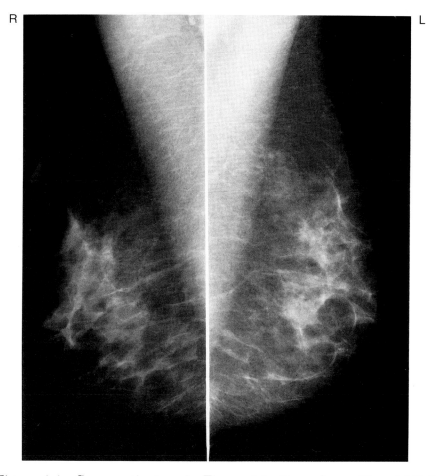

Figure 4-4. Same patient as in Figure 4-1. Properly positioned MLO images. MLO images show excellent positioning, with more pectoral muscle and deeper breast tissues included than in Figure 4-1.

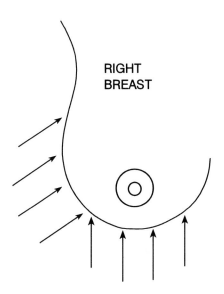

RIGHT
BREAST

Figure 4-5. Breast mobility. The lateral and inferior margins of the breast (arrows) are the mobile margins of the breast, while the upper and medial margins are relatively fixed and immobile.

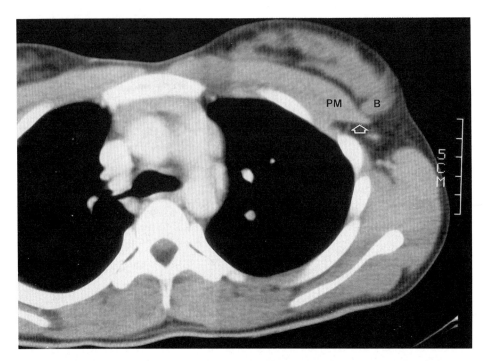

Figure 4-6. Breast mobility. CT scan of the chest shows the right breast and pectoral muscle (PM). Note that the lateral margin of the pectoral muscle is not attached to the chest wall (open arrow) and that glandular breast tissue (B) extends posterolaterally to the lateral margin of the muscle. The lack of muscle attachment to the chest wall gives the pectoral muscle and the overlying breast a substantial degree of medially directed mobility.

Question 16

Given unacceptable motion unsharpness on a mammogram taken with the parameters of 25 kVp, +1 density setting, 320 mAs, and 5-cm compression, corrective measures that would decrease the effects of motion include:

    (A) decreasing the density setting
    (B) decreasing the kVp
    (C) use of a manual technique of 27 kVp and 250 mAs
    (D) increasing compression
    (E) moving the photocell from under dense glandular tissue to under fatty tissue

Motion unsharpness or blurring results from (1) patient factors, such as the patient's inability to hold her breath or such physical problems as

Parkinson's disease or involuntary tremors that make it impossible for the patient to remain motionless during exposures; and from (2) technical factors, resulting in prolonged exposure times that magnify the effects of even the slightest patient motion. Patient factors are dealt with by shortening the exposure time, using better compression, and making the patient as comfortable and stable as possible. Technical factors that lead to prolonged exposure time include dense glandular tissue, poor compression, and low kVp when phototiming. All these situations require the delivery of more mAs (longer exposures) than usual to achieve the desired film density.

If we wish to shorten the exposure time and still maintain the optical density of the image while phototiming, we must increase the kVp. The phototimer regulates the number of photons reaching the film by adjusting the exposure time. By increasing the kVp, we deliver more penetrating photons, and thus the number of photons reaching the film per second is increased and less mAs is required. The phototimer responds to the increased kVp by shortening the exposure time.

When using manual techniques, we can adjust kVp and mAs independently. On most mammographic units there is no separate control for exposure time, so we reduce this parameter by reducing the mAs. However, to preserve the same optical density while decreasing the mAs, we must compensate for the loss in radiation by increasing the kVp (more photons reaching the film in less time). When phototiming, if we decrease the density setting, the phototimer responds by decreasing the exposure time, giving us less mAs **(Option (A) is true).** However, if we decrease the density setting without increasing the kVp, we can expect the optical density of our image to be lower (a lighter film). If we decrease the kVp while phototiming, the mAs and exposure time will increase to deliver the prescribed density, thus further increasing the potential for motion unsharpness **(Option (B) is false).** If we decrease the mAs while using manual techniques, the exposure time will decrease, regardless of which kVp was selected **(Option (C) is true).**

In a phototimed radiograph, the photocell is programmed to terminate the X-ray beam when a sufficient number of photons has been delivered to achieve the prescribed optical density. The duration of this exposure is influenced by the rate at which photons are delivered and by the objects between the X-ray source and the phototimer that may be absorbing photons or preventing photons from reaching the phototimer. If the photons must travel through thicker or more dense tissue before reaching the phototimer, more photons will be absorbed and fewer will reach the phototimer. To maintain proper optical density or film exposure under these circumstances, we have two options: (1) spend more time accumulating photons; or (2) deliver more photons to the image receptor per second. By decreasing tissue thickness with compression, fewer photons will be lost to tissue absorption, more photons will reach the phototimer in a given amount of time, and so less time will be required to collect the required number of photons **(Option (D) is true).**

Modern mammographic equipment allows the selection of various photocell locations. The photocell may be positioned to "read" under the anterior, middle, or posterior portion of the breast. If the photocell is positioned under fatty tissue, fewer photons will be required to achieve the same optical density as when the photocell is positioned under dense glandular tissue. Therefore, if the photocell "sees" less dense tissue, the exposure time will be shorter **(Option (E) is true).** However, although the exposure time is shortened in this circumstance, the overall exposure of the image may be unacceptably low.

In summary, we can shorten the exposure time by decreasing the phototimer density setting or by decreasing mAs by using a manual technique. However, to maintain the optical density (exposure) of our image, we must compensate by increasing kVp or by eliminating the need for a higher kVp by increasing compression.

Question 17

Concerning the phototimer in a mammographic unit,

   (A) it is located between the breast and the film
   (B) it senses the amount of radiation entering the breast
   (C) its primary function is to adjust the mA to achieve a specific film density for the selected kVp
   (D) it regulates the amount of radiation reaching the screen
   (E) its accuracy must be assessed every 6 months to meet American College of Radiology accreditation standards

Unlike the phototimer cell in conventional radiographic equipment, which is located between the object and the film, the phototimer cell in a mammographic unit is located behind the film cassette (Figure 4-7). Therefore, the X-ray beam must pass through the breast, film, and cassette before reaching the photocell **(Option (A) is false).** Hence, the phototimer senses the amount of radiation that already has passed through the breast and cassette **(Option (B) is false).** The phototimer exercises its control over the X-ray beam by adjusting the length of exposure, not the mA **(Option (C) is false).** In other words, it controls mAs, not mA. By regulating the exposure time, the phototimer in effect regulates the amount of radiation reaching the screen **(Option (D) is true)** and hence the exposure of the film.

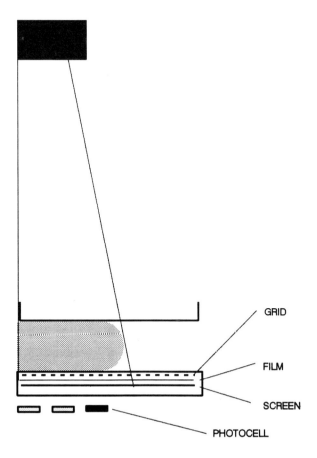

Figure 4-7. Location of the photocell during phototimed exposures. On most mammographic units there are three choices for photocell location. In this illustration the photocell (solid rectangle) is positioned to sense radiation passing through the anterior one-third of the breast. Note that if the breast were twice as large, the anterior photocell would be positioned closer to the center of the breast. If the breast were half the size illustrated, the most anterior photocell would "see" radiation passing through the air in front of the breast. Also note that the photocell is positioned under the breast, grid, film, and screen, thus sensing radiation that has already passed through all these objects.

The accuracy of the phototimer is tested whenever phototimed images of a phantom are made in a quality control program, because this tests not only the imaging system as a whole and the film processor but also phototimer performance. If standard sensitometry strips show no apparent abnormality in the function of the film processor, and if phototimed images of the phantom show a noticeable change in exposure (opti-

Table 4-1: ACR mammography quality control minimum test frequencies

Quality control check	Daily	Weekly	Monthly	Quarterly	Semiannually
Darkroom cleanliness	●				
Processor quality control	●				
Screen cleanliness		●			
View box/viewing conditions		●			
Phantom images			●		
Visual check list			●		
Repeat analysis				●	
Fixer retention				●	
Darkroom fog					●
Screen-film contact					●
Compression					●

cal density) when compared with previous phantom images, the function of the phototimer is in question. Immediate service should be sought to correct the problem. Manual techniques may be used if the problem rests solely with the phototimer, but the need for repeat images is usually greater without the benefit of a reliable phototiming mechanism.

The American College of Radiology (ACR) recommends that a phantom test be performed monthly **(Option (E) is false).** Phantom tests should also be performed whenever a mammographic unit is serviced or whenever degradation in image quality is noted. Radiologists should familiarize themselves with all quality control tests and the minimum performance frequency recommendations of the ACR (Table 4-1).

G. W. Eklund, M.D.

SUGGESTED READINGS

1. Eklund GW, Pisano ED, McLelland R. Technical considerations in optimizing the mammographic image. ACR Symposium on Mammography. Reston, VA: American College of Radiology; 1991:23–38
2. Haus AG. Recent advances in screen-film mammography. Radiol Clin North Am 1987; 25:913–928
3. Hubbard LB. AAPM tutorial. Mammography as a radiographic system. RadioGraphics 1990; 10:103–113
4. Kimme-Smith C, Bassett LW, Gold RH. Evaluation of radiation dose, focal spot, and automatic exposure of newer film-screen mammography units. AJR 1987; 149:913–917
5. Kimme-Smith C, Bassett LW, Gold RH. Workbook for quality mammography. Baltimore: Williams & Wilkins; 1992
6. Kimme-Smith C, Rothschild PA, Bassett LW, Gold RH, Moler C. Mammographic film-processor temperature, development time, and chemistry: effect on dose, contrast, and noise. AJR 1989; 152:35–40
7. Radiologic technologist's manual. Hendrick RE (chair), Mammography quality control. Reston, VA: American College of Radiology; 1992:1–106
8. Tabar L, Haus AG. Processing of mammographic films: technical and clinical considerations. Radiology 1989; 173:65–69

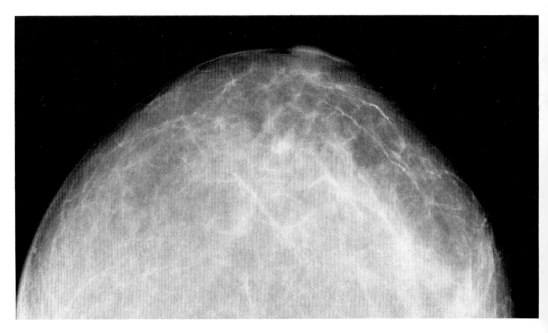

Figure 5-1. You are shown a CC view of the right breast of an 82-year-old woman, which was obtained with the following technical factors: 26 kVp, 2-cm compression, 0 density setting, resulting in 28 mAs.

Case 5: Mammographic Technique and Image Quality: Contrast and Optical Density

Question 18

Adjustments in technique that would result in an improved image include:

(A) reducing the kVp to 23
(B) increasing compression
(C) changing to a manual technique of 26 kVp with 80 mAs
(D) increasing density setting to +1

There are two important observations to make about the image quality of the test mammogram (Figure 5-1). First, it is underexposed (too light). Second, there is very poor contrast (too gray).

Image contrast refers to the differences in optical density between various radiographically identified entities on a given X-ray image. It is determined by a combination of inherent anatomic density differences, compression, the X-ray spectrum, and contrast characteristics of the X-ray film. Because the anatomic structures within the breast exhibit a narrow spectrum of atomic numbers, there is very little inherent density difference. In order to display these structures with sufficient differences in contrast to enhance differential perception and analysis, the other factors affecting contrast become very important.

The increase in Compton scatter that occurs with higher-energy photons (higher kVp) is primarily responsible for the degradation in contrast seen with high kVp use. Reducing the kVp decreases scatter radiation and improves the contrast **(Option (A) is true).** The phototimer will act to preserve the prescribed optical density by extending the exposure time, thus preventing further underexposure. The breast is already compressed to 2 cm; thus, it is unlikely that additional compression would produce a significant improvement in image quality **(Option (B) is false).** When compression can be increased, the ratio of scatter to pri-

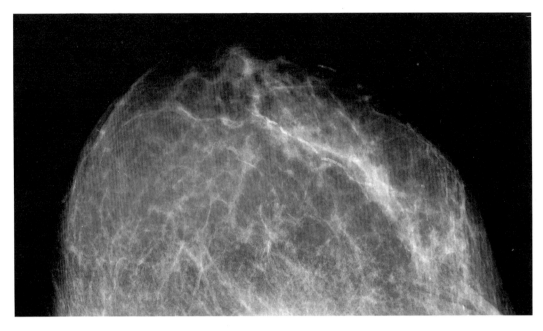

Figure 5-2. Same patient as in Figure 5-1. Effect of reducing the kVp and increasing the density setting on an underexposed, low-contrast image. This CC view was obtained with 23 kVp and +1 density setting. Note the significant improvement in image contrast and exposure.

mary radiation is reduced, thus increasing contrast. Proper compression is especially important with thick breasts. For example, when a 6-cm-thick phantom is exposed with a 10-cm-diameter image field, the intensity of scattered radiation reaching the film is about 80% of the intensity of the primary radiation. Note that scatter radiation degrades not only contrast but also image sharpness.

By using a manual technique, keeping the kVp the same, and increasing the mAs to 80, the film will receive approximately three times (300%) more radiation than in the test mammogram. This would cause significant overexposure (the image would be too dark) **(Option (C) is false).**

Density settings used with phototiming technique represent incremental changes in the amount of mAs delivered. Each step in the density setting represents a 10 to 20% change (average about 20%), depending on the equipment manufacturer. The mammographer should be aware of the change represented by each step on the density scale of the unit in use. A modest increase in mAs would correct the underexposure of the test case but would have no true effect on contrast. When comparing underexposed and properly exposed films, the eye will perceive the better-exposed film to have better contrast. An increase in the density setting from 0 to +1 represents approximately a 20% increase in radiation reaching the screen. This would increase the amount of fluorescent light exposing the film, and so the optical density of the film would increase without causing overexposure **(Option (D) is true)**.

Optimization of the image in the test patient requires both a reduction in kVp (to increase contrast) and an increase in the density setting (to increase the optical density of the film) (Figure 5-2).

Question 19

An increase in kVp with a fixed mAs would increase the:

(A) radiation dose
(B) exposure time
(C) scatter radiation
(D) image contrast
(E) optical density of the image

By maintaining a fixed mAs and increasing the kVp (higher energy photons), fewer photons will be absorbed by the breast tissue, resulting in more photons reaching the screen in the prescribed time. The lower the energy of photons entering the breast, the greater the tissue absorption of those photons. The net result of increasing the kVp and maintaining the mAs will be a reduction in radiation dose **(Option (A) is false)** and an increase in the optical density of the film **(Option (E) is true).** A fixed mAs means a fixed exposure time **(Option (B) is false).** The higher the energy of the entering photons (as occurs with higher kVp), the greater the amount of scatter **(Option (C) is true).** Image contrast can be expected to decrease as kVp and scatter radiation increase **(Option (D) is false).**

Question 20

An increase in mAs with a fixed kVp would increase the:

(A) radiation dose
(B) exposure time
(C) scatter radiation
(D) image contrast
(E) optical density of the image

An increase in mAs is actually an increase in exposure time **(Option (B) is true)**, which would result in increased radiation dose and optical density of the film **(Options (A) and (E) are true)**. Although it can be argued that a longer exposure time to a given energy of photons will cause more scatter radiation to reach the screen, the appreciable effect on image contrast will be minimal (and probably not recognizable) compared with the increased scatter and degradation of contrast that would result from an increase in kVp **(Options (C) and (D) are false)**.

Question 21

An increase in image contrast would be expected with the use of:

(A) a grid
(B) increased compression
(C) an increase in the density setting
(D) extended development time
(E) a smaller focal spot

Scatter radiation makes a significant contribution to decreased image contrast. The primary function of a grid is to decrease scatter radiation, thus improving image contrast **(Option (A) is true)**.

The more dense the breast tissue (higher atomic number), the greater the amount of scatter radiation. The greater the distance a photon has to travel through breast tissue, the greater the potential for photon absorption and scatter radiation. Compression spreads out dense breast tissue over a larger area and also reduces the distance that photons must travel to penetrate the breast. Therefore, scatter radiation is reduced for two reasons, producing improved image contrast **(Option (B) is true)**.

Increasing the phototimer density setting simply produces a darker film (more photons of the same energy) without significantly affecting contrast **(Option (C) is false)**. On the other hand, changes in the energy of the photons (kVp) will alter image contrast. The higher the energy of the photons striking molecules of breast parenchyma, the greater the amount of scatter radiation, thereby decreasing the image contrast. A lower kVp results in decreased scatter radiation and thus in enhanced contrast.

Mammographic film is incompletely developed in the 22 seconds that it is in contact with developer in most conventional 90-second film processors. Single-emulsion film contains the same amount of silver as double-emulsion film; however, the silver is contained in a single thicker emulsion. More time is required for developer chemistry to work through the thicker emulsion and convert silver bromide to metallic silver. Extending the developer immersion time to 43 seconds not only imparts more optical density to the film image but also increases image contrast **(Option (D) is true)**. Increased development time results in disproportionately more deposition of metallic silver on those areas of the film exposed to greater light intensity, compared with areas with less light exposure.

The use of a smaller focal spot can be expected to result in sharper image detail, but contrast will not be affected **(Option (E) is false)**.

Summary

When a single mammogram stands out as being underexposed (too light) when compared with other mammograms performed on the same day, possible explanations include:
1. Insufficient number of photons reaching the film
    a. Density setting set too low for the particular tissue being imaged
    b. Exposure terminated by the mAs limit
    c. Photocell positioned over fat or air, calling for fewer photons than were required to properly penetrate the glandular tissue
2. Film underdevelopment
    a. Drop in developer temperature
    b. Insufficient time for film contact with the developer solution
    c. Contamination of the developer by fixer

When a single mammogram exhibits poor contrast, possible explanations include:
1. High kVp
2. Low object contrast (uniform tissue density)
3. Film underdevelopment
4. Poor compression

When a single image shows unsharpness or "blur," the two most frequent causes are:

1. Motion (especially if only a single image is affected)
2. Geometric factors
   a. Large focal spot
   b. Subject-film distance too great

Technical image analysis should be included in every ongoing quality control program and should be part of every mammographic interpretation. Technologists should be alerted to deficiencies and should be taught to go through a standardized analytic process with every image they take. Even more important, previous images should be analyzed before any new images are taken; by understanding the deficiencies of a prior examination, corrective technical adjustments can be made to improve the new study. However, without knowing the kVp, mAs, centimeters of breast compression, and photocell location used for a given image, the technologist is substantially limited in making appropriate technical adjustments. Unfortunately, most mammographic facilities still do not record the technical factors used for each exposure. To overcome this problem, several of the newer mammographic units automatically record appropriate technical factors directly on each image. Alternatively, stick-on labels are available that provide space for recording technical factors by hand. Availability of this technical information provides the technologist with a distinct advantage in being able to obtain high-quality images.

G.W. Eklund, M.D.

SUGGESTED READINGS

1. Eklund GW, Pisano ED, McLelland R. Technical considerations in optimizing the mammographic image. ACR Symposium on Mammography. Reston, VA: American College of Radiology; 1991:23–38
2. Haus AG. Recent advances in screen-film mammography. Radiol Clin North Am 1987; 25:913–928
3. Haus AG (ed). Film processing in medical imaging. Madison, WI: Medical Physics Publishing; 1993
4. Hubbard LB. AAPM tutorial. Mammography as a radiographic system. RadioGraphics 1990; 10:103–113
5. Kimme-Smith C, Bassett LW, Gold RH. Evaluation of radiation dose, focal spot, and automatic exposure of newer film-screen mammography units. AJR 1987; 149:913–918
6. Kimme-Smith C, Bassett LW, Gold RH. Workbook for quality mammography. Baltimore: Williams & Wilkins; 1992

7. Kimme-Smith C, Rothschild PA, Bassett LW, Gold RH, Moler C. Mammographic film-processor temperature, development time, and chemistry: effect on dose, contrast, and noise. AJR 1989; 152:35–40
8. Radiologic technologist's manual. Hendrick RE (chair), Mammography quality control. Reston, VA: American College of Radiology; 1992
9. Tabar L, Haus AG. Processing of mammographic films: technical and clinical considerations. Radiology 1989; 173:65–69

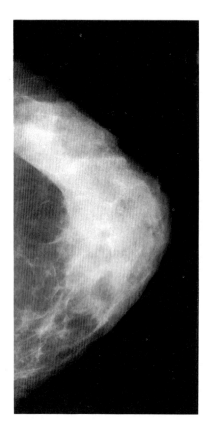

Figure 6-1. You are shown a photo-timed left CC mammogram of a 57-year-old woman.

Case 6: Mammographic Technique and Image Quality: Phototiming and Film Processing

Question 22

Which *one* of the following is the BEST explanation for the appearance of the test image?

    (A) mAs "cutoff" (tube limit exceeded)
    (B) Incompletely developed film
    (C) High kVp (>28)
    (D) Improper placement of the photocell
    (E) Parenchyma too dense for phototiming

Every mammographic unit with phototiming capability has a maximum allowable mAs that, when reached, will cause the exposure to be terminated. This safety feature prevents the flow of electrons from overheating or burning out the X-ray tube. The test mammogram (Figure 6-1) shows glandular tissue that is underexposed and fatty tissue that is appropriately exposed. If this exposure had been terminated by mAs cutoff (Option (A)), the fatty tissue would have been overexposed rather than being properly exposed. Therefore, this is a very unlikely possibility.

If Figure 6-1 had been underdeveloped (Option (B)), we would normally expect the fatty portion of the breast to appear underexposed. Only if the film had been both overexposed and underdeveloped would the fatty tissue appear properly exposed, as it does. However, given the apparently good contrast of Figure 6-1, such a scenario is highly unlikely.

High kVp (Option (C)) diminishes image contrast, but for a phototimed exposure, this should have no effect on under- or overexposure. Changes in kVp will affect film density only when the mAs remains fixed, with the use of a manual technique.

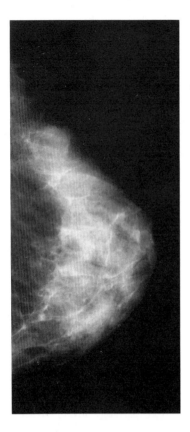

Figure 6-2. Same patient as in Figure 6-1. Effect on the mammographic image of changing the photocell placement. This is a phototimed CC mammogram of the breast shown in Figure 6-1, but with the photocell moved from under the retroglandular fat to under the dense parenchyma. There was no change in the density setting. In the mammograms in both Figures 6-1 and 6-2, the photocell produced what was asked of it, i.e., proper exposure of the tissue directly above the photocell.

The phototimer is not the limiting factor in imaging dense fibroglandular tissue (Option (E)). Both phototimed and manual techniques are capable of delivering radiation to the limit of the mammographic unit. If excessively dense parenchyma were to require more photons than the unit could deliver, the fatty tissue would appear burned out (overexposed) rather than being properly exposed.

We are left with the need to explain how the (phototimed) test mammogram displays proper exposure in one area and underexposure in another. The best explanation is that the phototimer did exactly what it was supposed to do. If the photocell had been positioned under the fatty tissue, we would expect the fatty tissue to have been properly exposed and areas of more dense tissue to have been underexposed **(Option (D) is correct)**.

During mammography the most important tissue to "see through" or penetrate with the X-ray beam is the dense fibroglandular tissue. For this reason, it is good practice to position the phototimer under the dense parenchyma (as determined by reviewing previous mammograms) or under the anterior one-third of the breast where dense parenchyma is most commonly found (if previous mammograms are not available). Figure 6-2 demonstrates the effect of moving the photocell from under the posterior fatty tissue to under the dense anterior glandular tissue. This produces adequate exposure of the dense parenchyma but also results in overexposure of fatty tissue, a disadvantage that can be overcome with the use of a high-intensity light. Unfortunately, use of a low-intensity light will not permit better visualization of underexposed tissues.

Question 23

Circumstances usually requiring the use of a manual technique, as opposed to phototiming, include:

    (A) imaging dermal calcifications in tangent to the skin
    (B) taking a standard MLO view of an augmented breast
    (C) ductography
    (D) a small breast with a 3-cm fibroadenoma
    (E) a large fibrofatty breast with a 3-cm lipoma

The use of a manual technique is required whenever it is necessary to position the phototimer under something that it is not supposed to "see," e.g., air, an implant, or any area that requires either higher or lower mAs than is needed to visualize a region of primary interest. When taking a spot-compression view of the subareolar region directly behind the nipple, a large portion of the area under the spot-compression paddle may be air anterior to the skin surface. Therefore, at least a portion of the photocell under the compression paddle can receive photons that have passed only through air, resulting in premature termination of the exposure and an underexposed film. The same is true of tangential-projection spot films of an area in or just under the skin **(Option (A) is true).**

If a portion of a breast implant overlies the photocell, this will result in an exposure with enough radiation to penetrate the implant, leading to mAs cutoff and overexposure of the native breast tissue. On standard CC and MLO views, no attempt is made to exclude the implant, which usually at least partially overlies the photocell **(Option (B) is true).**

On ductograms, the high-density contrast material within the ductal system usually does not cover a large enough portion of the photocell to affect the image density. Furthermore, the area of primary interest is within the opacified ducts, and so any resultant added mAs does not compromise the image quality **(Option (C) is false).**

The most important role of the phototimer is to ensure that the dense parenchymal areas of the breast are adequately penetrated. If a sizable mass within the breast is positioned directly over the photocell, as would probably occur when imaging a 3-cm fibroadenoma within a small breast, the probability of adequate penetration of the mass is enhanced **(Option (D) is false).**

It is conceivable that a 3-cm lipoma in a very dense breast could be positioned directly over the photocell and cause premature termination of exposure, resulting in inadequate penetration of the dense tissue. However, in a predominantly fibrofatty breast the presence of a lipoma should not have a substantial effect on exposure **(Option (E) is false).**

Question 24

Concerning single-emulsion film,

(A) it has as much silver as does double-emulsion film
(B) it requires a longer development time to achieve the same optical density obtained with double-emulsion film
(C) extended developer processing prolongs the life of the X-ray tube
(D) artifacts and scratches are more commonly seen than with double-emulsion film
(E) it should be developed at 33.3°C (92°F)

The silver content of single-emulsion film is the same as that of double-emulsion film **(Option (A) is true),** but this silver is contained within a thicker emulsion layer. A longer film immersion time is required for the developer to penetrate into and "develop" the silver in a thicker emulsion **(Option (B) is true).** Therefore, single-emulsion film is underdeveloped at the same development time used for double-emulsion film. It is important to understand that the development time is much shorter than the total processing time. Development time refers to the length of time the film is in actual contact with the developer solution. Processing time refers to the total time the film spends in the processor, including the time in the various processing solutions and the transport time to and between the solutions and the dryer. With standard 90-second processing of general radiographic film, the time of film contact with the developer solution usually is about 22 seconds. Extended developer processing (EDP) generally implies about 43 seconds of film contact with the developer.

With EDP, in addition to the major benefit of improved image contrast, greater optical density of the film can be produced with the same radiation dose required for conventional processing. Therefore, the use of

R   L

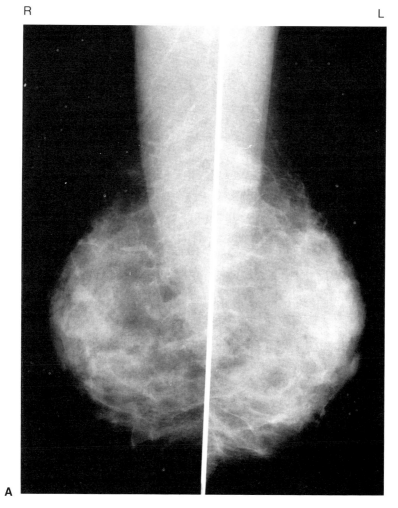

A

Figure 6-3. Effect of extended development film processing. (A) MLO
images obtained at 25 kVp and 0 density setting, with 90-second processing. The images appear rather gray (poor contrast). Note also that the
pectoral muscles appear well seen, until these images are compared with
the images in panel B, which were obtained with full attention to moving
the breasts and pectoral muscles medially before applying compression.
(B) MLO images obtained at 25 kVp and 0 density setting but processed
with an extended developer time of 43 seconds. Significantly better contrast is apparent in these images.

EDP effectively increases the speed of the film-screen system. However,
it is more likely that the radiologist will choose to obtain equivalent density by using a lower radiation dose (up to 40% less radiation) (Figure
6-3). The lower the radiation dose, the less heat is created in the anode,
thus prolonging the life of the X-ray tube **(Option (C) is true)** (Table

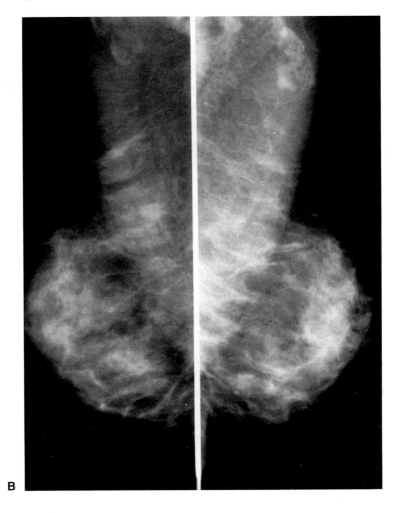

B

6-1). New high-contrast films, intended to be run in 90-second processors with 22-second developer time, offer an alternative to EDP; however, they exhibit a graininess that may be objectionable to some radiologists. These films do offer a definite advantage when used for localization or stereotactic biopsy procedures and for specimen radiography, in which speed is of great importance and graininess is of less concern.

With double-emulsion film, artifacts caused by dust particles or small scratches are not readily apparent because the image in the opposite emulsion surface masks the visibility of the artifact. With single-emulsion film, artifacts are much more easily seen because there is no image on the opposite surface to serve as a masking agent **(Option (D) is true).**

Table 6-1: Effect of increased mAs on heat generation in an X-ray tube, using techniques that result in comparable film optical density[a]

Processing type	(mAs) x (kVp) = Heat units (HU)
Standard	100 mAs x 25 kVp = 2,500 HU
Extended-development	50 mAs x 27 kVp = 1,350 HU

[a] Although both processing types result in comparable film optical densities, the standard method—with lower kVp and higher mAs—will result in a higher radiation dose to the patient and nearly twice the heat load on the X-ray tube.

The optimal development temperature for single-emulsion film varies with the manufacturer but is usually about 35°C (95°F) **(Option (E) is false).** Small variations in developer temperature can result in noticeable changes in mammographic image quality. For example, low developer temperature can result in underdevelopment, which not only leads to reduced image contrast but also lowers film speed (often compensated by longer exposure time and therefore increased patient exposure). The American College of Radiology specification for quality control testing of developer temperature is that the temperature be within ±0.5°F (±0.3°C) of that recommended by the manufacturer for the specific film-developer combination being used. When processors are modified for dual-speed operation to allow 90-second processing of conventional radiographic films and extended processing of mammographic film, it may be necessary to adjust exposure techniques for the general radiographic films to allow for processing at 95°F (if the temperature previously used was lower). Replenishment rates should also be adjusted if an increased number of films will be run through the processor.

Question 25

Concerning the tube limit or mAs "cutoff" when phototiming,

  (A) the Food and Drug Administration requires that mammographic units termi-
      nate exposure at 400 mAs
  (B) if mAs cutoff has occurred and the film was overexposed, lowering the kVp
      would result in a lighter film
  (C) if mAs cutoff has occurred and the film was underexposed, increasing the
      density by one step would result in a darker film
  (D) if mAs cutoff has occurred and the film was underexposed, increasing the
      kVp would result in a darker film

Every X-ray tube has a defined heat capacity; i.e., there is a threshold mAs level above which sufficient heat will be created that damage to
the tube is likely to occur. To protect the tube against such an overload,
the manufacturer builds a safety "cutoff" into the system, which automatically terminates an exposure when this threshold is reached. Most
mammographic units have a threshold of about 400 mAs; some may be
as low as 200 mAs, others as high as 600 mAs. This is not a Food and
Drug Administration requirement **(Option (A) is false).**

When cutoff occurs during a phototimed image, we can assume that
the system has been asked to deliver more photons than the X-ray tube
can withstand. We can also assume that the film did not receive as much
radiation as was prescribed with the density control. If we reduce the
kVp, the phototimer will attempt to compensate by lengthening the exposure time and delivering even more mAs in order to achieve the prescribed density. However, since mAs cutoff already has been reached, the
exposure time will remain the same. Fewer (reduced kVp) photons will
reach the film, and so the resultant image will be lighter **(Option (B) is
true).** Another, simpler method to obtain a lighter (more properly exposed) film would be to prescribe a decrease in the density setting. This
would result in a shorter exposure (reduced mAs), which would also
lessen the likelihood of motion.

Increasing the density setting simply calls for more mAs. If cutoff
occurs and an underexposed film results, we can conclude that the unit
cannot deliver more mAs at the set kVp. Therefore, increasing the density by one step would have no effect on the resultant film density
(Option (C) is false). The only option to penetrate underexposed tissue
properly if cutoff has occurred is to push more photons through per second; i.e., higher-energy photons (more kVp) must be used **(Option (D) is
true).** If we obtained cutoff at 400 mAs with 25 kVp, an increase in kVp
to 27 would deliver more photons to the film at the same mAs.

G. W. Eklund, M.D.

SUGGESTED READINGS

1. Eklund GW, Pisano ED, McLelland R. Technical considerations in optimizing the mammographic image. ACR Symposium on Mammography. Reston, VA: American College of Radiology; 1991:23–38

2. Haus AG. Recent advances in screen-film mammography. Radiol Clin North Am 1987; 25:913–928

3. Haus AG (ed). Film processing in medical imaging. Madison, WI: Medical Physics Publishing; 1993

4. Hubbard LB. AAPM tutorial. Mammography as a radiographic system. RadioGraphics 1990; 10:103–113

5. Kimme-Smith C, Bassett LW, Gold RH. Evaluation of radiation dose, focal spot, and automatic exposure of newer film-screen mammography units. AJR 1987; 149:913–917

6. Kimme-Smith C, Bassett LW, Gold RH. Workbook for quality mammography. Baltimore: Williams & Wilkins; 1992

7. Kimme-Smith C, Rothschild PA, Bassett LW, Gold RH, Moler C. Mammographic film-processor temperature, development time, and chemistry: effect on dose, contrast, and noise. AJR 1989; 152:35–40

8. Radiologic technologist's manual. Hendrick RE (chair), Mammography quality control. Reston, VA: American College of Radiology; 1992:1–106

9. Tabar L, Haus AG. Processing of mammographic films: technical and clinical considerations. Radiology 1989; 173:65–69

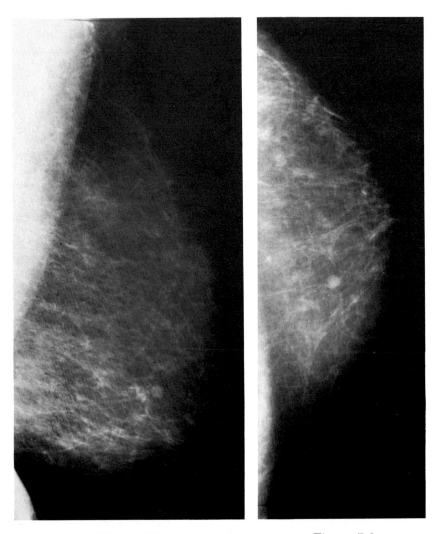

Figure 7-1   Figure 7-2

Figures 7-1 through 7-3. You are shown MLO (Figure 7-1), CC (Figure 7-2), and spot-compression magnification (Figure 7-3) views of the left breast from a baseline screening mammogram of a 59-year-old woman.

Case 7: Circumscribed Noncalcified Mass with Smooth Margins

Question 26

Which *one* of the following is the MOST appropriate next step?

(A) Clinical correlation
(B) Follow-up mammography in 3 months
(C) Follow-up mammography in 6 months
(D) Routine mammographic screening in 1 year
(E) Surgical biopsy

The standard MLO and CC views (Figures 7-1 and 7-2) show a smooth, noncalcified 5-mm mass in the medial aspect of the left breast (arrows in Figures 7-4 and 7-5). The spot-compression magnification view (Figure 7-3) was valuable in that it confirmed completely circumscribed borders and the lack of microcalcifications within the mass (arrow in Figure 7-6). This mass might represent a cyst; however, ultrasonography of a circumscribed mass this small and this deep within the breast would probably be indeterminate. A completely smooth, noncalcified mass less than 1 cm in diameter is almost always benign. Thus, obtaining follow-up mammography in 6 months would be the most appropriate step **(Option (C) is correct)**.

A 5-mm lesion in the location shown in the test images would not be expected to be palpable, regardless of its etiology, and therefore clinical correlation (Option (A)) would have little value. Most mammographers believe that close-interval mammographic follow-up is indicated for a lesion such as this that is considered "probably benign" after full mammographic examination. A complete evaluation including spot-compression magnification views is necessary to determine that all borders are truly smooth and that there are no microcalcifications before the lesion is classified as "probably benign." A lesion such as the one in the test patient would not be expected to be malignant, but periodic follow-up is needed because malignancy remains a remote possibility. There are no

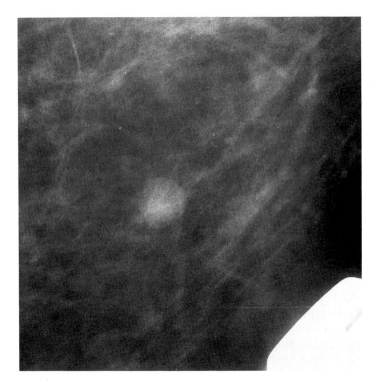

Figure 7-3

scientific studies that demonstrate the most effective follow-up protocol. A review of the literature, including a survey of practicing mammographers, shows that most experts use an initial 6-month follow-up examination. This is largely based upon a rough estimation of the growth rates of most breast cancers. A sufficient period must pass before any potential change is apparent; 3 months is too short an interval to expect change, unless an unusually aggressive carcinoma is present. Therefore, follow-up mammography in 3 months (Option (B)) is not the best management choice. Conversely, routine screening in 1 year (Option (D)) would be too long an interval for a lesion that does not have absolutely benign imaging features. Unless the woman is exceptionally anxious regarding mammographic follow-up of the lesion, surgical biopsy (Option (E)) would be too aggressive for a "probably benign" lesion. Most mammographers use a size threshold of 1.0 to 1.5 cm as a basis for recommending biopsy rather than follow-up of a completely circumscribed noncalcified mass (when no previous radiographs are available for comparison). This is not based upon experimental data; rather, it is the personal preference of the individual mammographer. Other factors affecting this decision include

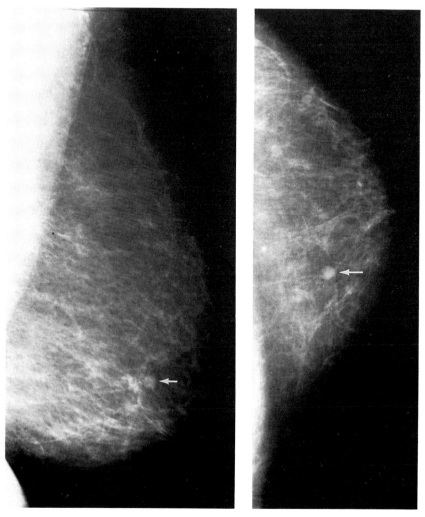

Figure 7-4　　　　　　　　　　　　Figure 7-5

Figures 7-4 through 7-6 (Same as Figures 7-1 through 7-3, respectively).
Well-defined noncalcified mass with smooth margins. The MLO (Figure
7-4) and CC (Figure 7-5) views show a 5-mm, round, completely smooth,
noncalcified mass in the medial aspect of the left breast (arrow). The
spot-compression magnification view (Figure 7-6) confirms that the mass
(arrow) has completely smooth borders and contains no microcalcifications.

the palpability of the lesion, the age of the woman, and personal or
strong family history of breast cancer.

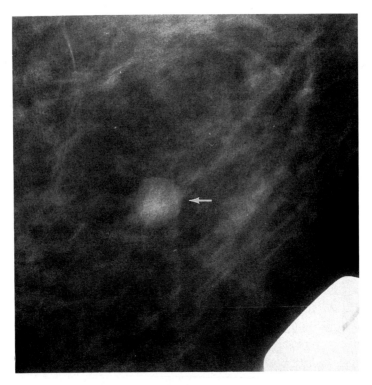

Figure 7-6

Question 27

The probability of carcinoma in a nonpalpable, completely smooth, noncalcified solid mass less than 1 cm in diameter is:

(A) 2%
(B) 5%
(C) 10%
(D) 20%
(E) 30%

In Sickles' large prospective study of 3,184 nonpalpable "probably benign" lesions, the overall probability of carcinoma was only 0.5%. For noncalcified, well-defined solid nodules, the probability of cancer was 2%. This is similar to the probabilities in published retrospective studies **(Option (A) is correct).** Because these types of lesions are so common yet so infrequently represent cancer, a conservative approach of close-interval follow-up mammography is used by most radiologists. However, compliance with follow-up protocols has been shown to be a problem. The radiologist must track these patients to ensure that they return for follow-up studies. For self-referred patients, the breast imaging facility must notify the patient of the need for follow-up, schedule the appointment, and then notify the patient and reschedule if she fails to keep the initial appointment. Physician-referred patients may be handled in the same way. If the facility relies upon the referring physician to schedule the follow-up appointment, then his or her office should be notified by phone or certified mail. If the woman fails to keep the follow-up appointment, the breast imaging center must notify the referring physician.

Question 28

Follow-up mammography in 6 months is MOST appropriate for which *one* of the following lesions?

(A) 1-cm cyst
(B) 7-mm completely smooth, noncalcified mass
(C) 3-cm smooth noncalcified mass
(D) 1.3-cm ill-defined noncalcified mass
(E) 1.5-cm smooth noncalcified mass with mixed fat and soft tissue density

Close-interval mammographic follow-up is appropriate only for lesions that are "probably benign," i.e., those that are not pathognomonically benign but that do not have common features of malignancy, such as indistinct or irregular borders, microcalcifications, or associated skin changes. Of the options given, the only lesion that fits this classification is the 7-mm completely smooth, noncalcified mass **(Option (B) is correct).**

If high-frequency ultrasound equipment is available and the size and location of a mass are appropriate, ultrasonography can be performed to determine whether the lesion is a cyst or a solid mass. Superficial cysts as small as 3 mm in diameter can be diagnosed by ultrasonography, but in most cases the lesion must be larger than approximately 6 to 8 mm for accurate determination of its internal matrix. Artifactual internal echoes are frequently seen within smaller cysts. Simple cysts and fat-containing circumscribed masses (Options (A) and (E)) are always benign, and therefore only routine screening mammography is required. When a circumscribed noncalcified mass 3 cm in diameter (Option (C)) is seen on baseline mammography, ultrasonography should be performed rather than a 6-month follow-up examination. If such a large lesion is solid, the probability of cancer may be somewhat greater than 2%, although this statement is based on anecdotal evidence. Nonetheless, most mammographers recommend needle or surgical biopsy for these large, smooth solid masses. A noncalcified mass with ill-defined borders (Option (D)) must be interpreted as being suspicious for malignancy, and either needle or surgical biopsy should be considered.

Valerie P. Jackson, M.D.

SUGGESTED READINGS

FOLLOW-UP OF "PROBABLY BENIGN" LESIONS

1. Adler DD, Helvie MA, Ikeda DM. Nonpalpable, probably benign breast lesions: follow-up strategies after initial detection on mammography. AJR 1990; 155:1195–1201
2. Brenner RJ. Follow-up as an alternative to biopsy for probably benign mammographically detected abnormalities. Curr Opin Radiol 1991; 3:588–592
3. Brenner RJ, Sickles EA. Acceptability of periodic follow-up as an alternative to biopsy for mammographically detected lesions interpreted as probably benign. Radiology 1989; 171:645–646
4. Cardenosa G, Eklund GW. Rate of compliance with recommendations for additional mammographic views and biopsies. Radiology 1991; 181:359–361
5. Datoc PD, Hayes CW, Conway WF, Bosch HA, Neal MP. Mammographic follow-up of nonpalpable low-suspicion breast abnormalities: one versus two views. Radiology 1991; 180:387–391
6. Hall FM, Storella JM, Silverstone DZ, Wyshak G. Nonpalpable breast lesions: recommendations for biopsy based on suspicion of carcinoma at mammography. Radiology 1988; 167:353–358
7. Helvie MA, Pennes DR, Rebner M, Adler DD. Mammographic follow-up of low-suspicion lesions: compliance rate and diagnostic yield. Radiology 1991; 178:155–158
8. Homer MJ. Nonpalpable mammographic abnormalities: timing the follow-up studies. AJR 1981; 136:923–926
9. Robertson CL, Kopans DB. Communication problems after mammographic screening. Radiology 1989; 172:443–444
10. Sickles EA. Periodic mammographic follow-up of probably benign lesions: results in 3,184 consecutive cases. Radiology 1991; 179:463–468
11. Varas X, Leborgne F, Leborgne JH. Nonpalpable, probably benign lesions: role of follow-up mammography. Radiology 1992; 184:409–414

MAMMOGRAPHIC INTERPRETATION OF MASSES

12. Feig SA. Breast masses. Mammographic and sonographic evaluation. Radiol Clin North Am 1992; 30:67–92
13. Marsteller LP, Shaw de Paredes E. Well defined masses in the breast. RadioGraphics 1989; 9:13–37

14. Moskowitz M. The predictive value of certain mammographic signs in screening for breast cancer. Cancer 1983; 51:1007–1011
15. Sickles EA. Mammographic features of 300 consecutive nonpalpable breast cancers. AJR 1986; 146:661–663
16. Sickles EA. Breast masses: mammographic evaluation. Radiology 1989; 173:297–303

BREAST ULTRASONOGRAPHY

17. Bassett LW, Kimme-Smith C. Breast sonography. AJR 1991; 156:449–455
18. Jackson VP. The role of US in breast imaging. Radiology 1990; 177:305–311
19. Jokich PM, Monticciolo DL, Adler YT. Breast ultrasonography. Radiol Clin North Am 1992; 30:993–1009
20. Sickles EA, Filly RA, Callen PW. Benign breast lesions: ultrasound detection and diagnosis. Radiology 1984; 151:467–470

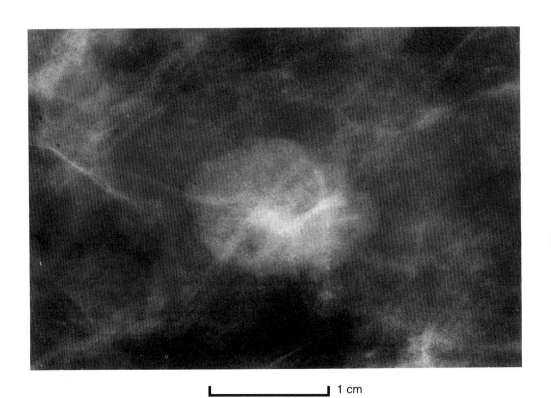

|_____| 1 cm

Figure 8-1. This 43-year-old woman presented with pain in the left breast. You are shown a spot-compression magnification CC view of the left breast. She has had no prior mammograms.

Case 8: Circumscribed Microlobulated Noncalcified Mass

Question 29

Which *one* of the following is the MOST likely diagnosis?

    (A) Phyllodes tumor
    (B) Fibroadenoma
    (C) Invasive ductal carcinoma
    (D) Ductal carcinoma *in situ*
    (E) Complex cyst

The test image (Figure 8-1) shows a 1.6-cm, circumscribed, noncalcified mass (Figure 8-2, arrows). The borders are microlobulated, with undulations of 2 to 4 mm in diameter. The lesion is classified as a low-density radiopaque mass because normal breast parenchymal markings are seen through the mass. Circumscribed margins and relatively low radiographic density are frequently signs of a benign lesion, but according to Kopans and to Moskowitz, the microlobulations on the test image should substantially increase the index of suspicion for malignancy. Thus, the most likely diagnosis is invasive ductal carcinoma **(Option (C) is correct).** When phyllodes tumors (Option (A)) and fibroadenomas (Option (B)) are lobulated, the undulations are usually large (Figure 8-3). Ductal carcinoma *in situ* (DCIS) (Option (D)) most commonly presents as microcalcifications, although noncalcified masses are occasionally seen. In Ikeda and Andersson's series, noncalcified circumscribed masses were found in 8% of DCIS cases, whereas in the study by Mitnick et al., less than 4% of DCIS cases presented as a circumscribed mass. Microcalcifications alone account for 62–72% of DCIS cases in published series. Because the vast majority of breast cancers are invasive ductal carcinoma, circumscribed invasive ductal carcinoma is much more common than circumscribed DCIS. Cysts, both simple and complex (containing internal echoes) (Option (E)) are usually round or oval, and when they

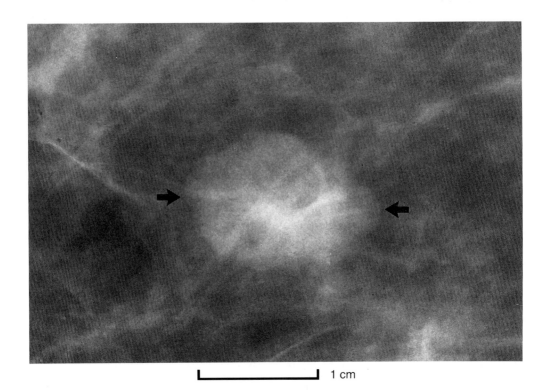

1 cm

Figure 8-2 (Same as Figure 8-1). Invasive ductal carcinoma. Left CC spot-compression magnification mammogram shows a completely well defined, 1.6-cm noncalcified mass (arrows) with microlobulated borders. The undulations are 2 to 4 mm in diameter.

are lobulated, the undulations are usually large because they are usually due to septations in the cyst or a cluster of cysts.

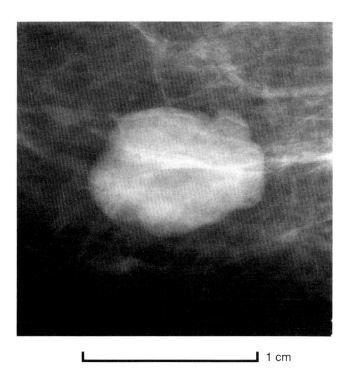

L————————————J 1 cm

Figure 8-3. Fibroadenoma. Mammogram shows a macrolobulated, circumscribed, noncalcified mass. Almost all of the undulations of the border of this 1-cm fibroadenoma are at least 5 mm in diameter.

Question 30

Which *one* of the following is the LEAST appropriate next step?

    (A) Routine screening mammography in 1 year
    (B) Follow-up mammography in 6 months
    (C) Ultrasonography
    (D) Fine-needle aspiration biopsy
    (E) Surgical biopsy

There are several acceptable ways to manage the test patient. The mass is circumscribed and thus could be a cyst; therefore, one might perform ultrasonography (Option (C)). If the mass were shown to be a simple cyst, no further workup, short-term mammographic follow-up, or biopsy would be necessary. If the mass were solid or complex (containing both cystic and solid elements) or if the lesion were not shown by ultrasonography (and therefore assumed to be solid), some form of biopsy, either fine-needle aspiration (Option (D)), core, or surgical (Option (E)), would be most appropriate. If one did not wish to be quite so aggressive, short-interval mammographic follow-up (Option (B)) might be considered, although this would be inadvisable for a microlobulated mass, which implies a substantial likelihood of malignancy. Finally, it would be totally unacceptable merely to recommend routine screening mammography in 1 year for a lesion such as that in the test patient **(Option (A) is correct)**.

Question 31

Concerning phyllodes tumor,

- (A) it usually presents as a large, rapidly enlarging mass
- (B) 5 to 10% of these tumors are malignant
- (C) its peak incidence occurs between the ages of 60 and 70 years
- (D) the mammographic appearance is similar to that of a large fibroadenoma
- (E) on ultrasonography, small fluid-filled spaces are occasionally seen within the tumor

Phyllodes tumor, also known as cystosarcoma phyllodes or phylloides, is an uncommon lesion, similar to fibroadenoma in that both epithelial and mesenchymal elements are present. Small phyllodes tumors are encountered, but the most common clinical presentation is that of a large, rapidly growing breast mass **(Option (A) is true)**. The vast majority of these tumors are completely benign, but approximately 5 to 10% contain areas of malignancy and can metastasize, usually hematogenously, to the lungs, pleura, and bones **(Option (B) is true)**. Local recurrence is much more common than metastasis and can occur with incompletely excised benign tumors as well as with malignant ones. Phyllodes tumors can occur at any age, but in most series the average age at diagnosis is in the early to mid forties **(Option (C) is false)**. This is somewhat older than the age of peak incidence for fibroadenoma, which is in the early thirties, and younger than that for carcinoma, which is in the fifties.

Mammographically, phyllodes tumors are usually large round, oval, or lobulated noncalcified masses with smooth borders (Figure 8-4A). As a rule, they are indistinguishable from large fibroadenomas **(Option (D) is true)**. The sonographic appearance is variable. Completely solid masses with low-level internal echoes are usually seen. Occasionally, small fluid-filled spaces are identified within the mass **(Option (E) is true)** (Figure 8-4B); these result from the cystic cavities filled with solid

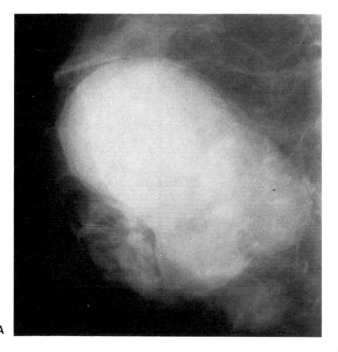

A

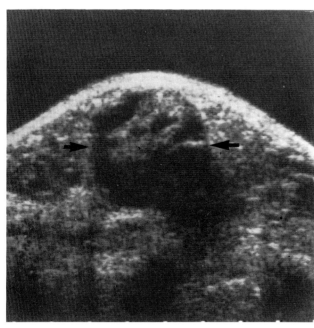

B

Figure 8-4. Phyllodes tumor. This 45-year-old woman presented with a rapidly growing right subareolar mass. (A) Her MLO projection mammogram shows a macrolobulated, smooth-contoured, circumscribed, noncalcified 4-cm mass. (B) Automated 7.5-MHz sonogram of the mass shows it to be a complex mass (arrows) with multiple anechoic fluid-filled spaces.

leaflike projections that give this tumor its name. Cole-Beuglet et al. identified a cystic space in one of their eight cases, whereas Buchberger et al. found intramural cysts in six of their ten cases. The discrepancy in the visualization of cystic spaces may be due to the improved resolution of the sonography equipment used in the latter study. Unfortunately, one cannot distinguish the benign and malignant forms of phyllodes tumor based on imaging features alone. Biopsy is necessary for a definitive diagnosis. Wide local excision is the preferred method of treatment.

Question 32

Concerning fibroadenomas,

   (A) they are multiple in approximately 15% of patients
   (B) they usually occur in women between the ages of 35 and 45 years
   (C) they usually develop coarse calcification after involution
   (D) they are associated with an increased risk for breast cancer
   (E) the frequency of carcinoma in fibroadenomas is approximately 5%

Fibroadenomas are the most common benign tumors arising in the female breast. They are multiple or bilateral in 15% of cases **(Option (A) is true).** Fibroadenomas develop in young women, although they can remain asymptomatic and undetected until years later. Haagensen found fibroadenomas to be the most common breast lesion in women under age 25, with a mean age at detection of 33.9 years **(Option (B) is false).** Fibroadenomas frequently undergo involution with hyalinization and development of calcification as a woman ages, particularly in the post-menopausal period. The calcifications are frequently peripheral; large, coarse "popcorn" calcifications are pathognomonic (Figure 8-5) **(Option (C) is true).**

Noncalcified fibroadenomas cannot be diagnosed with certainty by either mammography or ultrasonography. The typical mammographic appearance is a circumscribed oval or lobulated mass, and the typical sonographic appearance is a smooth oval or lobulated hypoechoic mass with relatively homogeneous internal echoes and occasional posterior acoustic enhancement (Figure 8-6). However, these features are not pathognomonic and carcinoma can have an identical appearance. Conversely, many fibroadenomas have "atypical" features on ultrasonography, such as irregular borders and inhomogeneous internal echoes. Therefore, either close-interval follow-up mammography or biopsy is necessary for the atypical cases, and proper management should be guided by the mammographic appearance of the lesion.

Fibroadenomas do not increase a woman's risk for subsequent development of breast carcinoma **(Option (D) is false).** Carcinoma within a fibroadenoma is also extremely rare **(Option (E) is false).** The prevalence of carcinoma arising in a fibroadenoma is unknown, but only 185

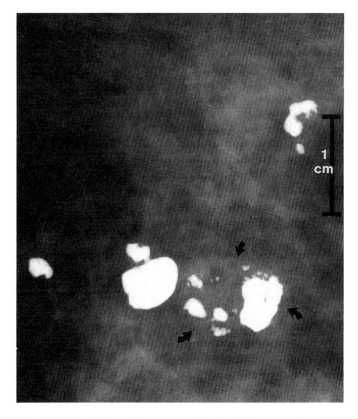

Figure 8-5. Calcified fibroadenomas. Typical "popcorn" calcifications in degenerated or involuted fibroadenomas. The residual soft tissue mass is visible for the largest lesion (arrows).

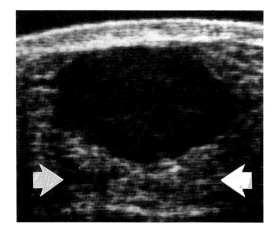

Figure 8-6. Sonogram of a "typical" fibroadenoma. This 2-cm oval mass is smooth, contains homogeneous internal echoes, and displays posterior acoustic enhancement (arrows).

cases have been reported in the world's literature. Deschenes reported carcinoma within a fibroadenoma in 0.02% of patients in a screened population. In most series, carcinomas "associated with" fibroadenomas are actually incidental *in situ* lesions located near, but not truly within, the fibroadenomas.

Question 33

Concerning circumscribed carcinoma,

    (A) invasive ductal carcinoma accounts for 20% of cases
    (B) magnification mammography often shows one or more indistinct borders
    (C) it can be reliably differentiated from a benign circumscribed mass by ultrasonography
    (D) papillary carcinoma typically appears as a circumscribed mass
    (E) cyst aspiration cytology is the most accurate way to diagnose intracystic carcinoma

Approximately 5% of breast carcinomas are circumscribed and have predominantly smooth borders. Most papillary, colloid, and medullary carcinomas are circumscribed **(Option (D) is true),** but these are unusual lesions. Invasive ductal carcinoma (not otherwise specified) is the most common type of breast cancer and accounts for most circumscribed carcinomas **(Option (A) is false).** These masses may appear to have completely or predominantly smooth borders and circumscribed margins on standard contact mammography; however, anecdotal reports indicate that spot-compression magnification mammography frequently demonstrates one or more indistinct borders (Figure 8-7; see also Case 9, Figures 9-4 and 9-5, page 109) **(Option (B) is true),** a clue to the true nature of the lesion. Ultrasonography is valuable for the evaluation of circumscribed masses in that it allows differentiation between cysts and solid masses. However, as discussed previously, it is not possible to reliably distinguish benign from malignant smooth solid masses sonographically **(Option (C) is false).** When a complex mass is seen by ultrasonography, aspiration with or without air injection (pneumocystography) can be helpful in demonstrating wall irregularity or an intramural nodule. However, cytologic evaluation of the aspirated fluid is frequently negative, even when malignancy is present. In the series of Tabar et al., only 27% of intracystic cancers were positive or suspicious by cytology **(Option (E) is false).** Therefore, surgical biopsy is the most accurate method for the diagnosis of intracystic carcinoma.

Valerie P. Jackson, M.D.

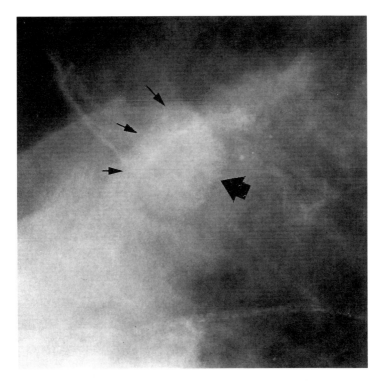

Figure 8-7. Circumscribed invasive ductal carcinoma. Right CC spot-compression magnification mammogram of a 1.2-cm noncalcified mass shows that most of the border is smooth (large arrow), but a segment of the border is indistinct (small arrows). Conventional mammography suggested the borders were circumscribed and smooth (not shown).

SUGGESTED READINGS

CIRCUMSCRIBED CARCINOMA

1. Kopans DB. Breast imaging. Philadelphia: JB Lippincott; 1989:76
2. Moskowitz M. The predictive value of certain mammographic signs in screening for breast cancer. Cancer 1983; 51:1007–1011
3. Moskowitz M. Circumscribed lesions of the breast. In: Moskowitz M (ed), Diagnostic categorical course in breast imaging. Oak Brook, IL: Radiological Society of North America; 1986:31–33
4. Sickles EA. Mammographic features of 300 consecutive nonpalpable breast cancers. AJR 1986; 146:661–663

PHYLLODES TUMOR

5. Browder W, McQuitty JT Jr, McDonald JC. Malignant cystosarcoma phylloides. Treatment and prognosis. Am J Surg 1978; 136:239–241

6. Buchberger W, Strasser K, Heim K, Müller E, Schröcksnadel H. Phylloides tumor: findings on mammography, sonography, and aspiration cytology in 10 cases. AJR 1991; 157:715–719
7. Cohn-Cedermark G, Rutqvist LE, Rosendahl I, Silfverswärd C. Prognostic factors in cystosarcoma phyllodes. A clinicopathologic study of 77 patients. Cancer 1991; 68:2017–2022
8. Cole-Beuglet C, Soriano R, Kurtz AB, Meyer JE, Kopans DB, Goldberg BB. Ultrasound, x-ray mammography, and histopathology of cystosarcoma phylloides. Radiology 1983; 146:481–486
9. D'Orsi CJ, Feldhaus L, Sonnenfeld M. Unusual lesions of the breast. Radiol Clin North Am 1983; 21:67–80
10. Feig SA. Breast masses. Mammographic and sonographic evaluation. Radiol Clin North Am 1992; 30:67–92
11. Haagensen CD. Diseases of the breast. Philadelphia: WB Saunders; 1986:284–312
12. Hawkins RE, Schofield JB, Fisher C, Wiltshaw E, McKinna JA. The clinical and histologic criteria that predict metastases from cystosarcoma phyllodes. Cancer 1992; 69:141–147
13. Pietruszka M, Barnes L. Cystosarcoma phyllodes: a clinicopathologic analysis of 42 cases. Cancer 1978; 41:1974–1983

FIBROADENOMAS

14. Baker KS, Monsees BS, Diaz NM, Destouet JM, McDivitt RW. Carcinoma within fibroadenomas: mammographic features. Radiology 1990; 176:371–374
15. Deschenes L, Jacob S, Fabia J, Christen A. Beware of breast fibroadenomas in middle-aged women. Can J Surg 1985; 28:372–374
16. Haagensen CD. Diseases of the breast. Philadelphia: WB Saunders; 1986:267–283
17. Yoshida Y, Takaoka M, Fukumoto M. Carcinoma arising in fibroadenoma: case report and review of the world literature. J Surg Oncol 1985; 29:132–140

DUCTAL CARCINOMA *IN SITU*

18. Dershaw DD, Abramson A, Kinne DW. Ductal carcinoma in situ: mammographic findings and clinical implications. Radiology 1989; 170:411–415
19. Holland R, Hendriks JH, Verbeek AL, Mravunac M, Schuurmans Stekhoven JH. Extent, distribution, and mammographic/histologic correlations of breast ductal carcinoma in situ. Lancet 1990; 335:519–522
20. Ikeda DM, Andersson I. Ductal carcinoma in situ: atypical mammographic appearances. Radiology 1989; 172:661–666
21. Mitnick JS, Roses DF, Harris MN, Feiner HD. Circumscribed intraductal carcinoma of the breast. Radiology 1989; 170:423–425
22. Stomper PC, Connolly JL, Meyer JE, Harris JR. Clinically occult ductal carcinoma in situ detected with mammography: analysis of 100 cases with radiologic-pathologic correlation. Radiology 1989; 172:235–241

23. Bassett LW, Jahanshahi R, Gold RH, Fu YS. Film-screen mammography: an atlas of instructional cases. New York: Raven Press; 1991
24. Kopans DB. Breast imaging. Philadelphia: JB Lippincott; 1989:62–133
25. Shaw de Paredes E. Atlas of film-screen mammography. Baltimore: Williams & Wilkins; 1992:131–232
26. Sickles EA. Breast masses: mammographic evaluation. Radiology 1989; 173:297–303

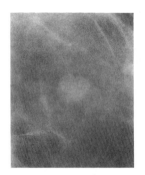

Figure 9-1. This 52-year-old asymptomatic woman was referred for her first mammographic screening after a recent normal breast physical examination. A 1-cm noncalcified mass in the upper outer quadrant of the left breast was seen. You are shown the portion of the MLO view that includes the mass.

Case 9:   Mass with Almost Completely Well Defined Margins

Question 34

Which *one* of the following is the LEAST likely diagnosis?

(A) Cyst
(B) Fibroadenoma
(C) Hamartoma
(D) Carcinoma
(E) Raised skin lesion

One of the most common abnormalities detected at mammographic screening is a solitary noncalcified mass. Initial evaluation involves identifying the lesion on both standard mammographic projections. This will verify that it is truly an abnormality rather than a summation shadow.

Figure 9-1 shows only a portion of the MLO view, but it is reasonable to infer that the lesion is a true abnormality because it is described as being located in the upper outer quadrant. A lesion can be triangulated only if it is seen on two different projections, thereby effectively excluding the diagnosis of summation shadow. Of course, the internal consistency checks comparing lesion depth and location on CC and MLO views would also have to be carried out (see the relevant discussion in Case 1, Question 3), but it is reasonable to assume that this has also been done.

The lesion in Figure 9-1 is oval in shape and appears to be more dense in the center than at its periphery. This combination of features convincingly indicates that it is a true mass, distinguishing it from asymmetric breast tissue, which is a normal variant that rarely harbors an underlying carcinoma. A true mass characteristically displays convex-outward margins and is volumetric rather than planar in aspect, whereas asymmetric breast tissue usually has concave-outward margins and appears to be interspersed with fat.

Figure 9-1 also shows that the mass has a relatively smooth contour and almost completely well defined margins. Its density approximates that of fibroglandular tissue, and it contains no calcifications either centrally or at its borders. It does not appear to cause any distortion of the adjacent parenchymal structures. The mammographic differential diagnosis includes a variety of lesions, the most important of which are discussed here.

Cysts (Option (A)) frequently display mammographic features identical to those seen in the test image. They are usually round or oval in shape and have smooth contours; they frequently have very well (circumscribed) defined margins except where obscured by adjacent dense fibroglandular tissue. However, occasionally the margins of a cyst are slightly indistinct, especially as seen on standard screening views. There may also be irregularities in contour, particularly when the mass is actually a multiloculated cyst or more than one contiguous cyst. Approximately 25% of solitary nonpalpable noncalcified masses are found to be cysts, with the likelihood of this diagnosis increasing further as the margins appear more and more well defined.

The mass seen in the test image also has a high probability of being a fibroadenoma (Option (B)). This is the most common benign solid tumor of the breast. It is characteristically oval in shape or gently lobular and has circumscribed (well-defined) margins when seen adjacent to fatty tissue. Many fibroadenomas display internal calcifications, especially those in women over 50 years old, but a substantial proportion remain noncalcified. It is usually impossible to distinguish between cyst and noncalcified fibroadenoma by mammography.

The typical mammographic features of a malignant mass do not resemble those of the mass in the test image. Most malignant masses have an irregular contour and indistinct margins, and some display characteristic fine spiculations radiating out from the borders of the mass. However, a small percentage present as circumscribed masses, similar in appearance to the mass seen in the test image. Therefore, carcinoma (Option (D)) must also be included in the differential diagnosis. The likelihood that a mostly well defined noncalcified mass will be malignant increases progressively with the age of the patient. For a woman over 50 years old, carcinoma is a major consideration if the mass has even slight irregularity in contour or indistinctness of margins.

Skin lesions often project over the breast parenchyma on both standard mammographic views because of the hemispheric shape of the breast and the manner in which compression distorts this geometry. If such a lesion were sufficiently thick to be seen by virtue of the added density that it imparts, and if its margins were circumscribed, it could readily simulate an intramammary mass with features similar to those observed in the test image. Thus, a raised skin lesion (Option (E)) must also be added to the differential diagnosis. These lesions are frequently

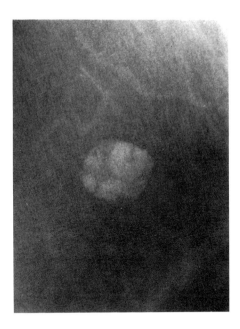

Figure 9-2. Raised skin lesion. This image is a portion of an MLO view of a raised skin lesion, superimposed over the the axillary tail region of the breast. The skin lesion appears to represent a noncalcified mass, but its margins are unusually well defined because the air adjacent to its borders produces even greater contrast than that produced by breast fat. Also note that some air is entrapped within the interstices of the mass, an appearance that is characteristic of a verrucous skin lesion.

recognized by their unusually well defined margins, which are seen so well because small amounts of air are entrapped at their edges during breast compression. A raised verrucous lesion, such as a seborrheic keratosis, often entraps some air not only at its margins but also within its interstices, producing an even more characteristic mammographic appearance (Figure 9-2). However, the fact that no air outlines the mass seen in Figure 9-1 does not exclude the possibility of a raised skin lesion.

A hamartoma is another benign solid tumor that can occur in the breast. It has fatty, fibrous, and glandular elements in various proportions. Some pathologists are more specific in naming these tumors, describing them by the relative amounts of their constituent elements (e.g., lipofibroadenoma, fibroadenolipoma). Histologic evaluation demonstrates a mixture of mature fat and dense connective tissue surrounding benign lobules and ducts. At mammography the hamartoma typically presents as a well-defined mass containing variable amounts of both fibroglandular and fatty density. In addition, if some of the fatty elements within the mass are located at its periphery and if there are also fatty tissues surrounding the mass, this will permit visualization of the thin fibrous capsule of the mass, a mammographic feature characteristic of all fat-containing lesions (Figure 9-3). Some small biopsy-proved hamartomas have been reported to show only dense fibroglandular tissue at mammography, but this is a very unusual occurrence. For this reason, and because hamartomas themselves are rare, the absence of any visible

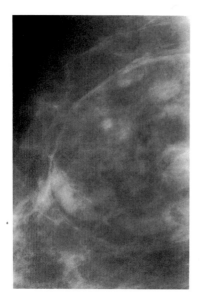

Figure 9-3. Hamartoma. This image is a portion of an MLO view showing the anterior part of a mass in the axillary tail region of the breast. There are areas of both fat and fibroglandular density within the mass, corresponding to the fatty, fibrous, and glandular elements within this benign tumor. This particular hamartoma is composed primarily of fatty tissues. Because fatty elements within the mass are adjacent to fatty tissues external to the mass, the thin fibrous capsule surrounding the mass is readily visible.

fatty component within the mass in the test image makes the diagnosis of hamartoma exceedingly unlikely **(Option (C) is correct).**

Questions 35 through 39

For each numbered nonpalpable lesion listed below (Questions 35 through 39), select the *one* lettered sequence of ultrasonography (US) and spot-compression magnification mammography (SM) (A, B, C, D, or E) that is MOST appropriate in conducting the imaging work-up. Each lettered work-up sequence may be used once, more than once, or not at all.

35. 1.2-cm fairly well defined upper outer right breast mass
36. 1-cm ovoid well-defined retroareolar left breast mass containing eight discrete calcifications
37. 1.6-cm spiculated upper outer left breast mass associated with focal skin thickening and retraction
38. 0.6-cm spiculated upper inner right breast mass
39. 1.3-cm fairly well defined round density identified in the outer aspect of the left breast only on the craniocaudal view

    (A)   US first, SM second
    (B)   SM first, US second
    (C)   US, no SM
    (D)   SM, no US
    (E)   Neither US nor SM first

The major role of ultrasonography in breast-imaging practice is to establish or exclude the diagnosis of simple benign cyst for nonpalpable masses detected at mammography. Virtually 100% accuracy can be achieved if strict sonographic criteria are utilized, including demonstration that a mass has smooth well-defined margins, increased through transmission of sound, and total lack of internal echoes. Thus, ultrasonography is frequently used as a first step in the imaging work-up of a nonpalpable mass, because confident diagnosis of a simple benign cyst obviates any further tests.

The principal role of spot-compression magnification mammography in the same clinical setting is to portray the margins of a mass more clearly and to search for additional subtle radiographic features (e.g., associated microcalcifications, architectural distortion) that may be useful in guiding subsequent management. As a result, demonstration of irregular margins or fine spiculations at the margins of a mass almost always prompts biopsy whereas portrayal of well-defined borders on fine-detail images usually leads to periodic follow-up.

Occasionally, practical considerations govern the sequence of imaging tests chosen by a radiologist in the work-up of a nonpalpable mammographically detected mass. If either ultrasonography or spot-compression magnification mammography is immediately available but the patient has to wait (or return at a later date) for the other examination, accessibility may be the deciding factor. However, much more frequently the work-up sequence will be determined by imaging considerations. As a general rule, it is more sensible to begin with ultrasonography for a mass judged likely to be cystic, because no further evaluation will be necessary if ultrasonography indeed proves the mass to be a simple benign cyst. On the other hand, spot-compression magnification mammography should be done first if the conventional mammographic features of the mass make cyst a very improbable diagnosis, because the clinical management of a solid (non-cystic) mass is usually based on its mammographic rather than sonographic characteristics.

For a 1.2-cm fairly well defined nonpalpable mass, cyst is a likely diagnosis. Therefore, ultrasonography should be the first step in the work-up. However, if sonography fails to result in the confident diagnosis of simple benign cyst, the work-up must proceed and spot-compression magnification mammography should be done next **(Option (A) is the correct answer to Question 35).** Fine-detail mammography will better define the border characteristics of the mass, thereby providing useful information to help the radiologist decide between recommending biopsy or periodic mammographic follow-up.

A 1-cm ovoid well-defined mass containing eight discrete calcifications is very unlikely to be a cyst, because of the presence of internal calcifications. Discrete calcifications are found only rarely within a cyst, and even then they are seen to sediment at the bottom of the cyst on MLO or 90° lateral views. For this reason, ultrasonography should not be included at all in the imaging work-up. On the other hand, spot-compression magnification mammography can be expected to aid substantially in the clinical management of the lesion, not only by more clearly portraying the margins of the mass but also by better demonstrating the shapes of the calcific particles **(Option (D) is the correct answer to Question 36).**

A spiculated mass associated with focal skin thickening and retraction almost certainly represents locally advanced invasive breast carcinoma. Ultrasonography can add little if anything to the management of such a lesion, which clearly is not a simple benign cyst. Furthermore, because of the high probability of locally advanced disease, mastectomy will be the likely treatment of choice for local cancer control, and therefore spot-compression magnification mammography will not affect subsequent management. The next step in the work-up should be to obtain a tissue diagnosis of carcinoma **(Option (E) is the correct answer to Question 37).**

A 0.6-cm spiculated nonpalpable mass is unlikely to be a simple benign cyst, so that ultrasonography has no place in the diagnostic imaging work-up. However, although such a lesion will probably be found to be malignant, its small size and impalpability make breast conservation surgery (lumpectomy) the likely choice for local cancer control. In this clinical setting, magnification mammography can provide valuable information in preoperative tumor staging because of its ability to determine the extent of disease and to identify possible multifocal or multicentric tumor deposits. Therefore, the first step in the work-up of such a lesion indeed should be magnification mammography **(Option (D) is the correct answer to Question 38).**

For a 1.3-cm fairly well defined round density seen only on one standard mammographic projection, the first step in the work-up is to distinguish between superimposition of normal structures and true breast mass (for a detailed discussion, see Case 2). This is accomplished effectively with spot-compression magnification mammography, which should be done in a shallow oblique projection to produce the most convincing results. Furthermore, it makes little sense to begin the work-up with ultrasonography, because even if this procedure identifies a true breast mass, additional mammography will be necessary to determine whether the lesion found at ultrasonography is indeed the same as the density seen at mammography. In the proper work-up sequence (i.e., starting with spot-compression magnification mammography), if the presence of a true mass is confirmed and if the mass continues to demonstrate a smooth contour and well-defined margins (findings that make cyst a distinct possibility), ultrasonography should be the next step in evaluation **(Option (B) is the correct answer to Question 39).**

Question 40

Spot-compression magnification mammography would prompt biopsy of a 1-cm fairly well defined mass seen on a standard mammogram by demonstrating:

- (A) the margins to be more well defined
- (B) the borders to be microlobulated
- (C) the contour to be more irregular
- (D) a few spiculations at the border
- (E) multiple tiny calcifications within the mass

Spot-compression magnification mammography produces fine-detail images that portray with greater than standard clarity all the radiographic features of breast masses. Consequently, the answers to this question depend primarily on the radiographic features themselves rather than on the ability of spot-compression magnification technique to demonstrate them.

Benign masses characteristically have circumscribed margins, whereas cancers are usually indistinct. Therefore, should the margins of a mass be seen to be more well defined on fine-detail images, the likelihood of malignancy decreases, sometimes sufficiently to prompt a recommendation of periodic mammographic follow-up instead of biopsy **(Option (A) is false).**

Benign breast masses not infrequently demonstrate lobulated borders, but these lobulations are usually relatively large and only a few are present. Thus, the presence of macrolobulations does not increase the likelihood of malignancy of a given mass. Most commonly, such lesions are fibroadenomas, intramammary lymph nodes, or cysts that are multiloculated or immediately adjacent to each other. However, as the number of lobulations in a mass increases, especially if the lobulations are small, the suspicion of malignancy does increase. Indeed, most radiologists will suggest biopsy rather than periodic mammographic follow-up for such a mass; therefore, when spot-compression magnification mammography demonstrates otherwise unsuspected microlobulated borders, biopsy is usually recommended **(Option (B) is true).**

Most benign breast masses are round or oval, and many intramammary lymph nodes have a reniform contour. In contradistinction, most malignant masses are irregular in contour. Therefore, if spot-compression magnification mammography shows the contour of a mass to be more irregular than was otherwise suspected, then the level of suspicion of malignancy increases and biopsy is likely to be recommended **(Option (C) is true).**

Spiculation is a mammographic hallmark of malignancy, although it is not sufficiently specific to be a pathognomonic sign. Therefore, the presence of only a few spiculations raises some suspicion of malignancy. However, most malignant masses do not exhibit spiculation, especially masses detected in women who regularly undergo mammographic screening. On occasion, a mass will demonstrate early spiculation only on spot-compression magnification mammography; in this circumstance, biopsy should be recommended because the likelihood of malignancy is relatively high **(Option (D) is true).**

Calcifications may be found in both benign and malignant masses. The benign mass that calcifies most frequently is the fibroadenoma, but to be considered characteristically benign, the calcific particles in such a mass should be relatively large and amorphous, often located near the periphery of the mass. Calcifications within a malignant mass are typically much smaller, although usually they are also variable in shape. When calcifications are seen within a mass only on spot-compression magnification mammography, the individual calcific particles must be so small as to approach the limits of mammographic resolution, i.e., much too small to be characteristic of fibroadenoma. Therefore, when fine-detail mammography demonstrates otherwise unsuspected tiny calcifica-

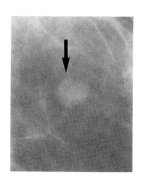

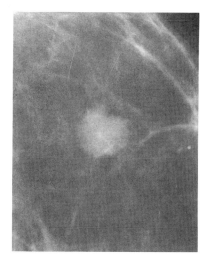

Figure 9-4   *Figure 9-5*

Figures 9-4 and 9-5. Mass with almost completely well defined margins. Figure 9-4 (same as Figure 9-1) is a portion of the standard MLO view of the test patient, showing a 1-cm ovoid noncalcified mass with a bilobed contour. The margins of the mass are almost completely well defined, except superiorly (arrow). Figure 9-5 is a spot-compression magnification view of the mass, also in the MLO projection, taken to obtain finer detail. The margins of the mass are now seen to be less well defined, and its contour is considerably more irregular. These changes in mammographic appearance raise some suspicion of malignancy. As a result, biopsy was done and the mass was found to be an invasive ductal carcinoma. Had the additional spot-compression magnification view not been obtained, interpretation of the standard mammography examination might have incorrectly categorized the mass as probably benign, leading to a recommendation for periodic mammographic follow-up instead of biopsy.

tions within a mass, the likelihood of malignancy increases and biopsy is usually recommended **(Option (E) is true)**.

Clearly, spot-compression magnification mammography can change the level of suspicion of malignancy for a mass already seen on standard mammograms. For the mass in the test patient, the screening images demonstrated almost completely well defined margins, a macrolobulated contour, and an oval in shape (Figure 9-4). These features strongly suggest that the mass is benign. However, because a "probably benign" diagnosis should not be made solely on the basis of standard (screening) images, additional spot-compression magnification mammograms were obtained (Figure 9-5). These show the margins of the mass to be less well defined and the contour to be considerably more irregular, features that raise some suspicion of malignancy. Biopsy was recommended, and this resulted in the diagnosis of invasive ductal carcinoma. The message from this case is clear: one should not consider a mass to be probably benign and one should not recommend periodic mammographic follow-up for a mass until appropriately benign findings are confirmed on fine-detail images.

Question 41

Types of carcinoma that are usually seen as fairly well defined masses at mammography include:

    (A) lobular carcinoma *in situ*
    (B) comedocarcinoma
    (C) colloid carcinoma
    (D) medullary carcinoma
    (E) invasive ductal carcinoma

Breast carcinoma presents as a fairly well defined mass in approximately 5% of cases. However, as indicated above, the term "well defined" may be a misnomer because fine-detail mammography often demonstrates that such a mass has subtle contour irregularities and somewhat indistinct margins that are difficult to appreciate on standard-technique mammograms.

Lobular carcinoma *in situ* (LCIS), otherwise known as lobular neoplasia, is the histologic diagnosis given to noninfiltrating neoplastic lesions that arise from the acinar epithelium within the breast lobule. It is generally believed that LCIS serves as a precursor to all cases of invasive lobular carcinoma, but only about 20 to 30% of women with LCIS develop invasive carcinoma within the next 15 to 20 years. Furthermore, the invasive tumors are almost as often ductal in origin as they are lobular, and they are found with equal frequency in both breasts. For these reasons, many researchers prefer to group LCIS together with the atypical hyperplasias rather than with the carcinomas, because its biologic behavior more closely parallels that of high-risk lesions. The mammographic features of LCIS are nonspecific, so much so that the great majority of lesions are not even seen. Indeed, LCIS is usually discovered by serendipity, located adjacent to rather than within areas of mammographic abnormality. Therefore, it is extremely rare for LCIS to present mammographically as a circumscribed mass **(Option (A) is false).**

Comedocarcinoma is a subtype of ductal carcinoma *in situ* that is characterized by abundant necrotic debris filling involved ducts. This debris frequently calcifies, and so the lesion usually presents mammographically as clustered calcifications, typically linear and branching-shaped particles that represent casts of the tiny peripheral neoplastic duct lumina within which they form. Often the calcifications of comedocarcinoma are so extensive as to appear segmental in distribution, because of the propensity of this lesion to spread throughout large areas within one or sometimes several adjacent duct systems. Uncommonly, comedocarcinoma forms a discrete tumor that may be seen mammographically as a circumscribed mass. However, this is the exception rather than the rule **(Option (B) is false).**

Colloid carcinoma is a well-differentiated subtype of invasive ductal carcinoma, in which the tumor cells secrete abundant quantities of mucin. Many invasive ductal carcinomas have a small proportion of mucin-producing cells, but pure colloid carcinoma is much more distinctive and carries a relatively favorable prognosis. Colloid cancers typically present mammographically as relatively well defined masses **(Option (C) is true),** usually with some contour irregularities and occasionally with microlobulated borders. However, not uncommonly the tumor masses have indistinct margins; only rarely do they have spiculation or contain calcifications.

Medullary carcinoma is another relatively well differentiated subtype of invasive ductal carcinoma. These lesions have characteristic histologic features, including abundant lymphocytic infiltration, extensive central necrosis, unusually large tumor cells, and an abrupt rather than infiltrating margin with surrounding benign breast tissues. They induce little if any desmoplastic stromal reaction and are therefore relatively soft to palpation, a property that often allows them to grow relatively large before detection. Mammographically, the typical medullary carcinoma presents as a circumscribed mass **(Option (D) is true).** However, especially on fine-detail views, the margins of the mass often appear somewhat indistinct and the contour slightly irregular.

Invasive ductal carcinoma is the most common type of breast cancer by far. Most of these neoplasms present mammographically as ill-defined masses having irregular contour. Calcifications are seen frequently, especially within areas of ductal carcinoma *in situ* that may be found inside the main tumor mass or in multifocal or multicentric tumor deposits. It is unusual for invasive ductal carcinoma to present mammographically as a circumscribed mass **(Option (E) is false).** However, because most breast cancers are invasive ductal lesions, a circumscribed carcinoma is just as likely, if not more likely, to be an invasive ductal cancer as it is to be one of the less commonly encountered but characteristically well-defined subtypes.

Edward A. Sickles, M.D.

SUGGESTED READINGS

MAMMOGRAPHIC ANALYSIS OF BREAST MASSES

1. Feig SA. Breast masses. Mammographic and sonographic evaluation. Radiol Clin North Am 1992; 30:67–92
2. Homer MJ. Imaging features and management of characteristically benign and probably benign breast lesions. Radiol Clin North Am 1987; 25:939–951
3. Homer MJ. Mammographic interpretation: a practical approach. New York: McGraw-Hill; 1991:30–34, 74–100
4. Kopans DB. Breast imaging. Philadelphia: JB Lippincott; 1989:68–81
5. Pisano ED, McLelland R. Mammographic analysis of breast masses. In: Sickles EA, Kopans DB (eds), Syllabus for the categorical course on breast imaging. Reston, VA: American College of Radiology; 1990:17–29
6. Sickles EA. Breast masses: mammographic evaluation. Radiology 1989; 173:297–303

HAMARTOMA

7. Andersson I, Hildell J, Linell F, Ljungqvist U. Mammary hamartomas. Acta Radiol [Diagn] (Stockh) 1979; 20:712–720
8. Crothers JG, Butler NF, Fortt RW, Gravelle IH. Fibroadenolipoma of the breast. Br J Radiol 1985; 58:191–202
9. Helvie MA, Adler DD, Rebner M, Oberman HA. Breast hamartomas: variable mammographic appearance. Radiology 1989; 170:417–421
10. Hessler C, Schnyder P, Ozzello L. Hamartoma of the breast: diagnostic observation of 16 cases. Radiology 1978; 126:95–98

ULTRASONOGRAPHY

11. Bassett LW, Kimme-Smith C. Breast sonography. AJR 1991; 156:449–455
12. Bassett LW, Kimme-Smith C, Sutherland LK, Gold RH, Sarti D, King W III. Automated and hand-held breast US: effect on patient management. Radiology 1987; 165:103–108
13. Hilton SV, Leopold GR, Olson LK, Willson SA. Real-time breast sonography: application in 300 consecutive patients. AJR 1986; 147:479–486
14. Jackson VP. The role of US in breast imaging. Radiology 1990; 177:305–311
15. Jellins J, Kossoff G, Reeve TS. Detection and classification of liquid-filled masses in the breast by gray scale echography. Radiology 1977; 125:205–212
16. Jokich PM, Monticciolo DL, Adler YT. Breast ultrasonography. Radiol Clin North Am 1992; 30:993–1009
17. Kopans DB. Breast imaging. Philadelphia: JB Lippincott; 1989:227–247
18. Mendelson EB. Breast sonography. In: Sickles EA, Kopans DB (eds), Syllabus for the categorical course on breast imaging. Reston, VA: American College of Radiology; 1990:31–45
19. Rubin E, Miller VE, Berland LL, Han SY, Koehler RE, Stanley RJ. Hand-held real-time breast sonography. AJR 1985; 144:623–627

20. Sickles EA, Filly RA, Callen PW. Benign breast lesions: ultrasound detection and diagnosis. Radiology 1984; 151:467–470

MAGNIFICATION MAMMOGRAPHY

21. Berkowitz JE, Gatewood OM, Gayler BW. Equivocal mammographic findings: evaluation with spot compression. Radiology 1989; 171:369–371
22. Faulk RM, Sickles EA. Efficacy of spot compression-magnification and tangential views in the mammographic evaluation of palpable breast masses. Radiology 1992; 185:87–90
23. Hall FM. Magnification spot compression of the breast (letter). Radiology 1989; 173:284
24. Sickles EA. Microfocal spot magnification mammography using xeroradiographic and screen-film recording systems. Radiology 1979; 131:599–607
25. Sickles EA. Magnification mammography. In: Feig SA, McLelland R (eds), Breast carcinoma: current diagnosis and treatment. New York: Masson; 1983:177–182
26. Sickles EA. Combining spot-compression and other special views to maximize mammographic information (letter). Radiology 1989; 173:571
27. Tabar L. Microfocal spot magnification mammography. In: Brunner S, Langfeldt B, Andersen PE (eds), Early detection of breast cancer. New York: Springer-Verlag; 1984:62–68

CIRCUMSCRIBED CARCINOMA

28. Hall FM, Storella JM, Silverstone DZ, Wyshak G. Nonpalpable breast lesions: recommendations for biopsy based on suspicion of carcinoma at mammography. Radiology 1988; 167:353–358
29. Helvie MA, Pennes DR, Rebner M, Adler DD. Mammographic follow-up of low-suspicion lesions: compliance rate and diagnostic yield. Radiology 1991; 178:155–158
30. Moskowitz M. The predictive value of certain mammographic signs in screening for breast cancer. Cancer 1983; 51:1007–1011
31. Moskowitz M. Circumscribed lesions of the breast. In: Diagnostic categorical course in breast imaging. Oak Brook, IL: Radiological Society of North America; 1986:31–33
32. Sickles EA. Mammographic features of 300 consecutive nonpalpable breast cancers. AJR 1986; 146:661–663
33. Sickles EA. Periodic mammographic follow-up of probably benign lesions: results in 3,184 consecutive cases. Radiology 1991; 179:463–468

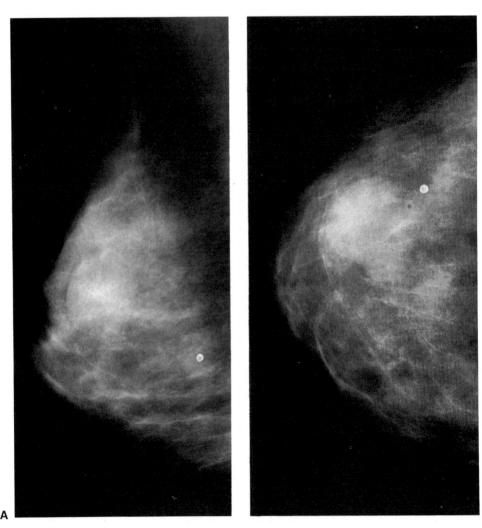

A   B

Figure 10-1. This 38-year-old woman has a palpable mass in the upper outer right breast. You are shown MLO (A) and CC (B) mammograms.

Case 10: Mass with Partial Halo Sign and Most Margins Obscured by Isodense Tissue

Question 42

Which *one* of the following is the MOST likely diagnosis?

(A) Cyst
(B) Medullary carcinoma
(C) Papilloma
(D) Intracystic carcinoma
(E) Hamartoma

The test images (Figure 10-1) show a large oval mass in the upper outer quadrant of the right breast (Figure 10-2, arrows). The posterior aspect of the lesion is obscured by adjacent fibroglandular tissue. The anterior aspect of the lesion demonstrates a "halo" sign (arrowheads). This sign is a nonspecific finding, which merely indicates that this margin of the lesion is circumscribed (smooth and sharply defined). The shape, density (low-density radiopaque), and lack of calcifications make a benign process such as cyst the most likely diagnosis **(Option (A) is correct).** Benign processes, such as cysts and fibroadenomas, are much more common than breast cancer as the cause of masses that display the halo sign. Cyst was indeed the diagnosis for the test patient, as shown in the sonogram in Figure 10-3. Medullary carcinoma (Option (B)) and intracystic carcinoma (Option (D)) are relatively rare, accounting for fewer than 5% and fewer than 2% of all cancers, respectively, thereby making these choices much less likely. Papillomas (Option (C)) are rarely seen mammographically, and when visible they are usually less than 1 cm in diameter, much smaller than the mass in the test patient. Hamartomas (Option (E)) are almost always mixed-density circumscribed masses, containing both fat and soft tissue density. The lesion seen in the

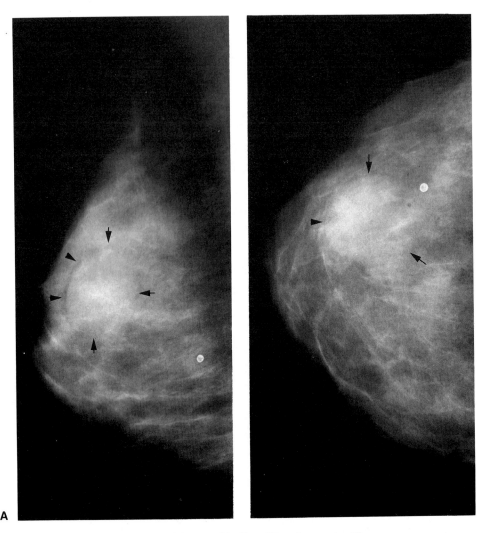

A

B

Figure 10-2 (Same as Figure 10-1). Simple cyst. The mammograms show a mass with a partial halo sign and most margins obscured by iso-dense tissues. The mass measures 3.0 by 2.5 cm and is seen in the upper outer quadrant of the right breast (arrows) on both MLO (A) and CC (B) mammograms. The posterior aspect of the lesion is obscured by adjacent fibroglandular tissue. Anteriorly, a halo sign (arrowheads) is seen on both projections.

test images is a low-density radiopaque mass and does not contain fat, making hamartoma a very unlikely diagnosis.

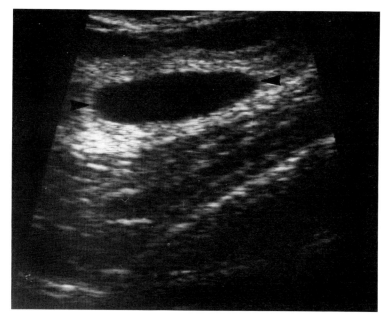

Figure 10-3. Same patient as in Figures 10-1 and 10-2. Simple cyst. This longitudinal 7.5-MHz real-time sonogram shows an oval, compressible, anechoic simple cyst (arrowheads) with posterior enhancement. In this case, the enhancement is seen only superiorly.

Question 43

Reliable methods for distinguishing a cyst from a sharply circumscribed solid mass include:

  (A) ultrasonography
  (B) needle aspiration
  (C) magnification mammography
  (D) pneumocystography
  (E) physical examination
  (F) MRI

Ultrasonography is a cross-sectional imaging modality that allows for accurate differentiation of fluid from solid material. It is the easiest way to make the diagnosis of a simple cyst when a nonpalpable circumscribed noncalcified mass is found by mammography **(Option (A) is true).** When a palpable circumscribed mass is present, needle aspiration can be performed instead of ultrasonography. Aspiration of clear, nonbloody fluid with resolution and non-recurrence of the palpable mass is

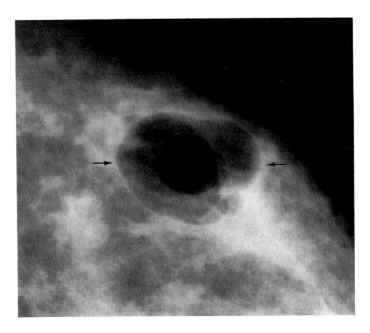

Figure 10-4. Pneumocystogram of a 2-cm cyst. ML view demonstrates smooth borders (arrows) and no evidence of intracystic tumor.

diagnostic of a simple cyst **(Option (B) is true)**. Pneumocystography involves replacement of the aspirated cyst fluid with air, followed by mammography. If smooth borders are seen in the air-filled space, as in Figure 10-4, the diagnosis of a simple cyst is made **(Option (D) is true)**. Some authorities believe that air insufflation of a cyst reduces the chance of recurrence by causing sclerosis of the cyst wall epithelium.

On either contact or magnification mammography, cysts and circumscribed solid masses vary from high- to low-density radiopaque, so that the use of density to predict etiology is unreliable. Indeed, many benign and malignant solid masses are identical to cysts in radiographic density. In addition, there is considerable overlap in the shape and border characteristics of benign and malignant masses; either mass may be round or oval and circumscribed. Therefore, one cannot accurately diagnose a cyst mammographically **(Option (C) is false)**.

Physical examination permits the detection of palpable abnormalities, and one might speculate that a palpable mass represents a cyst on the basis of its smooth, freely mobile, tender nature. However, physical examination is unreliable in the differentiation of cysts from solid masses **(Option (E) is false)**. Thus, needle aspiration may be attempted, rather than ultrasonography, once a mass has been palpated.

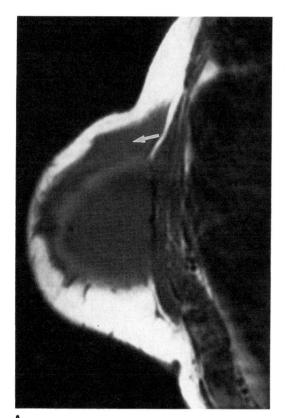
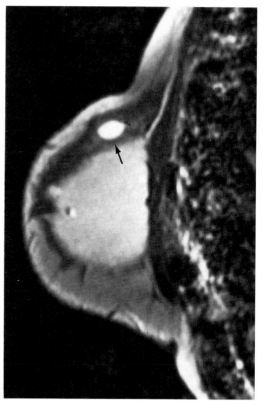

A

B

Figure 10-5. MR images of a simple cyst. On the T1-weighted image (A) of this woman with an implant, the cyst is not visible because, in this case, it has the same signal intensity as the surrounding breast tissue (arrow). On the T2-weighted image (B), the typical high signal intensity of the cyst is clearly seen (arrow). Ultrasonography confirmed that this lesion was a simple cyst. (Case courtesy of Handel E. Reynolds, M.D.)

Simple cysts have low signal intensity on T1-weighted MR images and high signal intensity on T2-weighted images (Figure 10-5); therefore, they can be distinguished from solid masses **(Option (F) is true).** While MRI is as reliable as ultrasonography for the diagnosis of cysts, MRI is rarely used for this purpose, principally because of its high cost relative to that of ultrasonography.

Question 44

Findings that preclude ultrasonographic diagnosis of a simple benign cyst include:

    (A) low-level internal echoes
    (B) compressibility
    (C) slightly irregular walls
    (D) acoustic enhancement behind the lesion
    (E) acoustic attenuation behind the lesion
    (F) edge refraction

The primary role of ultrasonography in breast imaging is to diagnose cysts, and its accuracy for this approaches 100% when strict criteria are used for interpretation. One should see smooth walls, no internal echoes, posterior acoustic enhancement, and no surrounding architectural distortion, as shown in Figure 10-6. Any other features would preclude the sonographic diagnosis of a simple cyst. When the gain is appropriately set, the presence of low-level internal echoes (except for reverberation artifact in the anterior portion of the cyst) indicates that the lesion is solid or is a complicated cyst (i.e., a cyst complicated by hemorrhage or infection) **(Option (A) is true).** Fluid-filled structures are characteristically more compressible than solid masses, and this feature can therefore be used to confirm the diagnosis of a cyst **(Option (B) is false).** If the walls of an anechoic mass are irregular, one cannot make the diagnosis of a simple cyst **(Option (C) is true).** Cysts occasionally have slightly irregular borders, but the visualization of wall irregularity should suggest a complicated cyst (Figure 10-7), abscess, or necrotic carcinoma. Posterior acoustic enhancement is one of the least consistently seen signs of a simple cyst, yet when present behind an anechoic mass, it serves as further evidence of the cystic nature of the lesion **(Option (D) is false).** However, enhancement may not be seen behind small cysts or with some types of sonographic equipment. In addition, posterior enhancement is often seen behind benign and malignant solid masses, so this feature alone should not lead to the diagnosis of a cyst. When posterior acoustic attenuation is seen, one should not make the diagnosis of a cyst **(Option (E) is true).** Edge refraction (or lateral shadowing) is commonly seen around any smooth curved reflector in the body, such as the wall of a cyst (Figure 10-8) **(Option (F) is false).**

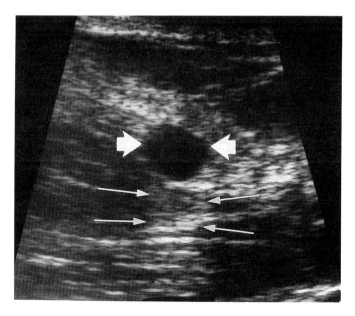

Figure 10-6. Simple cyst. This 7.5-MHz real-time transverse sonogram demonstrates the classic features of a simple cyst: smooth walls (wide arrows), no internal echoes, and posterior enhancement (thin arrows).

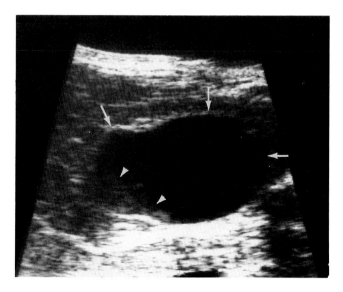

Figure 10-7. Complex cyst. Longitudinal 7.5-MHz real-time sonogram of a predominantly anechoic mass (arrows) shows an irregular solid projection (arrowheads) at the superior pole of the mass. This may be seen in intracystic benign or malignant tumors, necrotic carcinomas, or complicated cysts. In this case, it represented a blood clot within a hemorrhagic cyst.

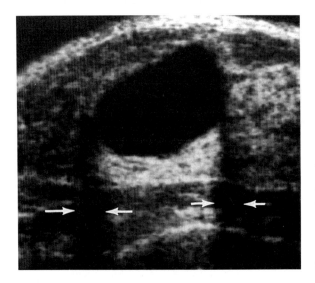

Figure 10-8. Simple cyst with edge refraction (lateral shadowing). These normal shadows (arrows) are seen at the edges of any smooth curved reflector.

Questions 45 through 48

For each numbered breast disorder listed below (Questions 45 through 48), select the *one* lettered sonographic finding (A, B, C, D, or E) that is MOST closely associated with it. Each lettered sonographic finding may be used once, more than once, or not at all.

45. Invasive ductal carcinoma
46. Hemorrhagic cyst
47. Intracystic papillary carcinoma
48. Hamartoma

    (A)   Heterogeneous solid smooth mass
    (B)   Smooth hypoechoic mass with low-level internal echoes
    (C)   Complex mass with solid projection into the anechoic area of the lesion
    (D)   Hyperechoic solid mass with lateral shadows
    (E)   Irregular hypoechoic mass with posterior attenuation

The classic sonographic appearance of an invasive ductal carcinoma is an irregular mass with heterogeneous internal echoes and posterior acoustic shadowing or attenuation **(Option (E) is the correct answer to Question 45).** Most sonographically visible invasive ductal carcinomas have these features, but some appear as circumscribed homogeneous solid masses. Similarly, some benign processes, such as scars, fibroadenomas, sclerosing adenosis, and fibrocystic changes, have an irregular, attenuating appearance. In addition, one must keep in mind

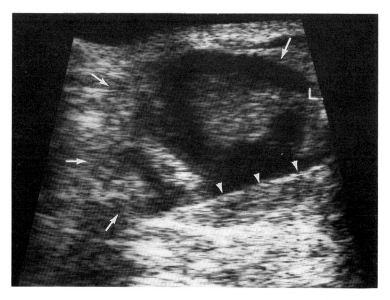

Figure 10-9. Intracystic papillary carcinoma. Longitudinal 7.5-MHz real-time sonogram of a palpable left breast mass shows a mass (arrows) that contains both fluid and solid components. A fluid-debris level (arrowheads) is present in the dependent portion of the mass.

that many small invasive ductal carcinomas are not visible by ultrasonography.

Simple cysts can undergo hemorrhage spontaneously or after trauma. In most cases, the cyst maintains its smooth walls and posterior enhancement but is filled with low-level internal echoes **(Option (B) is the correct answer to Question 46).** These internal echoes can be seen to move within the cyst during real-time examination. Occasionally, a blood clot forms that adheres to the cyst wall, producing wall irregularity or a solid projection into the cyst (Figure 10-7). Without demonstrating motion of internal echoes, one cannot make the diagnosis of a complicated cyst; needle aspiration or biopsy should be considered.

Intracystic papillary carcinoma is a rare cancer that has a better prognosis than invasive ductal carcinoma. Mammographically, this lesion frequently appears as a large, circumscribed mass. On ultrasonography, a complex mass is usually seen, with a solid projection into a cystic region of the lesion **(Option (C) is the correct answer to Question 47).** Hemorrhage is common within invasive papillary carcinoma, and fluid-debris levels are often seen within the cyst (Figure 10-9).

The diagnosis of a hamartoma can usually be made by mammography because of the typical features of both fat and fibroglandular density within an encapsulated smooth mass. Therefore, ultrasonography is not useful in the diagnosis of these typical cases. Ultrasonography of mammographically typical or atypical hamartomas can demonstrate a variety of findings. Most commonly, the appearance is that of a nonspecific smooth, solid mass. Internal echoes are frequently heterogeneous, with areas of hyperechogenicity from the fat within the mass **(Option (A) is the correct answer to Question 48).** However, the diagnosis of hamartoma cannot be made reliably by ultrasonography alone.

Question 49

Which *one of* the following is the MOST important meaning of the halo sign?

(A) The mass is benign
(B) The mass is malignant
(C) The border of the mass is smooth
(D) The mass is a cyst
(E) A partial halo sign is highly suggestive of an intracystic carcinoma

The halo sign is a narrow radiolucent line that surrounds all or part of the circumference of some circumscribed breast masses as seen on mammography. It has been described as a strong indicator of a benign lesion (Option (A)), such as a cyst (Option (D)) or fibroadenoma. However, it has been shown to be merely a Mach effect that can occur around any smooth mass and is also observed among some circumscribed malignancies (Option (B)). Because smooth masses are much more likely to be benign than malignant, the presence of the halo sign is not suggestive of intracystic carcinoma (Option (E)). In summary, because of its lack of specificity, the main value of the halo sign is simply to indicate that the margin of a lesion is smooth **(Option (C) is correct).**

Valerie P. Jackson, M.D.

SUGGESTED READINGS

HALO SIGN

1. Gordenne WH, Malchair FL. Mach bands in mammography. Radiology 1988; 169:55–58
2. Swann CA, Kopans DB, Koerner FC, McCarthy KA, White G, Hall DA. The halo sign and malignant breast lesions. AJR 1987; 149:1145–1147
3. Tabar L, Dean PB. Teaching atlas of mammography. New York: Thieme Stratton; 1985:18

MEDULLARY CARCINOMA

4. Kopans DB, Rubens J. Medullary carcinoma of the breast (letter). Radiology 1989; 171:876
5. Meyer JE, Amin E, Lindfors KK, Lipman JC, Stomper PC, Genest D. Medullary carcinoma of the breast: mammographic and US appearance. Radiology 1989; 170:79–82

PAPILLOMA

6. Cardenosa G, Eklund GW. Benign papillary neoplasms of the breast: mammographic findings. Radiology 1991; 181:751–755

INVASIVE PAPILLARY CARCINOMA

7. Mitnick JS, Vazquez MF, Harris MN, Schechter S, Roses DF. Invasive papillary carcinoma of the breast: mammographic appearance. Radiology 1990; 177:803–806

HAMARTOMA

8. Crothers JG, Butler NF, Fortt RW, Gravelle IH. Fibroadenolipoma of the breast. Br J Radiol 1985; 58:191–202
9. D'Orsi CJ, Feldhaus L, Sonnenfeld M. Unusual lesions of the breast. Radiol Clin North Am 1983; 21:67–80
10. Helvie MA, Adler DD, Rebner M, Oberman HA. Breast hamartomas: variable mammographic appearance. Radiology 1989; 170:417–421

ULTRASONOGRAPHY

11. Bassett LW, Kimme-Smith C. Breast sonography. AJR 1991; 156:449–455
12. Hilton SV, Leopold GR, Olson LK, Willson SA. Real-time breast sonography: application in 300 consecutive patients. AJR 1986; 147:479–486
13. Jackson VP. The role of US in breast imaging. Radiology 1990; 177:305–311
14. Jellins J, Kossoff G, Reeve TS. Detection and classification of liquid-filled masses in the breast by gray scale echography. Radiology 1977; 125:205–212
15. Sickles EA, Filly RA, Callen PW. Benign breast lesions: ultrasound detection and diagnosis. Radiology 1984; 151:467–470

PNEUMOCYSTOGRAPHY

16. Dyreborg U, Blichert-Toft M, Boegh L, Kiaer H. Needle puncture followed by pneumocystography of palpable breast cysts. A controlled clinical trial. Acta Radiol [Diagn] (Stockh) 1985; 26:277–281
17. Tabar L, Pentek Z. Pneumocystography of benign and malignant intracystic growths of the female breast. Acta Radiol [Diagn] (Stockh) 1976; 17:829–837
18. Tabar L, Pentek Z, Dean PB. The diagnostic and therapeutic value of breast cyst puncture and pneumocystography. Radiology 1981; 141:659–663

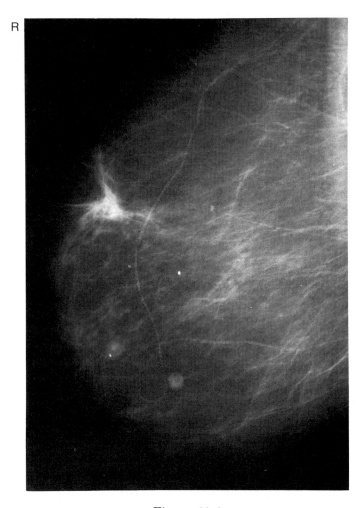

Figure 11-1

Figures 11-1 through 11-4. This 61-year-old woman has a palpable mass in the right breast. You are shown right MLO (Figure 11-1), left MLO (Figure 11-2), right CC (Figure 11-3), and left CC (Figure 11-4) baseline mammograms.

Case 11: Spiculated Lesion without a Central Area of Increased Density

Question 50

Which *one* of the following is the MOST likely diagnosis for the 1-cm smooth mass, containing a single coarse calcification, in the lower outer right breast?

(A) Medullary carcinoma
(B) Cyst
(C) Hamartoma
(D) Involuting fibroadenoma
(E) Lymph node

The differential diagnosis of a completely circumscribed mass, such as that in the test images (Figures 11-1 through 11-4), includes cyst, fibroadenoma, hamartoma, lymph node, and carcinoma. The most important clue to the diagnosis in the test images (Figures 11-5 and 11-6, curved arrows) is the coarse calcification within the mass. Involuting or degenerating fibroadenomas undergo hyalinization and calcification. Early calcification within a fibroadenoma can be less than 1 mm in diameter and can mimic malignant microcalcification. However, large or coarse calcifications are much more common and are typical for this benign tumor, especially when located at the periphery of the mass, as in the test patient **(Option (D) is correct)**.

Medullary carcinoma (Option (A)) frequently presents as a circumscribed mass, but calcifications are rare (Figure 11-7). In addition, if calcifications are present, they are generally microcalcifications rather than the large calcification seen in the test patient.

When calcifications are present within a cyst (Option (B)), they can be within the wall, producing a circumferential or "eggshell" calcification, or they can settle within the dependent portion of the cyst, producing "teacup" or meniscus-shaped calcifications on horizontal-beam

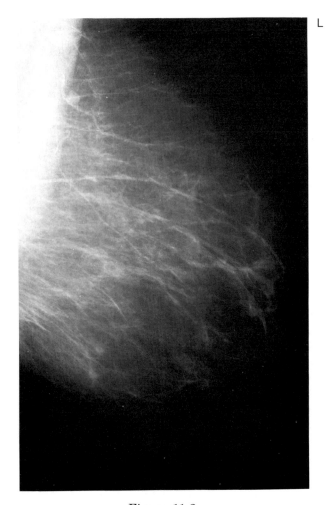

L

Figure 11-2

radiographs and rounded smudgelike densities on vertical-beam (CC projection) radiographs (Figure 11-8). A single coarse calcification would not be seen in a cyst.

Hamartomas (Option (C)) and lymph nodes (Option (E)) are mixed-density circumscribed lesions that contain fat, indicating that they are benign. Calcification in these two lesions is very uncommon.

R

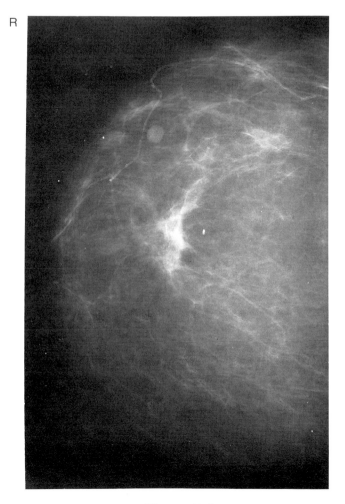

Figure 11-3

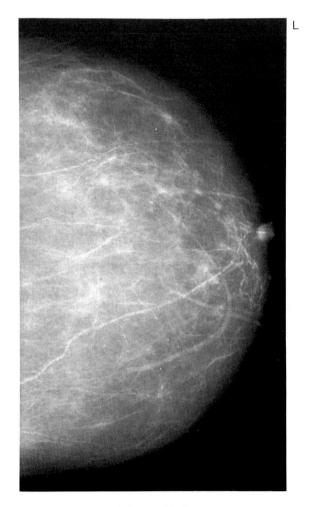

Figure 11-4

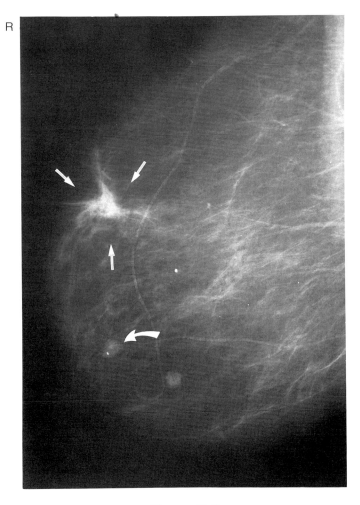

Figure 11-5

Figures 11-5 and 11-6 (Same as Figures 11-1 and 11-3, respectively). Circumscribed and spiculated masses in the right breast on MLO (Figure 11-5) and CC (Figure 11-6) mammograms. In the right lower outer quadrant, there is a 1-cm circumscribed mass (curved arrow) containing a single coarse calcification, typical of a calcified involuting fibroadenoma. In the upper central portion of the right breast, there is a 3-cm spiculated mass containing internal lucency (straight arrows), corresponding to the palpable mass. At biopsy, this was found to be invasive ductal carcinoma. The 8-mm circumscribed noncalcified nodule in the right lower outer quadrant appears to contain fat on the MLO view and most probably represents an intramammary lymph node.

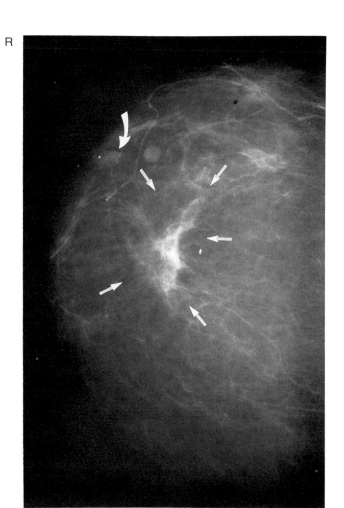

Figure 11-6

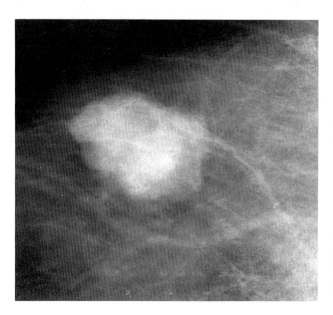

Figure 11-7 (left).
Medullary carci-
noma. Right CC
mammogram
demonstrating a
completely well-
defined 2.0-cm
mass. In this
case, the lesion is
macrolobulated.
There are no cal-
cifications within
the tumor.

132

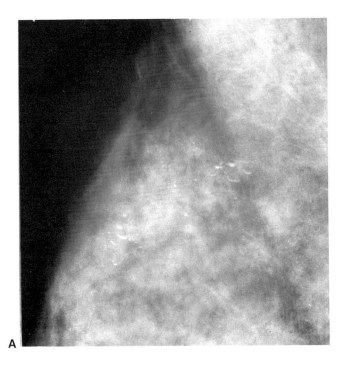

A

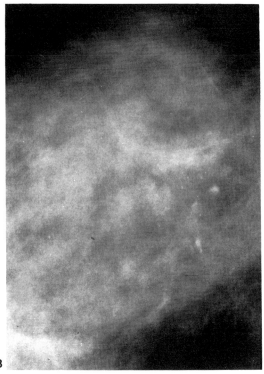

B

Figure 11-8. "Teacup" (semilunar) and meniscus-shaped calcifications from milk of calcium in tiny cysts. Magnification 90° mediolateral (A) and CC (B) mammograms show the characteristic change in the configuration of the calcifications. On the horizontal-beam mediolateral film (A), the milk-of-calcium forms layers in the dependent portion of the cysts, whereas on the vertical-beam film (B), the calcification takes on a rounded, smudgy, or amorphous appearance. The smallest pools of milk of calcium are not dense enough to visualize on the CC view.

Question 51

The single MOST important abnormality is:

(A) the 1-cm smooth mass, containing a single coarse calcification, in the lower outer right breast
(B) the 8-mm smooth noncalcified nodule in the lower outer right breast
(C) the ill-defined 3-cm asymmetric density with internal lucency in the upper central right breast
(D) the 2-mm calcification in the central right breast, 7 cm deep to the nipple

All but one of the mammographic findings in the test patient are either clearly or probably benign, including the calcified involuting fibro-adenoma (Option (A)); the 8-mm smooth nodule in the lower outer right breast (Option (B)), which likely is an intramammary lymph node, non-calcified fibroadenoma, or cyst; and the large calcification in the central right breast (Option (D)). The most important abnormality is the 3-cm asymmetric density in the upper central right breast (straight arrows, Figures 11-5 and 11-6) **(Option (C) is correct).** Recognizing this density is facilitated by comparison of the images of the right breast (Figures 11-1 and 11-3) with those of the normal left breast (Figures 11-2 and 11-4). This lesion corresponded to the woman's palpable abnormality. The differential diagnosis for this lesion based on its mammographic features includes asymmetric fibroglandular tissue, postsurgical or posttraumatic scar, carcinoma, and radial scar. The patient has no history of trauma or surgery; therefore, postsurgical or posttraumatic scar is not a serious consideration. This lesion has considerable architectural distortion, excluding the diagnosis of asymmetric fibroglandular tissue. Therefore, the most reasonable etiologies are invasive ductal carcinoma (IDC), invasive lobular carcinoma, and radial scar.

Question 52

The NEXT step should be:

(A) routine screening mammography in 1 year
(B) follow-up mammography in 6 months
(C) ultrasonography
(D) biopsy

The possibility that one of the abnormalities is malignant means that the proper next step is biopsy **(Option (D) is correct).** Routine screening mammography (Option (A)) would be indicated only for a normal or clearly benign finding. Follow-up mammography in 6 months

(Option (B)) should be recommended only for a "probably-benign" finding (see Case 7). Ultrasonography (Option (C)) is used to determine whether a circumscribed mass is cystic or solid. The spiculated opacity in the test images cannot be a simple cyst, and therefore ultrasonography has no role.

Question 53

Concerning spiculated lesions,

- (A) they most probably represent invasive lobular carcinoma
- (B) radial scar cannot be reliably differentiated from carcinoma by mammography
- (C) radial scar cannot be reliably differentiated from carcinoma by physical examination
- (D) postsurgical scar can be identical in appearance to breast carcinoma on mammography
- (E) ultrasonography reliably differentiates between asymmetric glandular tissue and breast carcinoma

Several processes produce spiculated breast masses. The differential diagnosis includes invasive carcinoma, postsurgical or posttraumatic scar, radial scar, and uncommon lesions such as granular cell myoblastoma and extra-abdominal desmoid. The mammographic features of these lesions are frequently similar, although correlation with the clinical history and physical examination can be helpful in determining the etiology.

Invasive lobular carcinoma is often very difficult to identify by mammography because the tumor cells tend to permeate normal breast tissue, producing little or no visible mass effect, architectural distortion, or microcalcification. Thus, a central tumor density is usually not seen and the lesion, when visible, is often an ill-defined area of asymmetric density with internal lucencies (Figure 11-9). Eventually, as the tumor grows to a considerable size, it develops spiculated margins and becomes mammographically suspicious for malignancy. However, invasive lobular carcinoma is much less common than IDC, which frequently presents as a spiculated mass **(Option (A) is false).** Occasionally, IDC contains internal lucency, as in the test patient (Figures 11-5 and 11-6).

Radial scar is a benign area of sclerosis and elastosis within the breast. It is not related to prior surgery or trauma; indeed, its cause is unknown. The mammographic appearance is that of a spiculated mass or area of architectural distortion that usually contains central lucency, as shown in Figure 11-10. However, radial scars can appear solid centrally

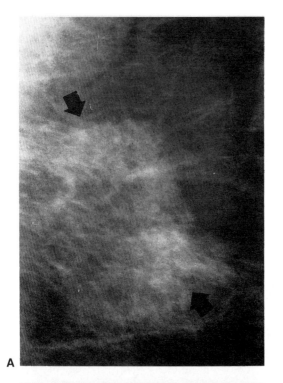

A

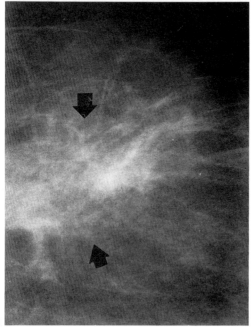

B

Figure 11-9. Invasive lobular carcinoma. Left MLO (A) and CC (B) mammograms show an ill-defined area of architectural distortion (arrows) with internal lucencies. This density was asymmetric (right mammograms are not shown).

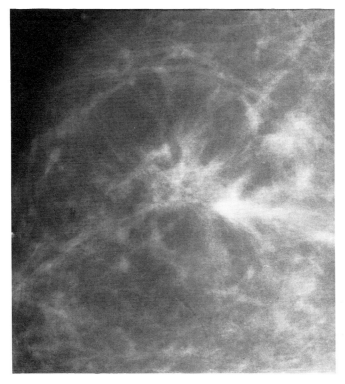

Figure 11-10. Radial scar. Mammogram shows a nonpalpable 4-cm spiculated mass containing central lucencies, very similar in appearance to the IDC in Figures 11-1 and 11-5.

and occasionally contain microcalcifications. The overlap in the mammographic appearances of carcinoma and radial scar means that it is not possible to differentiate these two lesions reliably without biopsy **(Option (B) is true).** Radial scars usually are not palpable, but the lack of a clinically palpable abnormality does not exclude a malignant lesion, which is also frequently impalpable. Thus, physical examination cannot reliably differentiate between carcinoma and radial scar **(Option (C) is true).** However, in the test patient, the presence of a corresponding palpable mass makes radial scar unlikely. Biopsy of a lesion subsequently determined histologically to be a radial scar should not be considered inappropriate, especially because some pathologists believe that this benign lesion is a high-risk marker or a precursor of tubular carcinoma.

Postsurgical scar frequently presents as a spiculated mass or area of architectural distortion on mammography. Central lucencies are commonly seen within the area of scar. As shown in Figure 11-11, the mammographic appearance is often identical to that of carcinoma **(Option**

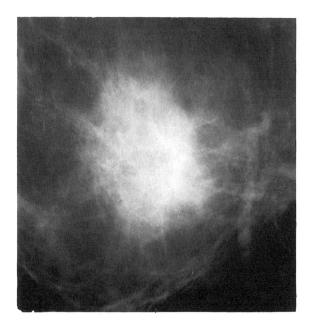

Figure 11-11. Postsurgical scar. Mammogram shows a 3-cm spiculated mass in an area of surgical biopsy performed 6 months earlier. The mammographic appearance of this scar is indistinguishable from that of carcinoma.

(D) is true). The key to correct diagnosis is a history of surgery at the site of the mammographic lesion. However, some surgeons make the skin incision at some distance from the lesion they remove, so that the location of the parenchymal "scar" may not correspond to the location of the skin scar. In these cases, it is very helpful to compare current and previous mammograms. The preoperative and needle localization (if performed) mammograms, including specimen radiographs, should allow determination of the surgical site. If these are not available but postsurgical scar is strongly suspected, a close-interval follow-up mammography examination (usually in 3 to 6 months) can be performed. The scar should remain stable or decrease in size; any enlargement should prompt biopsy.

Asymmetric densities are frequently found at mammography and often represent benign fibroglandular tissue. These findings require careful mammographic evaluation and correlation with physical examination. There should be no palpable abnormality associated with asymmetric fibroglandular tissue. Additional mammographic views, including spot-compression magnification views, may be necessary to evaluate for mass effect, architectural distortion, or microcalcifications. The presence of any of these mammographic findings or the identification of a palpable mass should lead to a suggestion of biopsy. If ultrasonography is performed, asymmetric fibroglandular tissue should not demonstrate cystic mass, solid mass, or architectural distortion. However, ultrasonography has a high false-negative rate for detection of breast cancer, and therefore a negative ultrasonographic examination does not rule out malignancy in an area of asymmetric density **(Option (E) is false).**

Question 54

Concerning medullary carcinoma of the breast,

    (A) it is the most common type of circumscribed carcinoma of the breast
    (B) calcifications are a common mammographic feature
    (C) internal necrosis is frequently found histologically
    (D) posterior shadowing on sonograms is common

Medullary carcinoma is a subtype of IDC that accounts for less than 5% of breast cancers. At mammography, it usually appears as a fairly well-circumscribed mass, frequently with lobulated contours (Figure 11-12). However, IDC "not otherwise specified" (NOS) also sometimes presents as a circumscribed mass. IDC NOS is by far the most common subtype of IDC and is therefore also the most common type of circumscribed carcinoma **(Option (A) is false).** Calcifications are usually not seen in medullary carcinomas **(Option (B) is false),** although these tumors frequently outgrow their blood supply, leading to areas of central necrosis **(Option (C) is true).** At ultrasonography, medullary carcinoma is usually a round, oval, or lobulated circumscribed mass that may be uniformly hypoechoic or contain anechoic areas (regions of necrosis). It frequently demonstrates posterior sonic enhancement because of its uniform cellular composition (Figure 11-13). Posterior shadowing is uncommon **(Option (D) is false).**

Valerie P. Jackson, M.D.

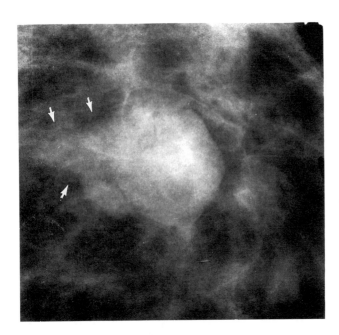

Figure 11-12.
Medullary carci-
noma. Mammo-
gram shows a 1.5-
cm lobulated cir-
cumscribed mass
with indistinct pos-
terior borders (ar-
rows).

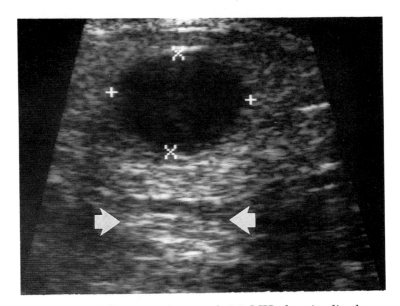

Figure 11-13. Medullary carcinoma. A 7.5-MHz longitudinal sonogram
of an oval circumscribed hypoechoic mass (calipers) is shown. There is
posterior acoustic enhancement (arrows). If the gain were not set appropriately, the low-level internal echoes would not be visible and the lesion
might be mistaken for a cyst. Histologically, the anechoic area at the
inferior aspect of the mass was an area of necrosis.

SUGGESTED READINGS

EVALUATION OF BREAST MASSES

1. Feig SA. Breast masses. Mammographic and sonographic evaluation. Radiol Clin North Am 1992; 30:67–92
2. Kopans DB. Breast imaging. Philadelphia: JB Lippincott; 1989:64–81
3. Sickles EA. Breast masses: mammographic evaluation. Radiology 1989; 173:297–303

ASYMMETRIC DENSITY

4. Kopans DB, Swann CA, White G, et al. Asymmetric breast tissue. Radiology 1989; 171:639–643

MEDULLARY CARCINOMA

5. Kopans DB, Rubens J. Medullary carcinoma of the breast (letter). Radiology 1989; 171:876
6. Meyer JE, Amin E, Lindfors KK, Lipman JC, Stomper PC, Genest D. Medullary carcinoma of the breast: mammographic and US appearance. Radiology 1989; 170:79–82

RADIAL SCAR

7. Adler DD, Helvie MA, Oberman HA, Ikeda DM, Bhan AO. Radial sclerosing lesion of the breast: mammographic features. Radiology 1990; 176:737–740
8. Ciatto S, Morrone D, Catarzi S, et al. Radial scars of the breast: review of 38 consecutive mammographic diagnoses. Radiology 1993; 187:757–760
9. Fisher ER, Palekar AS, Kotwal N, Lipana N. A nonencapsulated sclerosing lesion of the breast. Am J Clin Pathol 1979; 71:240–246
10. Linell F, Ljungberg O, Andersson I. Breast carcinoma. Aspects of early stages, progression and related problems. Acta Pathol Microbiol Scand Suppl 1980; 272:1–233
11. Mitnick JS, Vazquez MF, Harris MN, Roses DF. Differentiation of radial scar from scirrhous carcinoma of the breast: mammographic-pathologic correlation. Radiology 1989; 173:697–700
12. Orel SG, Evers K, Yeh I-T, Troupin RH. Radial scar with microcalcifications: radiologic-pathologic correlation. Radiology 1992; 183:479–482
13. Price JL, Thomas BA, Gibbs NM. The mammographic features of infiltrating epitheliosis. Clin Radiol 1983; 34:433–435

POSTSURGICAL SCAR

14. Sickles EA, Herzog KA. Intramammary scar tissue: a mimic of the mammographic appearance of carcinoma. AJR 1980; 135:349–352
15. Sickles EA, Herzog KA. Mammography of the postsurgical breast. AJR 1981; 136:585–588
16. Stigers KB, King JG, Davey DD, Stelling CB. Abnormalities of the breast caused by biopsy: spectrum of mammographic findings. AJR 1991; 156:287–291

HAMARTOMA

17. Crothers JG, Butler NF, Fortt RW, Gravelle IH. Fibroadenolipoma of the breast. Br J Radiol 1985; 58:191–202
18. D'Orsi CJ, Feldhaus L, Sonnenfeld M. Unusual lesions of the breast. Radiol Clin North Am 1983; 21:67–80
19. Helvie MA, Adler DD, Rebner M, Oberman HA. Breast hamartomas: variable mammographic appearance. Radiology 1989; 170:417–421

INVASIVE LOBULAR CARCINOMA

20. Hilleren DJ, Andersson IT, Lindholm K, Linnell FS. Invasive lobular carcinoma: mammographic findings in a 10-year experience. Radiology 1991; 178:149–154
21. Mendelson EB, Harris KM, Doshi N, Tobon H. Infiltrating lobular carcinoma: mammographic patterns with pathologic correlation. AJR 1989; 153:265–271
22. Sickles EA. The subtle and atypical mammographic features of invasive lobular carcinoma. Radiology 1991; 178:25–26

CALCIFICATION IN CYSTS

23. Linden SS, Sickles EA. Sedimented calcium in benign breast cysts: the full spectrum of mammographic presentations. AJR 1989; 152:967–971
24. Sickles EA, Abele JS. Milk of calcium within tiny benign breast cysts. Radiology 1981; 141:655–658

Notes

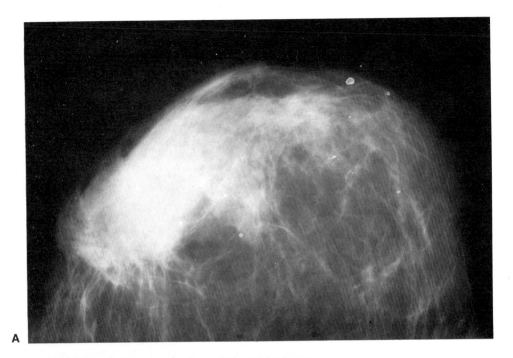

A

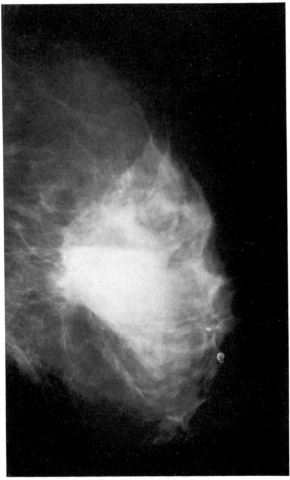

B

Figure 12-1. This 55-year-old woman has a palpable mass at 3 o'clock in the outer left breast. You are shown CC (A) and 90° lateral (B) views from her mammography examination.

144

Case 12: Fat-Containing Mass

Question 55

Which *one* of the following is the MOST likely diagnosis?

(A) Galactocele
(B) Hamartoma
(C) Hematoma
(D) Fat necrosis
(E) Sarcoma

The CC mammogram (Figure 12-1A) demonstrates a large, ill-defined density in the outer aspect of the left breast that correlates with the palpable mass (Figure 12-2A, arrows). The 90° lateral view (Figure 12-1B) demonstrates evidence of a fluid level within this mass (Figure 12-2B, arrows). There are also large benign-appearing calcifications scattered throughout the breast. Based on this appearance, hematoma is the most likely diagnosis **(Option (C) is correct).**

Hematoma of the breast can present as an ill-defined mass on mammography. The margins of the mass are sometimes obscured by surrounding soft tissue edema. As the hematoma starts to resolve, its contents liquefy and a fluid level may be demonstrated (Figures 12-2B and 12-3). On clinical inspection there may be bruising of the skin over the mass. The patient often has a history of trauma, such as a blow to the breast or recent surgery (which was the case in the test patient). A history of trauma is helpful in making this diagnosis, but the patient may not always recall the incident that resulted in hematoma formation. Likewise, a history of trauma can be serendipitous and should not lead one to rule out the possibility of cancer. Follow-up mammography at 6-month intervals for up to 2 years may be indicated to confirm resolution or stabilization of the hematoma.

A galactocele (Option (A)) commonly presents as a well-defined, mixed-density (both fat and fibroglandular density) mass in a young, lactating woman. The test patient is 55 years old and therefore does not fall into this category. A galactocele occasionally demonstrates a fluid level,

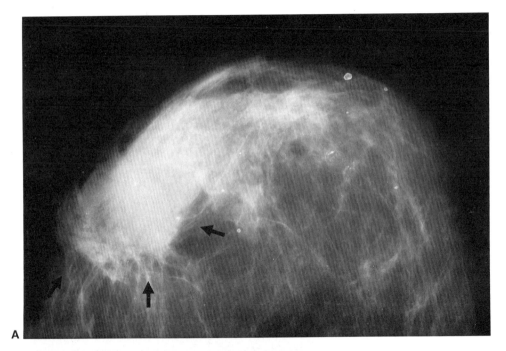

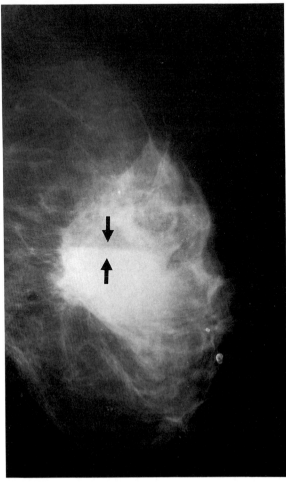

Figure 12-2 (Same as Figure 12-1).   Hematoma with fluid level. (A) A CC mammogram shows an ill-defined density in the outer portion of the left breast correlating with the palpable mass (arrows). (B) A 90° lateral mammogram demonstrates a fluid level in the palpable mass (arrows).

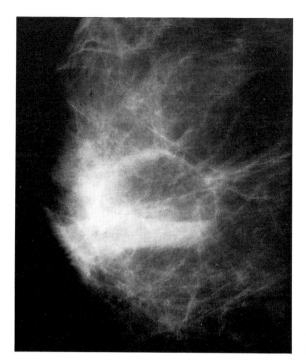

Figure 12-3. Hematoma. A 90° lateral spot-compression magnification mammogram demonstrates a fluid level.

but this is rare. Likewise, a hamartoma (also known as a fibroadenolipoma) of the breast (Option (B)) is a well-defined, mixed-density mass typically found in younger women. Mammography often shows hamartomas to be encased by a pseudocapsule, but they do not contain a fluid level on the 90° lateral view.

Fat necrosis (Option (D)) can be a sequela of trauma to the breast. The mammographic changes are not usually preceded by hematoma formation. Fat necrosis is discussed in more detail subsequently. The finding of an ill-defined mass with a fluid level is unlikely to represent fat necrosis; the mammographic presentation of the test patient is more consistent with hematoma.

Sarcoma of the breast (Option (E)) is a rare condition, accounting for fewer than 1% of breast neoplasms. It is a solid tumor and would not demonstrate a fluid level unless prior surgical intervention had taken place, with resultant hematoma formation. Sarcomas are also usually well defined. Differentiated sarcomas of the breast include hemangiosarcoma, malignant fibrous histiocytoma, liposarcoma, and lymphosarcoma. Undifferentiated types such as spindle cell, round cell, and polymorphous cell sarcoma have also been observed.

Question 56

Hamartomas of the breast:

    (A) have malignant potential
    (B) are characteristically firm on palpation
    (C) often result in asymmetric breast size
    (D) contain lobular and ductal epithelium
    (E) are occasionally anechoic on ultrasonography

Hamartomas of the breast are similar to hamartomas found elsewhere in the body in that they contain tissue elements normally found in the organ of origin. Therefore, the same fibrous, glandular, and fatty tissues normally found in the breast are present in hamartomas but are arranged in a disorganized fashion. Hamartomas are well defined on mammography because of the presence of a thin pseudocapsule. Typically, they have a mixed internal density, containing regions of both fat and fibroglandular density. Occasionally they display internal septations (Figure 12-4).

Hamartomas are invariably benign and do not have malignant potential **(Option (A) is false).** A characteristic appearance on mammography makes biopsy for confirmation unnecessary in most cases. However, not all hamartomas demonstrate a classic benign appearance, and in these cases biopsy is necessary to confirm the diagnosis. Hamartomas are often not discovered until the baseline mammography examination. They contain the same tissues as the surrounding breast parenchyma; therefore, it is common for them to be nonpalpable **(Option (B) is false).** However, when palpable, they are usually soft. Often hamartomas grow large, resulting in asymmetry in breast size **(Option (C) is true).** This may warrant removal for cosmetic reasons.

The breast contains both lobular and ductal epithelium, and therefore so do breast hamartomas **(Option (D) is true).** The haphazard arrangement of the different tissue elements within a hamartoma results in multiple acoustic interfaces. These interfaces cause low-level echoes within the mass during ultrasonography **(Option (E) is false).** The typical ultrasonographic appearance of a hamartoma is that of a well-defined hypoechoic mass without enhancement (Figure 12-5).

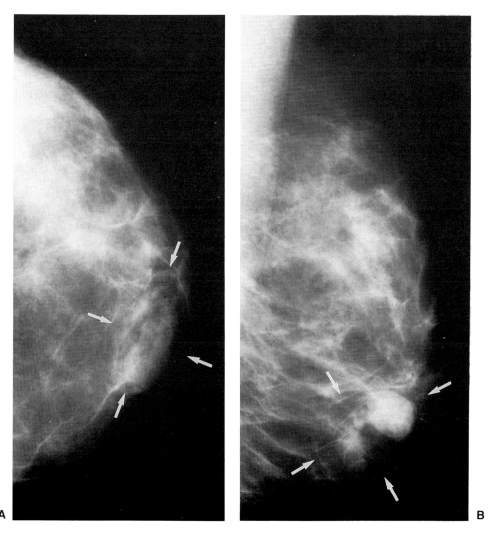

A

B

Figure 12-4. Hamartoma. CC (A) and MLO (B) mammograms show a well-defined mixed-density mass (arrows) in the lower inner quadrant of the left breast. Note the fatty and fibroglandular components of the mass. These findings are consistent with breast hamartoma. This mass was stable over a number of years.

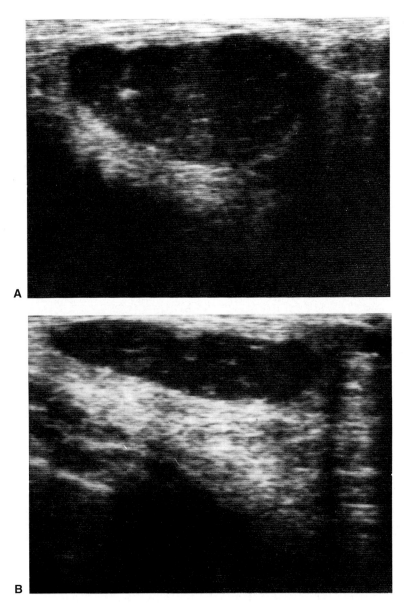

Figure 12-5. Hamartoma. Transverse (A) and longitudinal (B) sonograms demonstrate a hypoechoic mass with low-level internal echoes. This is the typical ultrasonographic appearance of a hamartoma.

Question 57

Concerning fat necrosis,

    (A) calcifications are linear and branching
    (B) history of a surgical biopsy is usually present
    (C) oil cysts are a mammographic manifestation
    (D) biopsy is usually necessary for confirmation of diagnosis
    (E) parenchymal distortion is occasionally an associated finding

According to Haagensen, fat necrosis is secondary to trauma. When fat necrosis first develops, an affected patient can present with overlying ecchymosis, erythema, or a superficial palpable mass. On pathologic specimens, there is usually hemorrhage within an indurated area of fat. The fat cells may have been injured by crushing or may have become ischemic and necrotic from hemorrhage. After 3 or 4 weeks, a rounded firm mass with a fibrous shell develops, containing liquefied fat or necrotic debris. The walls of the mass can calcify. This mass usually regresses and is replaced by fibrosis. The residual calcifications can present mammographically as coarse, nonlinear, irregular calcific particles that are usually larger than those associated with breast carcinoma **(Option (A) is false).**

The antecedent trauma can be surgical, and fat necrosis can therefore be found adjacent to scar tissue from a previous biopsy or from breast reduction or breast conservation procedures (Figure 12-6). However, most patients with fat necrosis cannot recall a history of trauma (surgical or otherwise), and the findings of fat necrosis are simply detected during routine mammography **(Option (B) is false).**

A very characteristic mammographic feature of fat necrosis is oil cyst formation **(Option (C) is true)** (Figure 12-7). Oil cysts are round or oval, encapsulated, radiolucent lesions that contain liquefied fat. As with other fat-containing masses in the breast, they are benign. The liquefied fat can be extremely viscous, and therefore aspiration can be unsuccessful, if attempted. Neither aspiration nor biopsy is necessary, however, since the characteristic mammographic appearance of the oil cyst is usually diagnostic **(Option (D) is false).**

Because fat necrosis is usually secondary to trauma, other findings associated with trauma are often seen in its presence. These include scarring, skin retraction, and skin thickening. Parenchymal distortion is also sometimes associated with fat necrosis **(Option (E) is true),** and careful evaluation including pertinent history and comparison with prior mammograms may be necessary to rule out a possible malignancy. Spontaneous fat necrosis is occasionally seen in patients with diabetes mellitus and collagen vascular disorders.

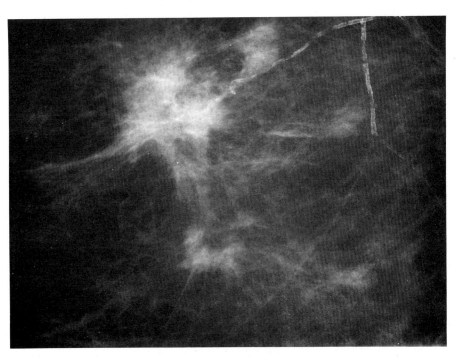

Figure 12-6. Fat necrosis. Spot-compression magnification mammogram of an area of fat necrosis that developed following percutaneous biopsy with a Tru-Cut needle approximately 2 years earlier. Scarring and low-density parenchymal distortion consistent with fat necrosis are present.

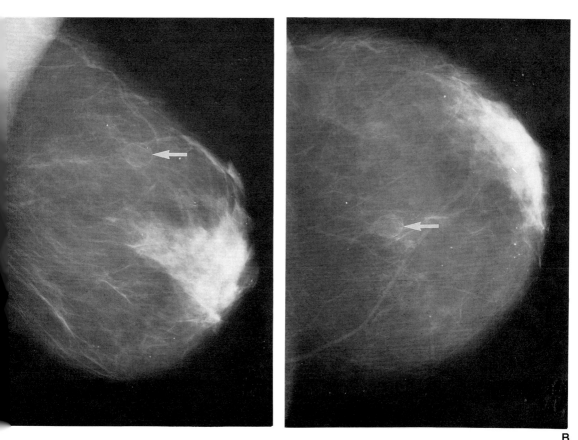

B

Figure 12-7. Fat necrosis. MLO (A) and CC (B) mammograms show an oil cyst (arrow) at a previous biopsy site.

Question 58

Concerning patients undergoing breast conservation therapy,

    (A) mammographic changes stabilize within 1 year
    (B) any new calcifications should be biopsied
    (C) most recurrent carcinomas develop 2 years or more after lumpectomy
    (D) 70% of recurrent carcinomas are detected only by mammography
    (E) a postlumpectomy mammography examination helps exclude residual tumor

Many patients with breast carcinoma who would previously have undergone mastectomy now select breast conservation therapy instead. Local excision (lumpectomy) and radiation therapy are the mainstays of this treatment for women with certain types of breast cancer. Because more and more women are undergoing breast conservation therapy, radiologists should be aware of the associated mammographic changes in the appearance of the breast. These include scarring with parenchymal distortion, fat necrosis, skin thickening, increased breast density secondary to edema, and postoperative hematoma. These changes tend to become less apparent with time, and many stabilize or return to normal, but usually not until 2 years after treatment **(Option (A) is false).** Any new areas of fibroglandular density should be viewed with suspicion and may warrant biopsy. On the other hand, many new calcifications simply represent fat necrosis, and the decision to perform a biopsy should be based on mammographic characteristics. Coarse, irregular calcifications consistent with fat necrosis do not warrant biopsy and should simply be monitored **(Option (B) is false).**

Protocols for mammographic follow-up after breast conservation therapy vary, but most authorities recommend evaluation at 6-month intervals for 2 to 5 years for the treated breast (yearly for the contralateral breast) and then bilateral mammography annually. The mammographic findings in the postlumpectomy breast have usually stabilized after this time; therefore, the development of any new irregular densities or suspicious microcalcifications indicates the need for rebiopsy. Most recurrent carcinomas develop at least 2 years after lumpectomy **(Option (C) is true)** (Figure 12-8). Unfortunately, because of the mammographic changes inherent in the postlumpectomy breast, recurrences may not be detectable by mammography, and most present with palpable findings **(Option (D) is false).** Therefore, close clinical follow-up is important in conjunction with mammography.

Follow-up mammography immediately after lumpectomy is advocated by many authors to help exclude residual tumor, especially when microcalcifications were present **(Option (E) is true).** This additional

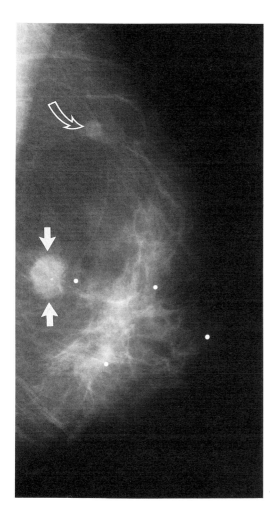

Figure 12-8. Recurrent carcinoma following lump-ectomy. MLO mammogram of the left breast in a patient 3 years after a lumpectomy. A spiculated mass adjacent to the lumpectomy site (solid arrows) was found to represent recurrent carci-noma. A smaller spiculated mass in the upper breast is a satellite lesion and also represents carcinoma (open arrow).

examination can be very helpful, but postoperative edema or hematoma can obscure a residual tumor mass or subtle microcalcifications. Spot-compression magnification mammography of the tumor bed postopera-tively and during routine mammographic follow-up is recommended. If there is any question of residual cancer, reexcision of the tumor bed is indicated.

Tracy L. Roberts, M.D.
Judy M. Destouet, M.D.

SUGGESTED READINGS

MIXED-DENSITY BREAST MASSES

1. Adler DD, Jeffries DO, Helvie MA. Sonographic features of breast hamartomas. J Ultrasound Med 1990; 9:85–90
2. Cole-Beuglet C, Soriano R, Kurtz AB, Meyer JE, Kopans DB, Goldberg BB. Ultrasound, x-ray mammography, and histopathology of cystosarcoma phylloides. Radiology 1983; 146:481–486
3. Haagensen CD. Diseases of the breast, 3rd ed. Philadelphia: WB Saunders; 1986:335–336
4. Helvie MA, Adler DD, Rebner M, Oberman HA. Breast hamartomas: variable mammographic appearance. Radiology 1989; 170:417–421
5. Langham MR Jr, Mills AS, DeMay RM, O'Dowd GJ, Grathwohl MA, Horsley JS III. Malignant fibrous histiocytoma of the breast. A case report and review of the literature. Cancer 1984; 54:558–563
6. Marsteller LP, Shaw de Paredes E. Well defined masses in the breast. RadioGraphics 1989; 9:13–17
7. Salvador R, Salvador M, Jimenez JA, Martinez M, Casas L. Galactocele of the breast: radiologic and ultrasonographic findings. Br J Radiol 1990; 63:140–142
8. Sickles EA. Breast masses: mammographic evaluation. Radiology 1989; 173:297–303
9. Sickles EA, Vogelaar PW. Fluid level in a galactocele seen on lateral projection mammogram with horizontal beam. Breast 1981; 7(2):32–33
10. Stigers KB, King JG, Davey DD, Stelling CB. Abnormalities of the breast caused by biopsy: spectrum of mammographic findings. AJR 1991; 156:287–291

FAT NECROSIS

11. Bassett LW, Gold RH, Cove HC. Mammographic spectrum of traumatic fat necrosis: the fallibility of "pathognomonic" signs of carcinoma. AJR 1978; 130:119–122
12. Bassett LW, Gold RH, Mirra JM. Nonneoplastic breast calcifications in lipid cysts: development after excision and primary radiation. AJR 1982; 138:335–338
13. Destouet JM, Monsees BS. Differential diagnosis of breast lesions on mammography. Curr Imaging 1989; 1:91–99
14. Evers K, Troupin RH. Lipid cyst: classic and atypical appearances. AJR 1991; 157:271–273

BREAST CONSERVATION THERAPY

15. Harris KM, Costa-Greco MA, Baratz AB, Britton CA, Ilkhanipour ZS, Ganott MA. The mammographic features of the postlumpectomy, postirradiation breast. RadioGraphics 1989; 9:253–268
16. Hassell PR, Olivotto IA, Mueller HA, Kingston GW, Basco VE. Early breast cancer: detection of recurrence after conservative surgery and radiation therapy. Radiology 1990; 176:731–735

17. Homer MJ, Schmidt-Ullrich R, Safaii H, et al. Residual breast carcinoma after biopsy: role of mammography in evaluation. Radiology 1989; 170:75–77

18. Libshitz HI, Montague ED, Paulus DD. Calcifications and the therapeutically irradiated breast. AJR 1977; 128:1021–1025

19. Locker AP, Hanley P, Wilson AR, et al. Mammography in the pre-operative assessment and post-operative surveillance of patients treated by excision and radiotherapy for primary breast cancer. Clin Radiol 1990; 41:388–391

20. Peters ME, Fagerholm MI, Scanlan KA, Voegeli DR, Kelcz F. Mammographic evaluation of the postsurgical and irradiated breast. RadioGraphics 1988; 8:873–899

21. Stein MA, Karlan M. Immediate postoperative mammogram for failed surgical excision of breast lesions. Radiology 1991; 178:159–162

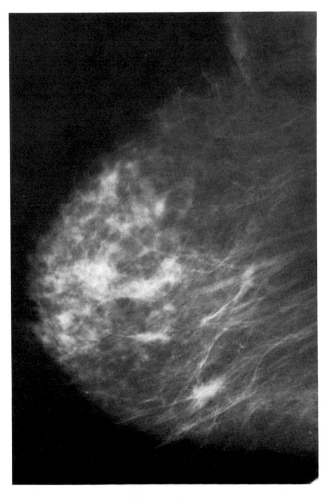

Figure 13-1

Figures 13-1 through 13-4. This 62-year-old asymptomatic woman underwent mammographic screening. She is on estrogen replacement therapy and has a negative family history for breast cancer. You are shown MLO (Figure 13-1) and CC (Figure 13-2) views of the right breast. You are also shown her MLO and CC right-breast mammograms from 2 years earlier (Figures 13-3 and 13-4, respectively).

Case 13: Developing-Density Sign

Question 59

Which *one* of the following BEST characterizes the mammographic findings?

    (A) Probably benign disease, unchanged
    (B) Probably benign disease, changed
    (C) Suspicious for malignant disease, unchanged
    (D) Suspicious for malignant disease, changed

Question 60

An abnormality requiring further evaluation appears in which *one* of the following locations?

    (A) Upper outer quadrant
    (B) Upper inner quadrant
    (C) Lower outer quadrant
    (D) Lower inner quadrant
    (E) Subareolar region

At approximately 7 o'clock in the lower outer quadrant of the right breast, there is a 2-cm spiculated noncalcified opacity (Figures 13-1 and 13-2; arrows in Figures 13-5 and 13-6). The prior study showed some ill-defined density in this region (Figures 13-3 and 13-4; arrows in Figures 13-7 and 13-8), but the degree of radiographic density has increased and the spiculation has appeared in the interval. These features are suspicious for malignancy **(Option (D) is the correct answer for Question 59, and Option (C) is the correct answer for Question 60).**

Mammograms of breasts with a moderate or large amount of fibroglandular density are often difficult to interpret. Comparison with prior mammograms is particularly helpful in these cases to detect subtle changes that may indicate malignancy. First, one must determine whether a developing radiographic density represents normal fibroglan-

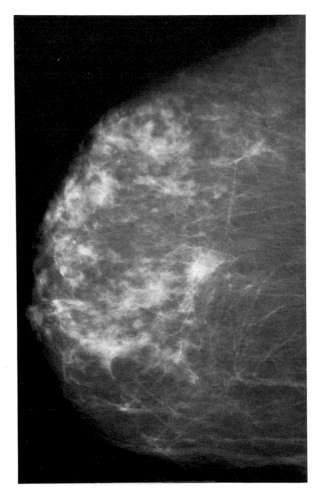

Figure 13-2

dular tissue or a mass. Fibroglandular tissue has scalloped, concave outward borders and frequently changes configuration from view to view. Any area with convex outward borders, spiculations, or architectural distortion must be further investigated to determine whether a mass is present. If a mass is seen, its size, radiographic density, shape, and border characteristics must be assessed to determine the proper work-up and management.

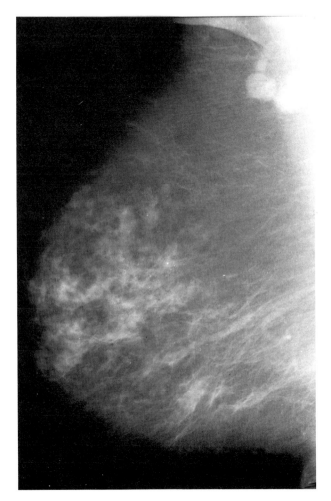

Figure 13-3

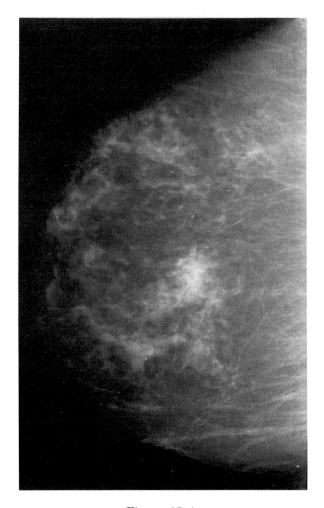

Figure 13-4

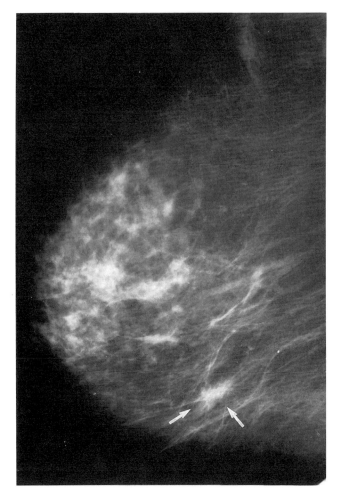

Figure 13-5

Figures 13-5 through 13-8 (Same as Figures 13-1 through 13-4, respectively). Developing density representing invasive ductal carcinoma. The current mammograms show a 2-cm spiculated opacity in the lower outer quadrant of the right breast (arrows in Figures 13-5 and 13-6), which has increased in size and density and has developed spiculation since the mammograms obtained 2 years earlier (arrows in Figures 13-7 and 13-8).

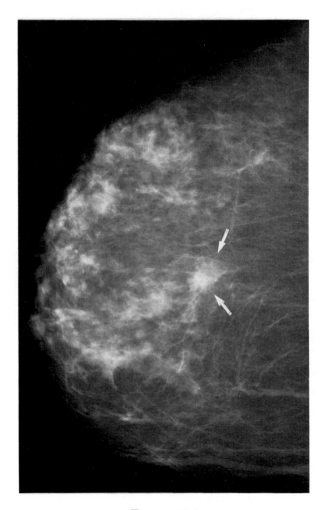

Figure 13-6

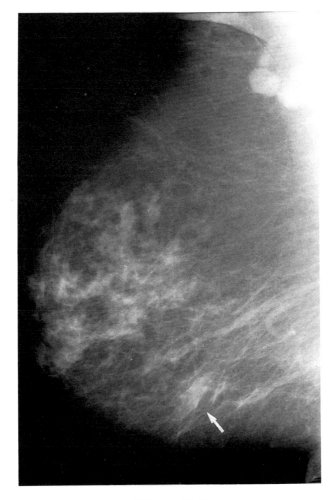

Figure 13-7

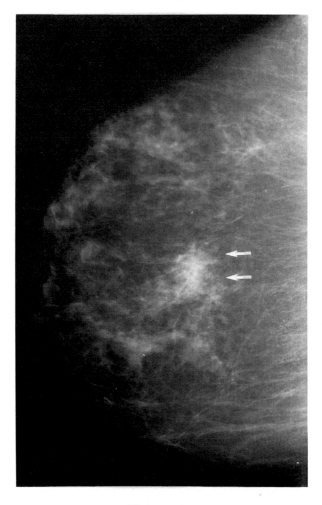

Figure 13-8

Question 61

Appropriate further imaging evaluation of the test patient includes:

(A) 90° lateral view
(B) spot-compression magnification view
(C) "nipple-in-profile" view
(D) ultrasonography

When a mass or microcalcifications are seen on standard mammograms, spot compression combined with magnification is most helpful to

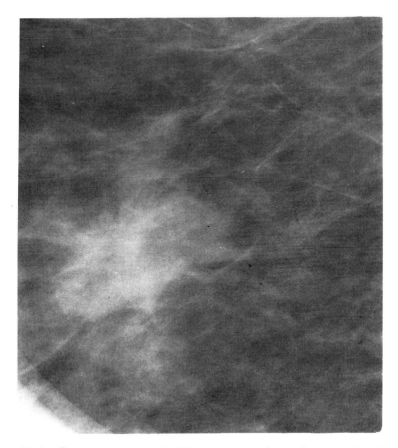

Figure 13-9. Same patient as in Figures 13-1 through 13-8. Developing density representing invasive ductal carcinoma. Spot-compression magnification right CC view confirms the presence of a spiculated mass, which contains two microcalcifications that were not visible on the standard mammograms.

better define the characteristics of the lesion **(Option (B) is true).** Spot compression gives increased compression in a focal area of the breast compared with the use of the standard whole-breast compression paddle. Thus, overlying densities tend to spread apart or shift away, allowing for improved visualization of the lesion. Magnification improves resolution and reduces system noise for better depiction of the borders of masses and shapes of calcific particles. The spot-compression magnification view obtained in CC projection for the test patient (Figure 13-9) shows the spiculated mass more clearly. On this radiograph the mass contains two microcalcifications, which were not visible on the original mammograms.

The 90° lateral view helps to determine the true location of a lesion already identified on CC and MLO projections. The mass in the test patient is lateral to the nipple and has therefore been projected falsely high on the MLO view. See Case 1 for a complete discussion of how to triangulate the location of a lesion by using the oblique view. An additional 90° lateral view would be useful for precise localization in the test patient **(Option (A) is true)**, but it has limited value in further characterization of mammographic features.

A "nipple-in-profile" view is useful for the evaluation of subareolar densities, particularly when there is concern that the nipple is not in profile and that it is the cause of a pseudolesion. The smooth 1-cm nodule seen in a subareolar location on the CC view in the test patient (Figure 13-6) is actually the nipple, which is not in profile. However, the suspicious spiculated mass is in the posterior half of the breast, far from subareolar location, and a nipple-in-profile view would be of no value **(Option (C) is false)**.

The main value of ultrasonography is in determining whether a mass is cystic or solid. A cyst is considered to be in the differential diagnosis of circumscribed masses or masses whose borders are obscured by isodense fibroglandular tissue. When a spiculated mass or area of architectural distortion is present, the lesion cannot be a simple cyst. Therefore, ultrasonography has no role in the test patient **(Option (D) is false)**.

Question 62

Concerning a developing density,

(A) a new density in a premenopausal woman is almost always an indication for biopsy

(B) a new density in a postmenopausal woman is almost always an indication for biopsy

(C) a new 1-cm smooth, noncalcified, nonpalpable mass should be evaluated by ultrasonography

(D) the most frequent cause is trauma to the breast

The most important role of comparison with prior mammograms is the identification of new or changed densities in the breasts. However, any area of mammographic change must be carefully evaluated to determine whether biopsy is indicated. Mammographic changes are common in premenopausal women, whose breasts remain under the cyclic influence of hormones. Thus, it is common to see increases in diffuse or focal areas of fibroglandular tissue, which should maintain the mammographic appearance of benign glandular tissue as described previously. In addition, cysts frequently develop in premenopausal women. Thus, many "neodensities" in premenopausal women will not require biopsy following careful imaging evaluation **(Option (A) is false).** New densities are less common in postmenopausal women and should cause more concern, but many can be shown to be benign by imaging studies and do not require biopsy as well **(Option (B) is false).** Again, any new or increasing opacity should be carefully evaluated by additional mammographic views and, if the lesion is smooth and noncalcified, ultrasonography should be performed to determine whether it is a simple benign cyst **(Option (C) is true).** The differential diagnosis for a new radiographic density includes hematoma from trauma to the breast, but this is less common than hormonal changes in fibroglandular tissue or the development of cysts or carcinoma **(Option (D) is false).**

Question 63

Concerning the effects of estrogen replacement therapy,

   (A) a diffuse increase in fibroglandular density develops in most patients
   (B) breast cysts develop in most patients
   (C) diffuse skin thickening usually develops
   (D) the relative risk of breast cancer is increased approximately threefold

Hormone replacement therapy is relatively common among postmenopausal women. In 17 to 24% of these patients, mammography demonstrates a diffuse or focal increase in fibroglandular density following institution of hormone replacement therapy **(Option (A) is false).** An example is shown in Figures 13-10 and 13-11. Only approximately 6% of treated women develop breast cysts **(Option (B) is false),** and these are often solitary. No other mammographic changes are seen with any frequency. The development of skin thickening suggests breast edema, mastitis, or carcinoma rather than hormonal changes **(Option (C) is false).**

There have been a number of studies evaluating the risk of breast cancer for women on hormone replacement therapy. Results have been conflicting. Hulka reviewed the literature on this subject and found that while some studies showed no effect from hormone replacement, most studies published prior to 1985 showed a small increase in the risk of breast cancer after many years of estrogen use. Recent larger studies of improved design have shown that there is no increase in the risk of breast cancer when analyzing "ever" versus "never" use of estrogens. However, for American women who have been placed on estrogens, there appears to be a slight increase in risk based upon the duration of use; the relative risk is approximately 1.5 after 15 or more years of use. European studies have shown a higher risk after shorter use, but this may be related to different types of estrogen and to the addition of progestins for

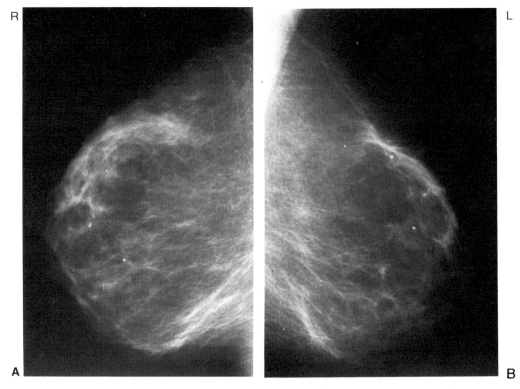

R L

A B

Figure 13-10

Figures 13-10 and 13-11. Benign mammographic changes resulting from hormone replacement therapy. Right MLO (A), left MLO (B), right CC (C), and left CC (D) views from screening mammograms obtained before (Figure 13-10) and 1 year after (Figure 13-11) initiation of hormone replacement therapy. In this case, there is a symmetric increase in fibroglandular density in the upper outer quadrants and retroareolar regions bilaterally.

replacement therapy. Thus, current evidence suggests that hormone replacement therapy has no effect on breast cancer risk or, if there is any increase in the risk, it is small and greatly outweighed by the advantages of preventing heart disease and osteoporosis that are provided by hormone replacement **(Option (D) is false).**

Valerie P. Jackson, M.D.

R

L

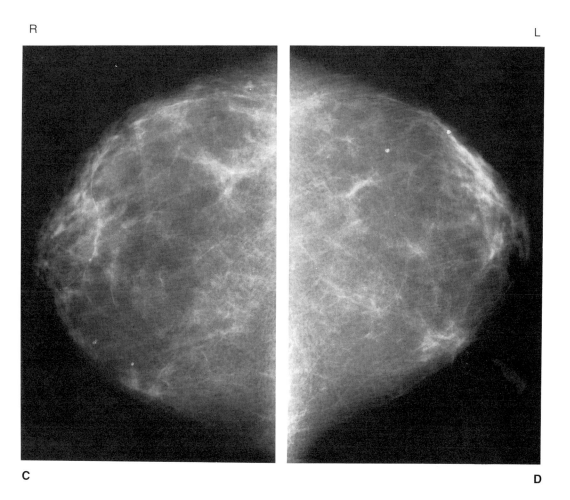

C

D

R

L

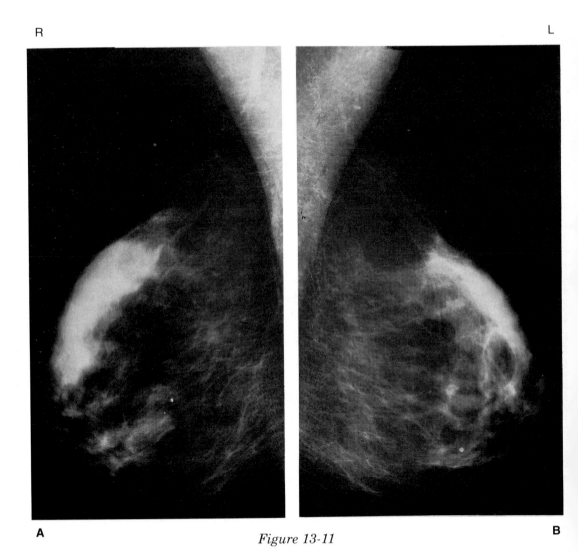

A

B

Figure 13-11

R

L

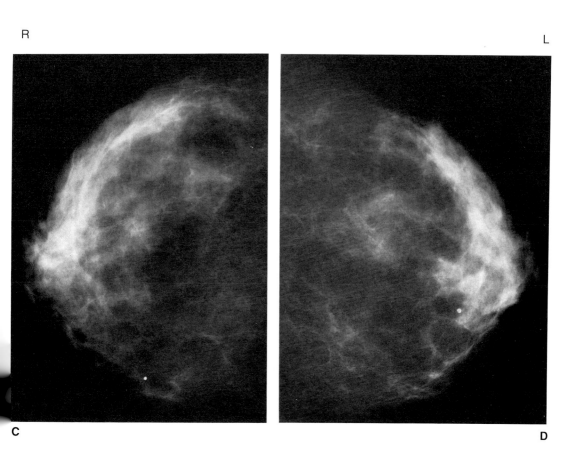

C

D

MAMMOGRAPHIC TECHNIQUE

1. Berkowitz JE, Gatewood OM, Gayler BW. Equivocal mammographic findings: evaluation with spot compression. Radiology 1989; 171:369–371
2. Faulk RM, Sickles EA. Efficacy of spot compression-magnification and tangential views in mammographic evaluation of palpable breast masses. Radiology 1992; 185:87–90
3. Sickles EA. Practical solutions to common mammographic problems: tailoring the examination. AJR 1988; 151:31–39
4. Sickles EA. Combining spot-compression and other special views to maximize mammographic information (letter). Radiology 1989; 173:571

ANALYSIS OF BREAST MASSES

5. Feig SA. Breast masses. Mammographic and sonographic evaluation. Radiol Clin North Am 1992; 30:67–92
6. Kopans DB. Breast imaging. Philadelphia: JB Lippincott; 1989:64–81
7. Sickles EA. Breast masses: mammographic evaluation. Radiology 1989; 173:297–303

INTERVAL BREAST CANCERS

8. Holland R, Mravunac M, Hendriks JH, Bekker BV. So-called interval cancers of the breast. Pathologic and radiologic analysis of sixty-four cases. Cancer 1982; 49:2527–2533
9. Ikeda DM, Andersson I, Wattsgård C, Janzon L, Linell F. Internal carcinomas in the Malmö Mammographic Screening Trial: radiographic appearance and prognostic considerations. AJR 1992; 159:287–294

HORMONE REPLACEMENT THERAPY

10. Bergkvist L, Adami HO, Persson I, Hoover R, Schairer C. The risk of breast cancer after estrogen and estrogen-progestin replacement. N Engl J Med 1989; 321:293–297
11. Berkowitz JE, Gatewood OM, Goldblum LE, Gayler BW. Hormone replacement therapy: mammographic manifestations. Radiology 1990; 174:199–201
12. Brinton LA, Hoover R, Fraumeni JF Jr. Menopausal oestrogens and breast cancer risk: an expanded case-control study. Br J Cancer 1986; 54:825–832
13. Colditz GA, Stampfer MJ, Willett WC, Hennekens CH, Rosner B, Speizer FE. Prospective study of estrogen replacement therapy and risk of breast cancer in postmenopausal women. JAMA 1990; 264:2648–2653
14. Ernster VL, Bush TL, Huggins GR, et al. Benefits and risks of menopausal estrogen and/or progestin hormone use. Prev Med 1988; 17:201–223
15. Hulka BS. Hormone-replacement therapy and the risk of breast cancer. CA—A Cancer Journal for Physicians 1990; 40:289–296

16. Kaufman Z, Garstin WIH, Hayes R, Michell MJ, Baum M. The mammographic parenchymal patterns of women on hormone replacement therapy. Clin Radiol 1991; 43:389–392

17. Kelsey JL, Gammon MD. The epidemiology of breast cancer. CA—A Cancer Journal for Clinicians 1991; 41:146–165

18. Stomper PC, Van Voorhis BJ, Ravnikar VA, Meyer JE. Mammographic changes associated with postmenopausal hormone replacement therapy: a longitudinal study. Radiology 1990; 174:487–490

19. Wingo PA, Layde PM, Lee NC, et al. The risk of breast cancer in postmenopausal women who have used estrogen replacement therapy. JAMA 1987; 257:209–215

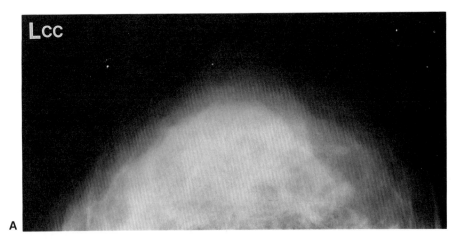

A

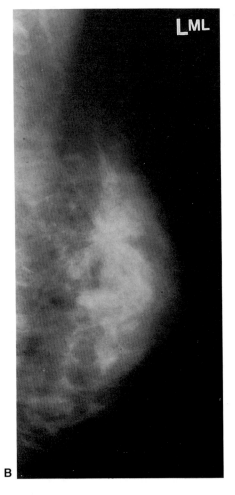

B

Figure 14-1. This 41-year-old woman underwent mammography after a 1-cm firm mobile mass was palpated in her upper outer left breast. You are shown the craniocaudal (A) and 90° lateral (B) views.

Case 14: Palpable Mass Obscured by Dense Fibroglandular Tissue with Mammographically Visible Mass in a Different Location

Question 64

Which *one* of the following BEST describes the mammographic findings with respect to the palpable mass?

    (A) No useful information
    (B) Cystic or solid benign mass
    (C) Probably benign mass
    (D) Mass, suspicious for malignancy
    (E) Mass, highly suspicious for malignancy

The CC and 90° lateral projection mammograms in Figure 14-1 demonstrate a considerable amount of dense fibroglandular tissue throughout the breast. The obvious abnormality is the spiculated mass in the upper inner quadrant of the breast (see Figure 14-2). This lesion is seen on both mammographic projections, is isodense compared with adjacent fibroglandular tissue, and has an irregular contour and spiculated margins. By standard mammographic interpretive criteria, it is highly suspicious for malignancy.

By history, however, there is also a 1-cm firm mobile mass palpable in the same breast, in the upper outer quadrant. No masses or areas of architectural distortion are seen in this region; however, there is an abundance of dense benign-appearing fibroglandular tissue, which could easily obscure a small benign or malignant lesion. Therefore, at this point in the work-up, the mammographic findings in the upper outer quadrant apparently provide no useful information about the palpable mass **(Option (A) is correct)**. It is neither appropriate nor even possi-

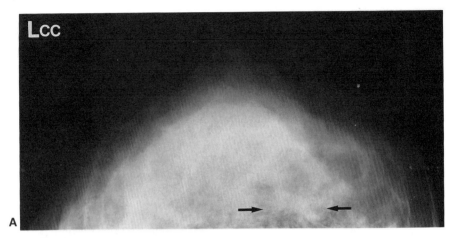

A

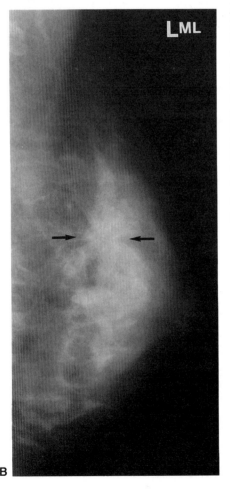

B

Figure 14-2 (Same as Figure 14-1). Palpable mass obscured by dense fibroglandular tissue with a mammographically visible mass in a different location. CC (A) and 90° lateral (B) views demonstrate a spiculated mass in the upper inner quadrant of the left breast (arrows). Physical examination identified a palpable mass in the upper outer quadrant of the same breast, at a site where the mammograms show only dense benign-appearing fibroglandular tissue.

ble to differentiate among benign (Option (B)), probably benign (Option (C)), and malignant (Options (D) and (E)) mammographic interpretations for a mass that is as yet unseen.

Question 65

Further imaging evaluation of the test patient should include:

    (A) review of the CC view to confirm proper placement of the "CC" marker
    (B) shallow oblique (from CC) view
    (C) spot-compression magnification views of the mammographic abnormality
    (D) CC and 90° lateral views with a metallic marker placed over the palpable mass
    (E) spot-compression tangential view of the palpable mass

The potentially confusing situation illustrated in the test images involves the presence of two different lesions, one that is palpable but mammographically occult and one that is detected on the mammograms but is clinically occult. Great care must be taken to verify that there has not been an error either in describing the location of the palpable mass or in the labeling of the films that indicate the location of the mammographic mass. Concerning film labeling, since the two suspect lesions are in the upper inner and upper outer quadrants, only the CC view need be evaluated **(Option (A) is true).** The most reliable error-checking method involves identifying the emulsion (dull, not shiny) side of the film and then mounting the film on a viewbox with the emulsion side facing away from the observer. In this manner, the film is viewed from the vantage point of the X-ray tube (during exposure, the emulsion side of the film faces away from the breast because X-ray photons pass completely through the film before illuminating the intensifying screen). Thus, for a CC view of the left breast that is oriented horizontally, with the base of the breast at the bottom of the image, the "CC" marker should be seen in the upper left corner of the film.

Assuming that it is determined with certainty that the mammographic and palpable masses are located in different quadrants and are therefore different lesions, the radiologist must then consider additional imaging procedures to evaluate each of these lesions.

Shallow oblique views are used to establish or exclude the diagnosis of summation shadow when a finding is seen on only one of the two standard mammographic projections. Consequently, there is no reason to obtain a shallow oblique view in the test patient, since the mammographic mass is seen on both views and the palpable mass is not seen on either view **(Option (B) is false).**

The mammographic mass can be interpreted as being highly suspicious for malignancy on the basis of the two standard views alone; however, there is still good reason to obtain spot-compression magnification views of this lesion as well as of other areas of the ipsilateral breast **(Option (C) is true)**. These additional fine-detail mammograms occasionally demonstrate otherwise unsuspected evidence of more extensive tumor involvement, which can have a major effect on subsequent therapeutic decisions. Usually, this occurs when one or several areas of tiny calcifications are seen only on the magnification views, either extending for a considerable distance from the tumor mass or as non-contiguous multifocal tumor deposits.

Additional mammographic imaging is also helpful in further evaluating the as yet unseen palpable mass. The first step would be to repeat the CC and 90° lateral views with a metallic marker placed over the palpable mass **(Option (D) is true)**. This subject will be discussed fully below in the answer to Question 66.

If the palpable lesion is still not seen despite these marker-guided views, the radiologist should then consider obtaining one final extra exposure, a spot-compression tangential view of the palpable mass **(Option (E) is true)**. This subject will be discussed fully below in the answer to Question 67.

Question 66

Use of a metallic marker for evaluation of a palpable mass:

    (A) requires the mammography technologist to place the marker over the single point on the breast at which the mass is most readily palpable
    (B) often interferes with mammographic interpretation
    (C) indicates whether the palpable mass is included in the mammographic image
    (D) indicates whether the palpable mass and a mammographically identified mass are one and the same

Placement of a metallic marker to evaluate a palpable mass during mammography can aid the radiologist in identifying the mammographic correlate of the palpable lesion. The goal is to have the marker superimposed over the palpable mass on two images, preferably CC and 90° lateral views (Figure 14-3). Implementation of this approach requires the mammography technologist to place the marker separately for each projection, depending on the palpable location of the mass while the breast is being positioned for that exposure. Therefore, the marker is placed over a somewhat different area of the breast for each view, rather than at

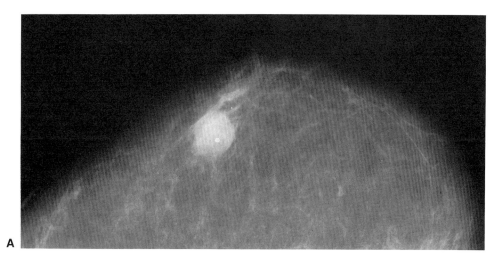

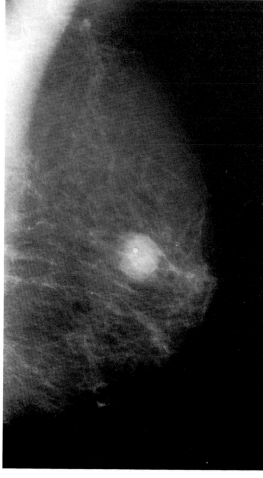

Figure 14-3. Use of metallic markers to indicate the site of a palpable mass at mammography. CC (A) and 90° lateral (B) projection mammograms, with a metallic marker placed overlying a palpable upper outer quadrant left breast mass, demonstrate that the palpable mass corresponds to a 2.4-cm mass seen at mammography (biopsy-proved invasive ductal carcinoma).

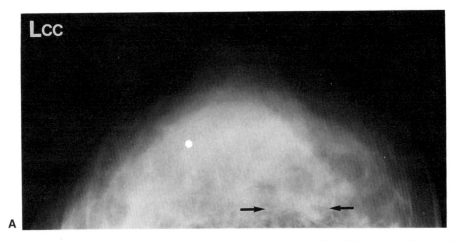

Figure 14-4 (Same as Figures 14-1 and 14-2). Palpable mass obscured by dense fibroglandular tissue with a mammographically visible mass in a different location. CC (A) and 90° lateral (B) views demonstrate that the palpable mass (not seen, but indicated by a metallic marker) indeed is in a different location than the spiculated mammographic mass (arrows). Subsequently, both lesions were removed by excisional biopsy. The palpable mass was a fibroadenoma, and the mammographic mass was an invasive ductal carcinoma.

the single point on the breast at which the mass is most readily palpable **(Option (A) is false)**. In most cases, tiny spherical metallic markers 1.5 mm in diameter are used. These markers are sufficiently large to be readily visible but small enough not to obscure substantial portions of the palpable mass. As a result, a metallic marker will interfere with mammographic interpretation only very rarely, if ever **(Option (B) is false)**.

There are two important reasons to use a metallic marker for evaluation of a palpable mass. First, this approach will confirm that the palpable mass has indeed been included on both images, further directing the radiologist to focus attention on the correct location within the suspect breast quadrant **(Option (C) is true)**. Second, if there is any uncertainty about whether the palpable mass and any visible mammographic mass are truly different lesions, these additional views will convincingly solve the problem by indicating that the metallic marker does or does not overlie the mammographic mass (Figure 14-4) **(Option (D) is true)**.

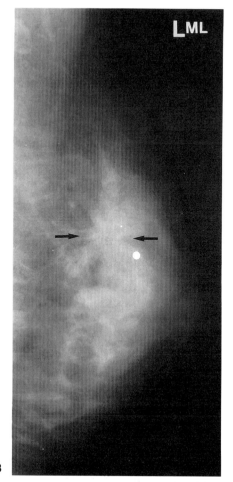

B

Question 67

Appropriate reasons for obtaining a spot-compression tangential view for evaluation of a palpable mass include:

    (A) determining whether the mass is within the skin
    (B) determining whether there is associated skin thickening
    (C) better defining the features of the margins of the mass
    (D) demonstrating a mass not seen on routine views

    A palpable lesion is often superficial, and therefore part of its borders may actually abut the subcutaneous fat; alternatively, the lesion may distort the usually scalloped interface between subcutaneous fat and fibroglandular tissue. In a dense breast, these findings may be visible only if the mass is imaged tangentially, when it is projected as close as possible to the skin surface. When taking such a tangential view, spot-compression magnification mammography should be used to spread apart as much overlying dense fibroglandular tissue as possible. Positioning the breast in the tangential projection is aided by placing a metallic marker directly over the single point on the skin at which the mass is most readily palpable, since that usually indicates the most superficial location of the lesion; the technologist then makes an exposure at the precise degree of obliquity that projects the marker tangentially.

Such a tangential view will indicate whether the palpable mass is or is not within the skin; however, it is unnecessary to use mammography for this differentiation **(Option (A) is false).** Rather, physical examination of a palpable mass is usually sufficient; one simply determines by palpation whether the mass moves along with the skin separately from the underlying parenchymal tissues or whether the skin moves freely over the palpable mass.

However, there are indeed several valid reasons for obtaining a spot-compression tangential projection mammogram of a palpable mass. When the overlying skin is imaged tangentially, a focal area of nonpalpable skin thickening may become evident **(Option (B) is true).** An additional spot-compression tangential view can also more effectively portray the margins of a palpable mass that had been partially obscured on standard views, by projecting these margins adjacent to the subcutaneous fat **(Option (C) is true).** Finally, the spot-compression tangential approach is the sole method of visualizing an otherwise mammographically occult palpable mass in approximately 10% of patients (Figure 14-5) **(Option (D) is true).** Even though this is only a small percentage, the mammographic information obtained from the extra tangential view may be useful in guiding the work-up of the palpable mass.

Edward A. Sickles, M.D.

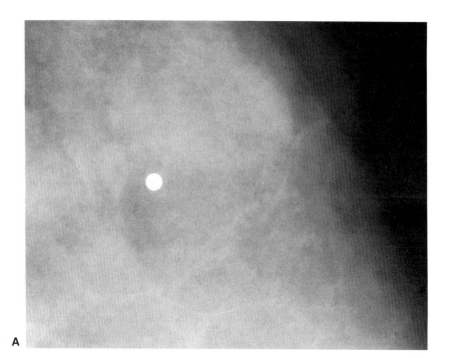

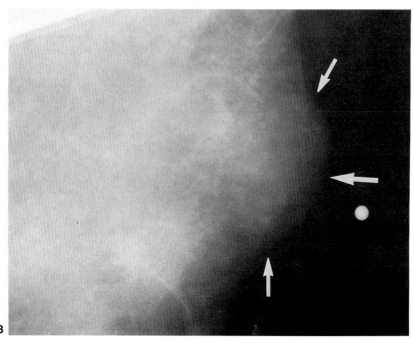

Figure 14-5. Value of tangential view in demonstrating an otherwise obscured palpable mass. This 38-year-old woman had a palpable upper outer quadrant left breast mass that could not be seen on standard projection mammograms. (A) A spot-compression magnification 90° lateral view, taken with a metallic marker placed overlying the palpable mass on that projection, still fails to demonstrate the mass. (B) However, after repositioning the metallic marker at the site where the mass was most readily palpable, a spot-compression magnification mammogram taken tangential to the metallic marker now shows the mass (arrows). It is ovoid in shape, with somewhat indistinct margins. Subsequent biopsy proved the mass to be an invasive ductal carcinoma.

SUGGESTED READINGS

1. Eklund GW. Problem-solving mammography. In: Sickles EA, Kopans DB (eds), Syllabus for the categorical course on breast imaging. Reston, VA: American College of Radiology; 1990:69–75

2. Eklund GW, Cardenosa G. The art of mammographic positioning. Radiol Clin North Am 1992; 30:21–53

3. Faulk RM, Sickles EA. Efficacy of spot compression-magnification and tangential views in the mammographic evaluation of palpable breast masses. Radiology 1992; 185:87–90

4. Homer MJ. Mammographic interpretation: a practical approach. New York: McGraw-Hill; 1991:4–7

5. Kopans DB. Breast imaging. Philadelphia: JB Lippincott; 1989:51–56

6. Logan WW, Janus J. Use of special mammographic views to maximize radiographic information. Radiol Clin North Am 1987; 25:953–959

7. Logan WW, Janus JA. Breast carcinoma: the work-up of the symptomatic patient. In: Diagnostic categorical course in breast imaging. Oak Brook, IL: Radiological Society of North America; 1986:67–70

8. Sickles EA. Practical solutions to common mammographic problems: tailoring the examination. AJR 1988; 151:31–39

9. Sickles EA. Combining spot-compression and other special views to maximize mammographic information (letter). Radiology 1989; 173:571

10. Sickles EA. Tailoring the mammogram: problem solving and special views. In: Thrall JH (ed), Current practice of radiology. Philadelphia: BC Decker/Mosby; 1993:393–402

Notes

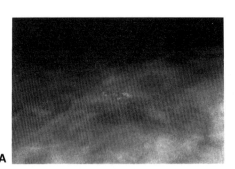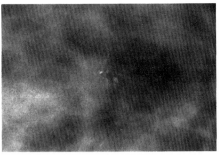

Figure 15-1. This 44-year-old asymptomatic woman with a normal breast physical examination underwent mammographic screening, which revealed an isolated cluster of tiny calcifications. You are shown photographic enlargements from the CC (A) and MLO (B) views.

Case 15: Isolated Cluster of Tiny Calcifications

Question 68

Which *one* of the following is the BEST interpretation of the test images?

(A) Sedimented calcium in tiny benign cysts
(B) Benign skin calcifications
(C) Incompletely evaluated calcifications
(D) Probably benign calcifications
(E) Calcifications suspicious for malignancy

One of the most common abnormalities detected at mammographic screening is an isolated cluster of tiny calcifications. Initial evaluation involves identifying the calcifications on both standard mammographic projections at a similar depth from the nipple and in a location on the MLO view that is consistent with the observed location on the CC view (see the discussion of internal consistency checks in Case 1, Question 3). This will verify that the calcifications truly are very close to each other rather than fortuitously being superimposed on only one view. Demonstration of grouped calcifications on two different projections also excludes the possibility that the tiny particles represent artifactual shadows produced by dust or dirt on the film or intensifying screen.

In the test patient, a cluster of approximately 15 calcifications is indeed seen on both CC and MLO views (Figure 15-1). In addition, the calcifications are sufficiently tiny (smaller than 0.5 mm) and numerous (at least five particles within a 1-cm^3 volume) to meet the minimum criteria of possible malignancy. However, it would be premature to interpret these calcifications as being suspicious for malignancy, thus effectively mandating an invasive tissue-sampling procedure. First, one should exclude from the differential diagnosis, by using additional mammographic views if necessary, benign types of calcification that may appear as isolated clusters on standard CC and MLO views.

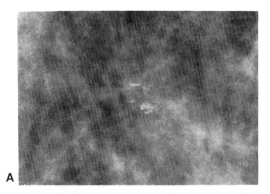

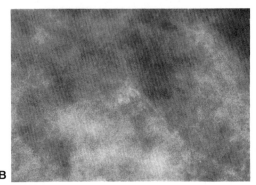

Figure 15-2. Milk of calcium within tiny benign cysts. Spot-compression magnification mammograms in 90° lateral (A) and CC (B) projections, showing a cluster of microcalcifications appearing to sediment to the bottom of small cysts (unseen). On the 90° lateral view, the shapes of the calcific particles resemble teacups, menisci, or thin lines oriented parallel to the horizontal plane, whereas on the CC view they are much less readily apparent and are visible only as ill-defined smudges of calcific density. This highly characteristic difference in calcification shape as seen on 90° lateral and CC projections is diagnostic of milk of calcium within tiny benign cysts.

Figure 15-2

Sedimented calcium within tiny benign cysts (Option (A)) occasionally mimics the clustered microcalcifications associated with breast cancer. Sedimented calcific particles are similar in size to malignant calcifications, and although the sedimented deposits are usually scattered throughout both breasts, they are seen as an isolated cluster in approximately 20% of cases. The vast majority of these calcifications are milk of calcium. This condition characteristically appears as linear, curvilinear, and semilunar particles (with a flat contour at the top) on the 90° lateral view, which is taken with a horizontal X-ray beam directed along the plane of the fluid-calcium levels (Figure 15-2A). An equally typical feature of milk of calcium is the smudgy and indistinct shape of its particles as seen on the CC projection, which is taken with a vertical X-ray beam (Figure 15-2B). Fine-detail views are usually necessary to portray the shapes of clustered microcalcifications with sufficient clarity to permit confident diagnosis of milk of calcium. However, the calcific particles shown on the CC view of the test patient (Figure 15-1A) appear too distinct and well defined to be consistent with this diagnosis. Rarely, dis-

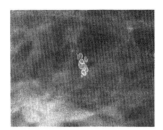

Figure 15-3. Isolated cluster of skin calcifications. Spot-compression magnification mammogram of a cluster of skin calcifications, projected over the breast parenchyma. Most of the calcific particles have radiolucent centers and are round, oval, or polygonal. They are so close to each other that some appear to overlap. This constellation of findings is so typical of benign skin calcifications that an additional tangential view is not needed to verify intradermal location.

crete sandlike calcifications are visualized settling to the bottom of cysts, so that sedimented calcium does remain a remote possibility in the diagnosis of the test patient.

Skin calcification (Option (B)) can present as an isolated cluster of calcific particles, although it is also usually bilateral and widespread. The great majority of clustered skin calcifications are seen to have radiolucent centers, the individual particles being round, oval, or polygonal and often so close together that they appear to be in contact with each other (Figure 15-3). However, a small percentage of dermal calcifications have neither lucent centers nor this very tightly clustered distribution, and they could appear similar to the features in the test images. Therefore, skin calcification must be considered in the differential diagnosis, although it is unlikely.

Other benign types of calcifications rarely mimic those of malignancy. Arterial calcification, when visualized very early in development, may display just a few calcific particles along only one wall of the artery, thereby confounding the correct diagnosis. The zinc or aluminum compounds in skin deodorant, skin powder, or skin ointment also may appear similar to microcalcifications; it is exceedingly unusual for these compounds to be present on only a single patch of skin that is not imaged tangentially, thereby simulating an isolated cluster of parenchymal calcifications.

Certain clustered microcalcifications may also display features that indicate such a low probability of malignancy (less than 1%) that periodic mammographic surveillance is recommended instead of an invasive procedure for the purpose of tissue diagnosis. These "probably benign" calcifications (Option (D)) are discrete round or oval particles of uniform and equal density allowing for differences in size (Figure 15-4). Fine-detail images are usually required to demonstrate characteristic particle shapes. The calcifications shown in the test images, although seen as dis-

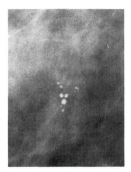

Figure 15-4. Isolated cluster of probably benign calcifications. Spot-compression magnification mammogram of a cluster of tiny calcifications, each of which is round or oval. The densities of the individual calcific particles appear to be similar, allowing for differences in particle size. These mammographic features should prompt a probably benign diagnosis, since the likelihood of malignancy is less than 1%.

crete particles, are not seen clearly enough to permit a probably benign diagnosis.

The best interpretation of the screening examination in the test patient is that the calcifications are incompletely evaluated **(Option (C) is correct).** Additional mammographic views are needed to further assess for sedimented calcium, skin calcifications, other even less likely benign calcifications, and probably benign calcifications. Only if these possibilities had already been excluded from consideration would it be appropriate to interpret the calcifications as being suspicious for malignancy (Option (E)).

Question 69

Which *one* of the following is the MOST appropriate next step?

 (A) Routine mammographic screening in 1 year
 (B) Follow-up mammography in 6 months
 (C) Tangential views
 (D) Spot-compression magnification views
 (E) Preoperative needle localization

Routine mammographic screening in 1 year (Option (A)) would be correct only if a confidently benign interpretation could be made from the two screening views. Similarly, follow-up mammography in 6 months (Option (B)) would be appropriate management if the calcifications were interpreted as probably benign. Preoperative needle localization (Option (E)) would be warranted if the interpretation was suspicious for malignancy. However, as discussed above, the standard CC and MLO views do not portray the clustered microcalcifications with sufficient clarity to support any of these interpretations confidently.

Tangential views (Option (C)) would be useful primarily in assessing for skin calcifications, which is only one of several differential diagnostic possibilities and a relatively unlikely one at that. Tangential views of skin deodorant, powder, or ointment would provide the correct diagnosis; however, these are even less likely, and a more effective imaging approach would be to repeat one of the standard mammographic views after the patient washes the skin of her breast.

The next step in the mammographic work-up should be to obtain spot-compression magnification views in both CC and 90° lateral projections **(Option (D) is correct)**. This will provide useful additional information to evaluate for several of the differential diagnoses, including the two most likely interpretations: probably benign and suspicious for malignancy. Fine-detail images are usually required to establish the diagnoses of sedimented calcium in tiny benign cysts, very early arterial calcification, and probably benign calcifications. They may also be helpful in portraying the radiolucent centers of some skin calcifications. Furthermore, the heterogeneous sizes, densities, and shapes of some malignant microcalcifications can be seen only on spot-compression magnification views.

Question 70

When undertaking further imaging evaluation of an isolated cluster of tiny calcifications, useful information is likely to be provided by:

    (A) tangential projection mammography
    (B) 90° lateral projection mammography
    (C) spot-compression mammography
    (D) magnification mammography
    (E) shallow oblique (from any standard) projection mammography

Additional mammographic projections are often used to further evaluate an isolated cluster of microcalcifications in order to determine the extent and precise location of the lesion and to portray the shapes of its individual calcific particles with greater clarity.

The tangential view is done to project superficially located structures as close as possible to the skin. In the evaluation of clustered calcifications, tangential projection mammography is used whenever it is necessary to establish or exclude the possibility that the calcifications are located within the skin **(Option (A) is true).** This is an important clinical distinction, because dermal calcifications are invariably benign; therefore, no further work-up is needed once calcifications are shown to be intradermal. Most commonly, tangential views are obtained when a cluster of calcifications displays some features of dermal particles but when these features are not sufficiently convincing to confirm the mammographic diagnosis. This subject is discussed in greater detail in Case 16, Question 73.

The use of 90° lateral projection mammography is usually reserved for the nonpalpable cluster of microcalcifications that has already been judged to be suspicious for malignancy, if the cluster has been imaged only on CC and MLO projections. In this circumstance, the additional 90° lateral view permits a description of the three-dimensional location of the calcifications that is more accurate than the estimate derived from the triangulation methods discussed in Case 1, Question 3 **(Option (B) is true).** Another less commonly used but also important role for 90° lateral projection mammography is the demonstration of the fluid-calcium levels within tiny benign cysts that are partially filled with milk of calcium, as discussed above (Figure 15-2A).

Spot-compression mammography improves image quality by more effectively applying compressive force to a small area of interest. This reduces geometric blur (unsharpness) by bringing the lesion closer to the film and minimizes motion blur by better immobilizing the radiographed area and by decreasing exposure time. Therefore, the use of spot-compression mammography as an adjunct to standard imaging can be expected to provide additional useful radiographic information in the evaluation of an isolated cluster of calcifications **(Option (C) is true).**

Direct radiographic magnification also improves the imaging of clustered calcifications, principally by increasing resolution and thereby portraying the number, extent, and shapes of calcific particles with greater clarity **(Option (D) is true).** Large-scale clinical studies have actually validated the use of magnification mammography for this task.

The purpose of the shallow oblique view is to provide a slightly different imaging perspective with which to display an already-detected mammographic finding. There are two major indications for using shallow oblique projection mammography. First, it is often effective in establishing the diagnosis of summation shadow (superimposition of normal structures) when a finding is seen on only one standard mammographic projection; this is discussed more fully in Case 1, Question 4. Second, it may be useful in projecting away from overlying dense fibroglandular tissue the otherwise obscured margins of a breast mass. However, shallow oblique projection mammography has little if any role in the evaluation of an isolated cluster of calcifications, because the distribution of calcific particles is virtually identical on shallow oblique images **(Option (E) is false).**

Question 71

Concerning magnification in mammography,

(A) it is best performed by combining conventional mammographic imaging with the use of a powerful magnifying lens

(B) images demonstrate both increased spatial resolution and reduced system noise

(C) the nominal size of the X-ray focal spot should be ≤0.3 mm

(D) the simultaneous use of spot-compression and magnification techniques usually provides more mammographic information than the use of either technique alone

(E) the use of an oscillating grid usually improves the mammographic image

Magnification mammography has gained widespread acceptance as an adjunct to conventional mammography by virtue of its ability to provide additional radiographic information not available on standard images. Clinical success with magnification mammography requires specialized equipment and a thorough understanding of the principles on which magnification imaging is based.

Optical enlargement of mammograms is an inherent part of standard interpretation procedure, since viewing the image through a magnifying lens makes more readily apparent the smallest visible intramammary structures, such as clustered microcalcifications. However, this procedure enhances perceptibility only by image enlargement, not by improving image quality itself. Truly fine-detail imaging techniques, such as direct radiographic magnification, are needed whenever conventional mammography results in incomplete or indeterminate interpretation. Therefore, magnification is best performed by using direct radiographic magnification rather than optical enlargement of conventional mammograms **(Option (A) is false).**

Laboratory studies demonstrate that direct radiographic magnification improves several of the basic characteristics of the mammographic image. Spatial resolution is increased, as shown by the ability to resolve finer-wire-mesh test objects and by quantitative measurement of modulation transfer functions. System noise is reduced, as indicated by increased visibility of low-contrast test objects and by quantitative measurement of Wiener spectra. The increased resolution and smoother background noise pattern of magnification images permit superior visualization of detail **(Option (B) is true).**

Spatial resolution is improved with radiographic magnification because of the wider distribution of the X-ray input pattern relative to the inherent blur (unsharpness) of the recording system. In addition, because radiographic magnification requires the use of a very small X-ray focal spot, there also is reduced geometric blur. However, if the focal spot is not sufficiently small, the geometric blur of magnification images may actually be greater than that of conventional mammograms, resulting in a substantial degradation of the overall image quality. For a magnification factor of 1.4x, it has been determined in the laboratory that the measured focal spot must be ≤0.3 mm to produce improved resolution; the focal spot must be even smaller for the greater degrees of magnification currently used in most dedicated mammography units. Furthermore, equipment manufacturers specify the *nominal* size of the focal spot, which often is as much as 50% larger than the measured size. Therefore, a nominal focal spot size of ≤0.3 mm is too large for current magnification techniques **(Option (C) is false).** Almost all focal spots now supplied for magnification mammography have a nominal size of 0.1 mm.

The major advantage of magnification technique is its ability to produce enlarged and inherently finer-detail images. Spot-compression technique, on the other hand, improves the mammographic image primarily by providing more effective compression, thereby minimizing motion blur and spreading apart overlapping areas of isodense fibroglandular tissue. Since the operating principles of spot-compression and magnification are different, and since the two techniques do not both require the same limiting resource (e.g., longer exposure time), the simultaneous use of spot-compression and magnification usually produces more mammographic information than the use of either technique alone **(Option (D) is true).** Indeed, spot-compression mammography should almost always be done by using magnification technique, just as magnification mammograms should almost always be taken by using a spot-compression device.

This is illustrated convincingly by comparing the conventional CC projection mammogram of the test patient's clustered microcalcifications (Figure 15-5) with both spot-compression (Figure 15-6) and spot-compression magnification (Figure 15-7) CC projection mammograms. Spot-compression mammography portrays the microcalcifications with slightly increased clarity compared with standard techniques, but the shapes of the individual calcific particles still cannot be resolved; therefore, biopsy would be the next step. Only the combination of spot compression and magnification provides sufficiently fine image detail to demonstrate that the calcifications are all round, permitting the "probably benign" diagnosis that averted biopsy.

Not all combinations of enhanced imaging techniques operate synergistically. Most mammographic exposures are taken with the use of an oscillating grid to increase the ratio of primary to scattered radiation and hence improve image contrast. Magnification technique also increases contrast, by air-gap elimination of scattered radiation. It is reasonable to

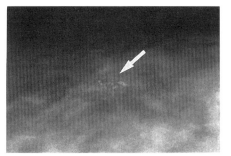

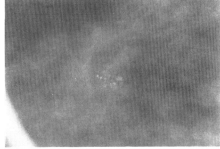

Figure 15-5   *Figure 15-6*

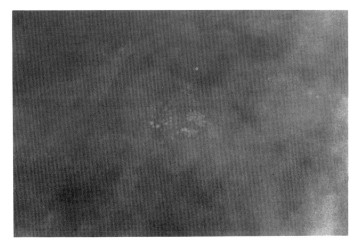

Figure 15-7

Figures 15-5 through 15-7. Value of the combination of spot-compression and magnification techniques in fine-detail mammography. In Figure 15-5 (same as Figure 15-1A), the standard CC view shows the isolated cluster of microcalcifications (arrow) in the test patient. Figure 15-6, a spot-compression view, also in the CC projection, spreads apart the calcifications slightly and indicates the presence of a few more calcific particles but still does not display the shapes of the individual calcifications with sufficient clarity to avert biopsy. However, the spot-compression magnification view in the same projection (Figure 15-7) does provide sufficient image detail to demonstrate that the calcifications are round and regular in shape, thereby leading to a "probably benign" diagnosis. As a result, periodic mammographic follow-up was undertaken instead of biopsy.

assume that the combination of grid enhancement and magnification will result in even more scatter reduction (and therefore even higher image contrast) than either technique alone. However, both grid use and magnification require substantially longer exposures to produce adequate film blackening. As a result, the combination of these techniques frequently requires such a prolonged exposure time that the overall image quality is compromised, either by motion blur or because the film remains underexposed even when the longest permissible exposure is used. Therefore, use of an oscillating grid usually does not improve the magnification mammography image **(Option (E) is false).**

Question 72

Potential explanations for blurring of a magnification mammogram by comparison with a standard image include use of a:

(A) faster screen-film combination
(B) longer X-ray exposure
(C) higher kVp
(D) 0.1-mm focal spot
(E) 2x magnification tray

As noted in the preceding discussion, to produce proper film blackening, magnification technique requires much longer exposures than those used for standard mammography. As a result, a major reason for blurring of magnification mammograms is motion of the breast during exposure. Moreover, any change in technique that further prolongs X-ray exposure can be expected to increase the chance of breast motion and therefore to contribute substantially to blurring of the magnification image **(Option (B) is true).** However, use of a faster screen-film combination has the potential to correct this problem, by permitting shortened exposure times, thereby reducing the likelihood of motion blur **(Option (A) is false).** Similarly, use of a higher-kVp technique results in increased penetration of the X-ray beam, which also allows for shorter duration exposures and therefore reduces motion blur **(Option (C) is false).**

The other major cause of blurring of magnification mammograms is geometric unsharpness. The larger the size of the X-ray focal spot, the greater is the likelihood of geometric blur. Focal spots that measure 0.1 mm are sufficiently small to produce sharp images at any degree of magnification up to and including 2x, and even most nominal 0.1-mm focal spots are also adequate, provided that the magnification factor is no greater than 1.7x **(Option (D) is false).** However, among the nominal 0.1-mm focal spots, those that actually measure close to or larger than 0.15 mm routinely produce clinically evident geometric blur when 2x magnification is used **(Option (E) is true).**

Blurring of magnification exposures can completely negate the several imaging advantages of magnification technique, limiting the ability to produce fine-detail images of the breast. As a general rule, if one encounters such blurring only occasionally, the usual cause is breast motion and the proper solution involves the use of increased compression, higher kVp, or a faster screen-film combination. On the other hand, if the magnification mammograms produced by an X-ray unit are always blurry, the underlying problem is usually geometric unsharpness. In this circumstance, reducing the magnification factor to 1.5x is a less expensive and longer-lasting solution than replacing the X-ray tube with one that has a smaller measured focal spot size.

Edward A. Sickles, M.D.

SUGGESTED READINGS

MAMMOGRAPHIC ANALYSIS OF BREAST CALCIFICATIONS

1. Bassett LW. Mammographic analysis of calcifications. Radiol Clin North Am 1992; 30:93–105
2. Homer MJ. Mammographic interpretation: a practical approach. New York: McGraw-Hill; 1991:34–47
3. Ikeda DM. Mammographic analysis of breast calcifications. In: Sickles EA, Kopans DB (eds), Syllabus for the categorical course on breast imaging. Reston, VA: American College of Radiology; 1990:47–55
4. Kopans DB. Breast imaging. Philadelphia: JB Lippincott; 1989:86–96
5. Lanyi M. Diagnosis and differential diagnosis of breast calcifications. Berlin: Springer-Verlag; 1986
6. Sickles EA. Breast calcifications: mammographic evaluation. Radiology 1986; 160:289–293

SEDIMENTED CALCIUM IN TINY BENIGN CYSTS

7. Homer MJ, Cooper AG, Pile-Spellman ER. Milk of calcium in breast microcysts: manifestation as a solitary focal disease. AJR 1988; 150:789–790
8. Lanyi M. Differentialdiagnose der Mikroverkalkungen. Die verkalkte mastopathische Mikrocyste. Radiologe 1977; 17:217–218
9. Linden SS, Sickles EA. Sedimented calcium in benign breast cysts: the full spectrum of mammographic presentations. AJR 1989; 152:967–971
10. Pennes DR, Rebner M. Layering granular calcifications in macroscopic breast cysts. Breast Dis 1988; 1:109–112
11. Sickles EA, Abele JS. Milk of calcium within tiny benign breast cysts. Radiology 1981; 141:655–658

SKIN CALCIFICATIONS

12. Berkowitz JE, Gatewood OM, Donovan GB, Gayler BW. Dermal breast calcifications: localization with template-guided placement of skin marker. Radiology 1987; 163:282
13. Homer MJ, Marchant DJ, Smith TJ. The geographic cluster of microcalcifications of the breast. Surg Gynecol Obstet 1985; 161:532–534
14. Homer MJ, Smith TJ, Safaii H. Prebiopsy needle localization. Methods, problems, and expected results. Radiol Clin North Am 1992; 30:139–153
15. Kopans DB, Meyer JE, Homer MJ, Grabbe J. Dermal deposits mistaken for breast calcifications. Radiology 1983; 149:592–594

PROBABLY BENIGN CALCIFICATIONS

16. Adler DD, Helvie MA. The "probably benign" breast lesion: work-up and management. In: Sickles EA, Kopans DB (eds), Syllabus for the categorical course on breast imaging. Reston, VA: American College of Radiology; 1990:57–61
17. Brenner RJ. Follow-up as an alternative to biopsy for probably benign mammographically detected abnormalities. Curr Opin Radiol 1991; 3:588–592
18. Brenner RJ, Sickles EA. Acceptability of periodic follow-up as an alternative to biopsy for mammographically detected lesions interpreted as probably benign. Radiology 1989; 171:645–646
19. Datoc PD, Hayes CW, Conway WF, Bosch HA, Neal MP. Mammographic follow-up of nonpalpable low-suspicion breast abnormalities: one versus two views. Radiology 1991; 180:387–391
20. Hall FM, Storella JM, Silverstone DZ, Wyshak G. Nonpalpable breast lesions: recommendations for biopsy based on suspicion of carcinoma at mammography. Radiology 1988; 167:353–358
21. Helvie MA, Pennes DR, Rebner M, Adler DD. Mammographic follow-up of low-suspicion lesions: compliance rate and diagnostic yield. Radiology 1991; 178:155–158
22. Lanyi M. Microcalcifications in the breast—a blessing or a curse? A critical review. Diagn Imaging Clin Med 1985; 54:126–145
23. Sickles EA. Periodic mammographic follow-up of probably benign lesions: results in 3,184 consecutive cases. Radiology 1991; 179:463–468
24. Sigfusson BF, Andersson I, Aspegren K, Janzon L, Linell F, Ljungberg O. Clustered breast calcifications. Acta Radiol [Diagn] (Stockh) 1983; 24:273–281
25. Tabar L, Dean PB. Teaching atlas of mammography. New York: Thieme-Stratton; 1983:138–203

MAGNIFICATION MAMMOGRAPHY

26. Faulk RM, Sickles EA. Efficacy of spot compression-magnification and tangential views in mammographic evaluation of palpable breast masses. Radiology 1992; 185:87–90
27. Hall FM. Magnification spot compression of the breast (letter). Radiology 1989; 173:284

28. Muntz EP, Logan WW. Focal spot size and scatter suppression in magnification mammography. AJR 1979; 133:453–459

29. Sickles EA. Microfocal spot magnification mammography using xeroradiographic and screen-film recording systems. Radiology 1979; 131:599–607

30. Sickles EA. Further experience with microfocal spot magnification mammography in the assessment of clustered breast microcalcifications. Radiology 1980; 137:9–14

31. Sickles EA. Mammographic detectability of breast microcalcifications. AJR 1982; 139:913–918

32. Sickles EA. Magnification mammography. In: Feig SA, McLelland R (eds), Breast carcinoma: current diagnosis and treatment. New York: Masson; 1983:177–182

33. Sickles EA. Combining spot-compression and other special views to maximize mammographic information (letter). Radiology 1989; 173:571

34. Sickles EA, Doi K, Genant HK. Magnification film mammography: image quality and clinical studies. Radiology 1977; 125:69–76

35. Tabar L. Microfocal spot magnification mammography. In: Brünner S, Langfeldt B, Andersen PE (eds), Early detection of breast cancer. New York: Springer; 1984:62–68

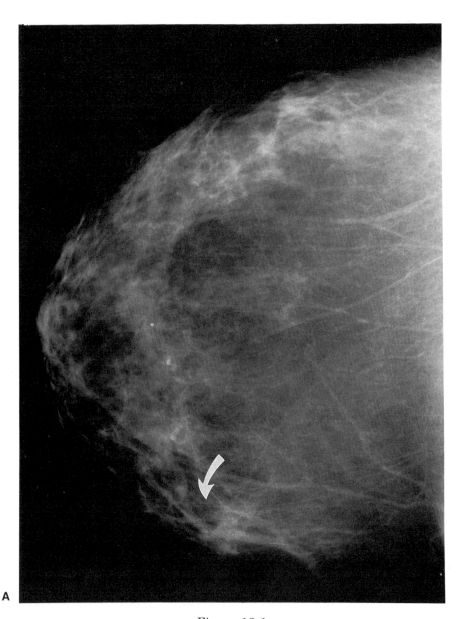

A

Figure 16-1

Figures 16-1 and 16-2. A 57-year-old asymptomatic woman underwent her first screening mammography examination. You are shown CC (A) and MLO (B) views of the right breast (Figure 16-1) demonstrating an isolated cluster of calcifications (arrows), which was further evaluated on a spot-compression magnification MLO view (Figure 16-2).

Case 16: Localized Dermal Calcifications

Question 73

The NEXT step should be:

    (A) follow-up mammography in 6 months
    (B) tangential view
    (C) 90° lateral view
    (D) needle localization

The CC and MLO views of the right breast (Figure 16-1) demonstrate an isolated cluster of calcifications. The magnified MLO view (Figure 16-2) shows it to be a cluster of approximately 30 calcifications in a 1-cm^2 area. The calcific particles vary in size, and some are linearly arrayed. Although these characteristics could indicate malignancy and so suggest the need for biopsy following needle localization (Option (D)), this approach should not be the next step because several other features suggest that the calcifications are benign. First, they are very close together; many are "tightly packed" and almost apposed. Second, they have well-defined, smooth borders. Third, they appear to be round or oval rather than irregular in shape.

The CC view (Figure 16-1A) shows that the calcifications are in the far medial breast, projected 1 to 2 cm from the skin surface. On the MLO view (Figure 16-1B), they are in the upper aspect of the breast, apparently about 5 cm from the skin surface. Since the MLO view is obtained at a 30° to 60° angle from the vertical and is projected from the supero-medial to the inferolateral breast, the principles of parallax indicate that an object in the medial breast projects lower than its actual position on an MLO view (see Case 1, Figure 1-13). Therefore, the calcifications should actually be higher (and also much closer to the skin surface) than indicated on the MLO view.

Based on an assessment of the CC and MLO views, the calcifications could actually be in the skin rather than in the breast parenchyma. Mak-

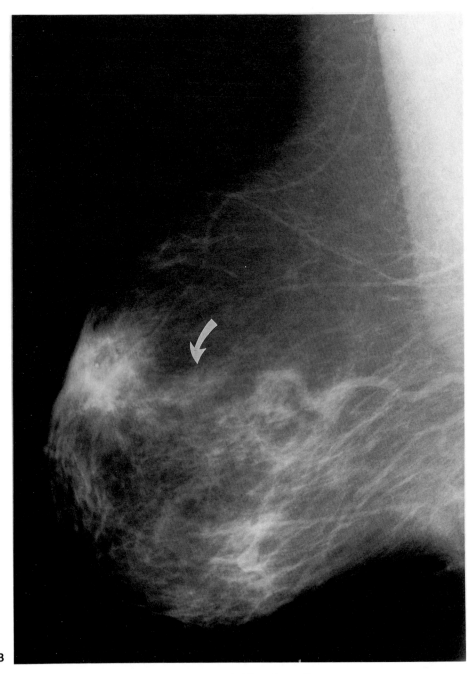

B

Figure 16-1 (Continued)

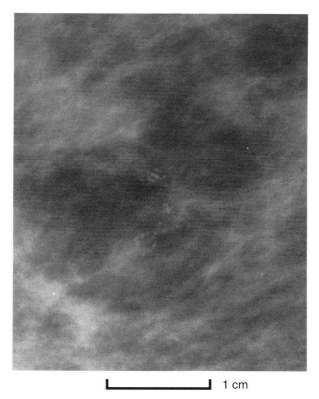

_____ 1 cm

Figure 16-2

ing this distinction is important because dermal calcifications are invariably benign and therefore do not require biopsy. For this reason, the next step in the work-up should be to obtain a tangential view so as to project truly dermal calcifications within the skin surface **(Option (B) is correct).**

Although the calcifications in the test patient happen to project much closer to the skin surface on the 90° lateral view (Option (C)) (Figures 16-3 and 16-4) than on the MLO view, the 90° lateral view is generally much less likely than a tangential view to project calcifications within the skin. Follow-up mammography (Option (A)) would not likely produce further information regarding the dermal location of the calcifications and would not be appropriate until there is a high degree of confidence that the calcifications are benign. Thus, this is not the best next step in the imaging evaluation.

To obtain the appropriate tangential view, a mammogram should be obtained with an alphanumeric-cutout compression plate placed over the skin surface believed to contain the calcifications (Figure 16-5). This

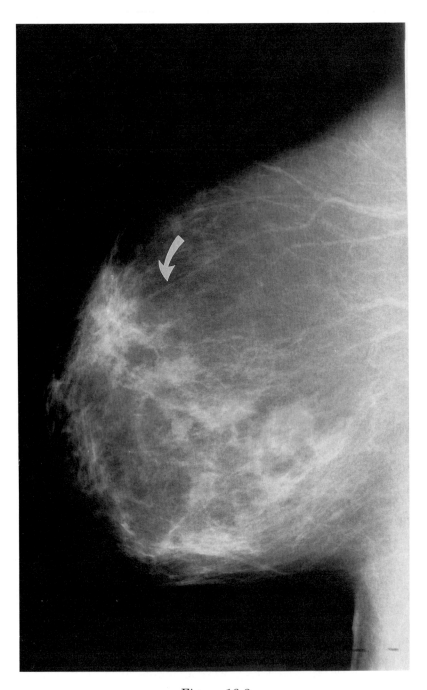

Figure 16-3

Figures 16-3 and 16-4. Same patient as in Figures 16-1 and 16-2. Sebaceous calcifications. A 90° mediolateral view (Figure 16-3) shows that the calcifications (arrow) are projected closer to the skin surface of the upper breast than is seen on the MLO view. Figure 16-4 is a photographic enlargement of the area of calcifications.

Figure 16-4

would be a CC view for calcifications in the upper breast, a caudocranial view for calcifications in the lower breast, a 90° mediolateral view for calcifications in the medial breast, or a 90° lateromedial view for calcifications in the outer breast. The breast is kept in compression while the film is developed, so that the relationship of the calcifications to the compression-plate grid system remains unchanged. A metallic marker is then placed over the calcification site as determined from the mammographic location of the calcifications relative to these coordinates (Figure 16-6). Breast compression is removed, and a view tangential to the skin beneath the metallic marker is then obtained. To optimize visualization of the calcifications, this view is best taken underexposed, using spot-compression magnification technique (Figure 16-7).

Skin calcifications usually appear to be solid or hollow spheres, 1 to 2 mm in diameter. Less commonly, they can have irregular margins or can even be punctate or rod-shaped (Figure 16-8). Skin calcifications are found within the sebaceous glands. They are most often found in the periareolar, axillary, and medial breast areas, the three areas that contain the highest concentrations of sebaceous glands. Skin calcifications

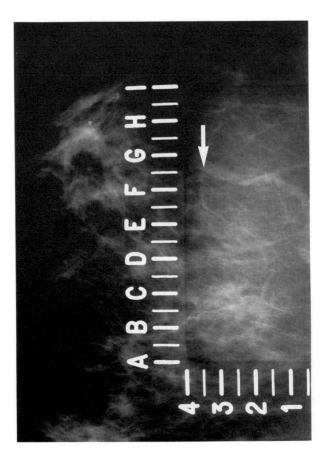

Figure 16-5

Figures 16-5 through 16-7. Same patient as in Figures 16-1 through 16-4. Sebaceous calcifications. Figure 16-5 is a 90° mediolateral view imaged through an alphanumeric-cutout compression plate to obtain coordinate measurements for the calcifications (arrow). Figure 16-6 is a photographic enlargement of the area of calcifications on the 90° mediolateral view taken through the alphanumeric plate after placement of a metallic skin marker at the coordinate intersection site. Figure 16-7 is a view tangential to the skin beneath the metallic marker and documents that the calcifications are in the skin.

are usually projected overlying the breast tissue rather than tangentially within the skin itself on routine views. They are commonly bilateral and have a scattered distribution, although occasionally they can appear as a single localized cluster.

Certain mammographic findings suggest that clustered calcifications are in the skin rather than in the parenchyma. These findings include

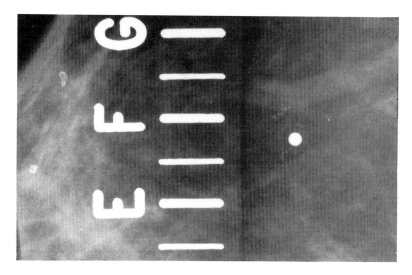

Figure 16-6

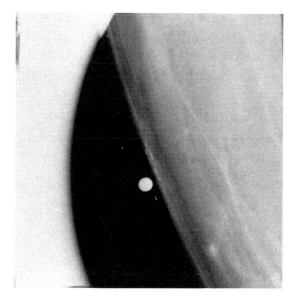

Figure 16-7

projection in a superficial location (frequently in the subcutaneous tissues), especially in the periareolar, axillary, or medial portions of the breast. In addition, the presence of one or more tiny hollow spherical calcifications within a cluster also suggests skin calcifications (Figures 16-9 and 16-10). Another suggestive finding is the presence of calcifications that appear to be arrayed on a surface rather than in a volumetric distribution, i.e., they appear as a plaquelike grouping on one view and in a linear arrangement on another.

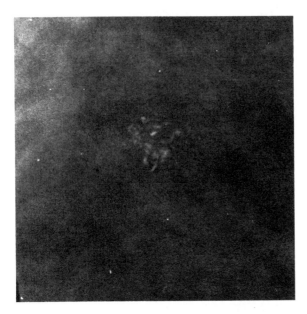

Figure 16-8 (left). Localized skin calcifications. Rod-shaped and irregular calcifications are seen. For this lesion, the correct diagnosis was made by projecting the calcifications within the skin surface on a tangential view (not shown) rather than on the basis of particle morphology.

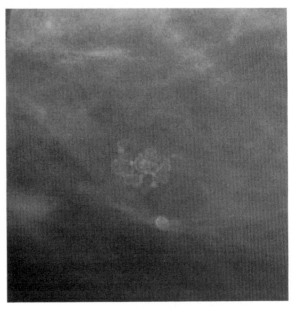

Figure 16-9 (right). Localized skin calcifications. Most of the calcifications in this cluster have hollow centers, a mammographic feature that suggests the correct diagnosis.

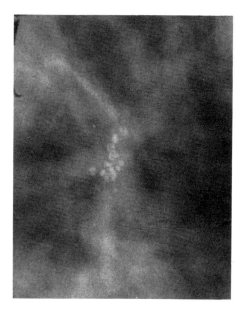

Figure 16-10. Localized skin calcifications. The hollow centers are less apparent and are seen in only some of the calcifications.

Question 74

In a patient with nonspecific calcifications, a change to a more specific mammographic appearance over 6 months is MOST likely with:

(A) fat necrosis
(B) sebaceous gland calcification
(C) sclerosing adenosis
(D) milk of calcium in cysts
(E) arteriosclerosis

Of the options given in this question, only fat necrosis is likely to be associated with calcifications that evolve from a nonspecific to a specific appearance over a 6-month interval **(Option (A) is correct).** The classic appearance of fat-necrosis calcifications develops over a period of months or years (Figure 16-11). An initial traumatic event such as blunt trauma, surgery, or radiation therapy results in the development of a round or oval radiolucent oil cyst or a less well defined area of saponified fat. The margins of either of these areas of fat may eventually calcify, producing the pathognomonic appearance of a hollow spherical calcification or a plaquelike area of calcification. During the development phase, these calcifications can have a nonspecific appearance that can be confused with malignancy. However, there are several management alternatives that

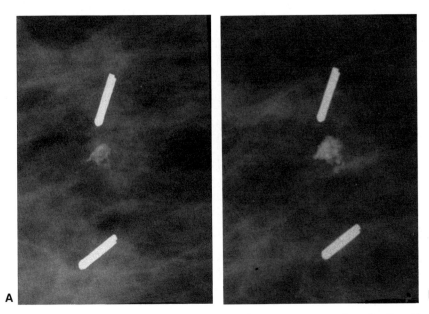

A   B

Figure 16-11. Fat necrosis secondary to lumpectomy and radiation therapy. Note the slow development of calcifications over a 2-year period: 1987 (A), 1988 (B), and 1989 (C and D). The 1989 study shows the typical coarse shell-like calcifications.

are usually preferable to biopsy. Among these alternatives are spot-compression magnification views and other supplementary views to better establish the typical appearance of peripheral "eggshell" calcifications or plaquelike calcifications seen *en face*, or to demonstrate a clear relationship of the calcifications to lucent areas of fat. Another alternative is close mammographic follow-up to document the evolution of the calcifications into a more typical form.

The calcifications of sclerosing adenosis (Option (C)) (see Case 18) and in sebaceous glands (Option (B)) (see Question 73) occasionally have an indeterminate appearance resembling that in the test images. However, change to a more specifically benign mammographic appearance over time has not been demonstrated. Similarly, the mammographic appearance of milk of calcium in cysts (Option (D)) (see Case 19) is typically benign at initial detection and should be evaluated with supplementary views rather than with follow-up mammography.

Since arteriosclerotic calcifications (Option (E)) represent a chronic disease process rather than a response to trauma, they evolve more slowly and are unlikely to show change over 6 months. Arteriosclerotic calcifications are usually easily identified, but although early findings can occasionally mimic linear malignant calcifications, further evalua-

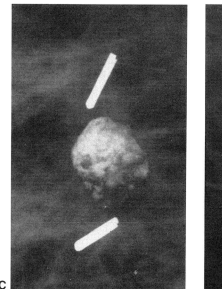
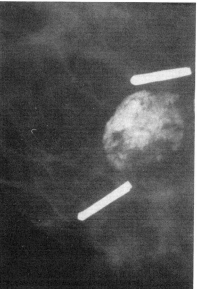

C

D

tion should be done with supplementary mammographic views and not by follow-up.

Question 75

Magnification views are LEAST helpful in evaluating which *one* of the following types of calcifications?

(A) Arteriosclerotic
(B) Secretory
(C) Sebaceous gland
(D) Milk of calcium
(E) Sclerosing adenosis

Magnification mammography is extremely useful in demonstrating characteristically benign or malignant features of calcifications that appear indeterminate or subtle on initial nonmagnification studies. Not only does magnification produce larger images in which features are more easily seen, but it can reveal some very tiny calcifications not otherwise shown. There will also be increased image clarity due to an increase in resolution and a decrease in image mottle (noise). Magnification is rarely useful in the evaluation of secretory calcifications, since these calcifications are relatively large and have well-defined borders **(Option**

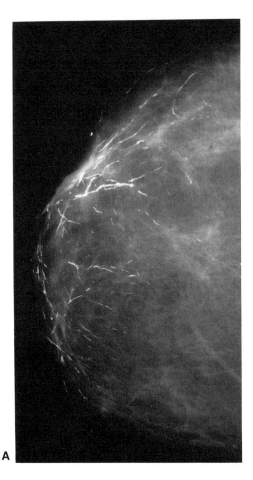

Figure 16-12. Secretory calcifications. (A) A CC view demonstrates typical long, well-defined cylindrical calcifications extending back from retroareolar location in an arclike distribution. (B) A photographic enlargement effectively shows the shapes and well-defined borders of these large calcifications, so that magnification imaging is not needed for further evaluation.

(B) is correct) (Figure 16-12). Also, the diagnosis of secretory calcifications is based on a typical and often bilateral pattern of distribution rather than on any subtle characteristics of individual particles that can be better demonstrated with magnification technique.

Although most arteriosclerotic calcifications (Option (A)) have a characteristic appearance, magnification may be helpful in some cases by establishing the proximate relationship of the calcifications to a noncalcified vascular structure not well seen on the initial nonmagnified view.

Magnification can also be helpful in revealing the correct identity of clustered sebaceous gland calcifications (Option (C)) by demonstrating the presence of benign features such as smooth borders and lucent centers (Figure 16-2). Magnification views in a tangential projection can help document the location of the calcifications within the skin.

Magnification is often extremely helpful in distinguishing milk of calcium in tiny cysts (Option (D)) from nonspecific clustered calcifica-

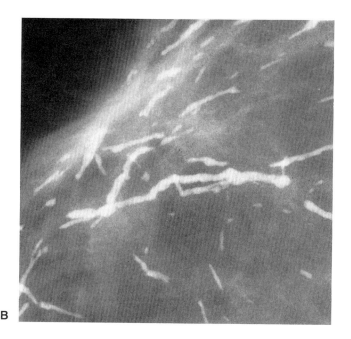

B

tions. It helps by clearly showing teacup-shaped, meniscus-shaped, or
linear calcific particles on the lateral projection but smudgy and much
less readily apparent calcifications on the CC view (Figure 16-13).

In the case of sclerosing adenosis (Option (E)), magnification can be
helpful in establishing the absence of suspicious morphologic features for
the calcific particles and in more accurately demonstrating their usual
round or oval (benign) shapes (see Case 15).

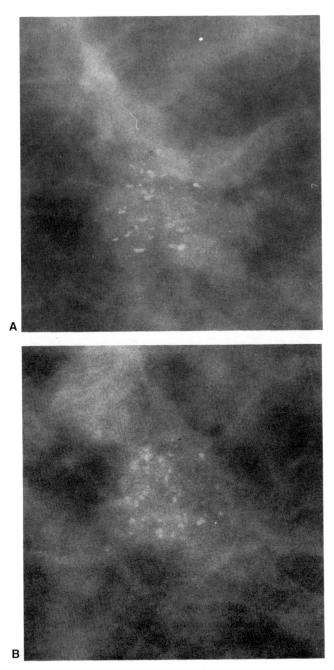

Figure 16-13. Milk of calcium in clustered microcysts. Calcific particles are meniscus shaped on the lateral view (A) but are less dense, appear smudgy, and lack the meniscus shape on the CC view (B).

Question 76

Dermal calcifications are associated with:

- (A) keloids
- (B) raised nevi
- (C) tattoos
- (D) trichinosis
- (E) burns

To avoid mistaking a skin lesion for a calcified (or noncalcified) parenchymal lesion, the location of any skin lesions should be marked on a diagram of the breast that accompanies the mammographic images when they are interpreted by the radiologist. When necessary, a metallic marker should be placed over the skin lesion. Tangential views should then be obtained to establish or exclude a dermal location of the lesion.

Keloids are large tumorous scars that protrude above the skin surface. These lesions are due to the formation of excessive collagen in areas of connective tissue repair and occur almost exclusively in blacks. On mammography, keloids appear as oval and elongated circumscribed densities that can mimic masses within the breast when projected *en face*. Calcification in keloids is uncommon, but when present can be coarse, dense, irregular, or ringlike **(Option (A) is true).**

Dermal nevi that are not elevated above the skin surface cannot be seen on mammography, but raised dermal nevi appear as round or oval masses and may have a characteristic mosaic or cauliflower pattern if the nevus is fissured (see Case 9, Figure 9-2 [page 103]). Nevi can entrap radiopaque powders within such crevices and can also calcify themselves **(Option (B) is true).**

A tattoo is produced by embedding various pigment particles into the skin. Metallic salts are used to provide the coloring of the pigment in most instances. Occasionally, these salts are seen on mammograms as a calcific pattern **(Option (C) is true).** However, the distribution of particles, echoing the pattern of the tattoo, usually suggests the correct diagnosis. Tangential views will show that these particles are within the skin.

Infection with the roundworm *Trichinella spiralis* results from eating raw or improperly cooked or processed meat or meat products, usually pork, that contain encysted larvae (trichinae). Once ingested, the larvae reach the axial skeletal muscles, where they penetrate individual fibers to produce a myositis. The larvae encyst within the muscles and calcify after they die. Trichinosis does not involve the breast or skin **(Option (D) is false),** but its calcifications are seen within the pectoral muscles on mammograms.

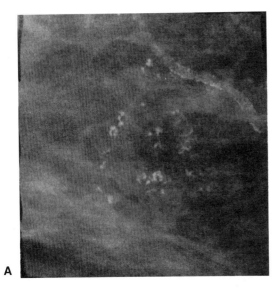

Figure 16-14. Dystrophic calcifications in the skin. These calcifications are due to a previous biopsy of this patient's breast, as shown on spot-compression CC (A) and tangential (B) views. Arteriosclerotic vascular calcification is also seen on the CC view.

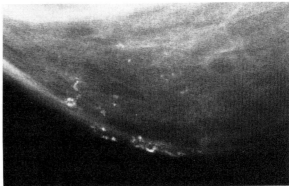

Dystrophic calcifications are usually found within the breast parenchyma, where they form after biopsy and other types of trauma. However, dystrophic calcification can also develop within the breast skin, most commonly resulting from thermal burns or surgery such as reduction mammoplasty **(Option (E) is true).** These can be solid or hollow round calcifications or irregular calcifications (Figure 16-14).

Stephen A. Feig, M.D.

SUGGESTED READINGS

SEBACEOUS GLAND CALCIFICATIONS

1. Berkowitz JE, Gatewood OM, Donovan GB, Gayler BW. Dermal breast calcifications: localization with template-guided placement of skin marker. Radiology 1987; 163:282
2. Kopans DB, Meyer JE, Homer MJ, Grabbe J. Dermal deposits mistaken for breast calcifications. Radiology 1983; 149:592–594

OTHER SKIN CALCIFICATIONS

3. Brown RC, Zuehlke RL, Ehrhardt JC, Jochimsen PR. Tattoos simulating calcifications on xeroradiographs of the breast. Radiology 1981; 138:583–584
4. DeParedes ES. Atlas of film-screen mammography, 2nd ed. Baltimore: Williams & Wilkins; 1993:300, 340
5. Ikeda DM, Sickles EA. Mammographic demonstration of pectoral muscle microcalcifications. AJR 1988; 151:475–476
6. Miller CL, Feig SA, Fox JW IV. Mammographic changes after reduction mammoplasty. AJR 1987; 149:35–38
7. Reeder M. Tropical diseases of the soft tissues. Semin Roentgenol 1973; 8:47–53
8. Sickles EA. Breast calcifications: mammographic evaluation. Radiology 1986; 160:289–293

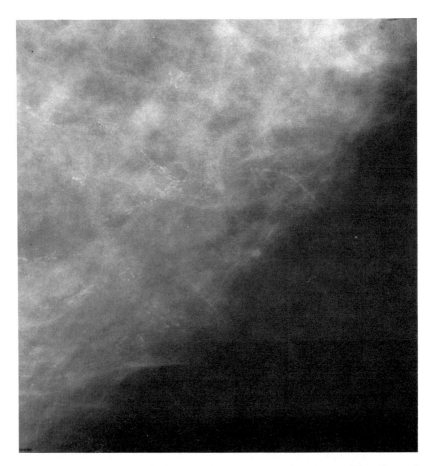

Figure 17-1. You are shown a spot-compression magnification view obtained following the first screening mammography examination of a 50-year-old asymptomatic woman.

Case 17: Ductal Calcifications

Question 77

The NEXT step should be:

  (A) excisional biopsy
  (B) fine-needle aspiration biopsy
  (C) follow-up mammography in 3 months
  (D) follow-up mammography in 6 months
  (E) follow-up mammography in 1 year

The punctate calcifications seen in Figure 17-1 have the appearance of a "string of pearls." This linear arrangement suggests that they are within the ductal system even though they do not have the classic rod shape, which more obviously indicates an intraductal process. Ductal distribution is also less apparent since the calcifications are arranged not in a straight line but rather in a sinuous line. Although this pattern might be mistaken for arteriosclerotic calcification, the arrangement of the calcifications in this case differs from that of vascular calcifications (Figure 17-2) in two respects. First, the calcifications are not associated with any vascular markings, which would be expected to branch into smaller vessels as they extend anteriorly toward the nipple. Rather, the distribution of calcifications in the test patient follows the ductal system, which branches into smaller ducts from the nipple toward the posterior breast. Second, there is no "railroad track" appearance of calcification on both sides of a blood vessel wall.

Although ductal calcifications can be due to either benign or malignant disease, their appearance, with the notable exception of secretory calcifications, is nonspecific. Thus, since there is a reasonable chance of malignancy in this 50-year-old woman, excisional biopsy should be performed **(Option (A) is correct)**. Moreover, the presence of multiple crossing bands of calcification producing the lacelike appearance seen in Figure 17-1 is much more likely to represent malignancy than is a single band of calcifications.

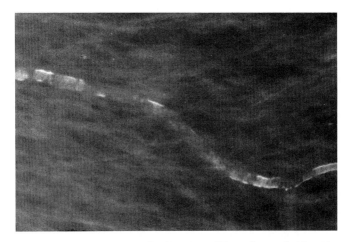

Figure 17-2. Arteriosclerotic calcification. Vascular calcifications appear as two parallel but interrupted lines of calcifications that are continuous with a noncalcified tubular density that represents the remainder of the blood vessel.

Since the calcifications appear to be within the ducts and there is no evidence of a mass or parenchymal invasion, fine-needle aspiration biopsy (Option (B)) might result in a sampling error, producing an "insufficient specimen" or a false-negative result. At present, there is no substantial body of data specifically assessing the accuracy of fine-needle aspiration biopsy for diagnostic evaluation of calcifications alone.

Short-term follow-up in 3 months (Option (C)) for calcifications would probably be misleading, since many clusters of malignant calcifications do not change in appearance even over much longer intervals. Follow-up in 6 months (Option (D)) and in 1 year (Option (E)) would similarly be inappropriate, since follow-up mammography should be reserved for lesions that are probably benign and not for lesions considered suspicious for malignancy.

Question 78

Calcifications are found predominantly within ducts in:

(A) ductal hyperplasia
(B) secretory disease (plasma cell mastitis)
(C) comedocarcinoma
(D) Paget's disease of the nipple
(E) sclerosing adenosis

A variety of benign and malignant conditions are associated with calcifications that are found primarily in the ducts. Among these is ductal hyperplasia (e.g., epitheliosis and papillomatosis), a benign proliferation of epithelial cells in the terminal ductal-lobular unit **(Option (A) is true)**. Ductal hyperplasia may be mild, moderate, or florid and may progress to atypical ductal hyperplasia, which in turn may evolve into ductal carcinoma *in situ* (Figure 17-3). Women with moderate or florid ductal hyperplasia are at increased risk (1.5x to 2x) for breast cancer; those with atypical ductal hyperplasia are at even greater risk (4x). Some studies also suggest that the risk of subsequent cancer is further increased (6.5x) in women with ductal hyperplasia if histologically or mammographically evident calcifications are present. Ductal hyperplasia is frequently associated with lobular hyperplasia so that calcifications are present in both ducts and lobules. Ductal hyperplasia itself does not have any clinical manifestations. However, it may occur in association with gross cysts, which may result in palpable nodules, masses, and breast pain. Ductal hyperplasia may be seen at any age but is less common after menopause.

Secretory disease (otherwise known as plasma cell mastitis or benign duct ectasia) is characterized by inspissated secretions, dilated ducts, and chronic inflammation of the intermediate and larger ducts. The calcifications associated with secretory disease (Figure 17-4) occur in the duct lumen or within the duct wall so that they are seen at mammography as long solid cores or long hollow cylinders, respectively **(Option (B) is true)**. Secretory calcifications usually have a characteristic appearance that is easily distinguishable from malignant linear calcifications; secretory calcifications have greater length and width, as well as variation in width in a single calcification. Common symptoms of secretory disease include pain, nipple discharge, and nipple retraction. Although secretory calcifications are frequently seen at mammography, clinically evident disease is relatively infrequent. The overwhelming majority of women with clinical symptoms are near menopause or past it.

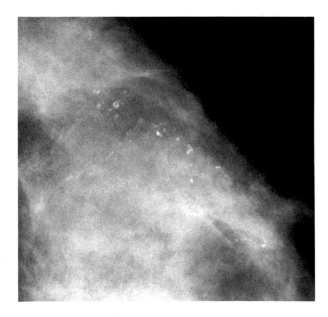

Figure 17-3. Ductal hyperplasia. The calcifications seen in benign ductal hyperplasia have a linear distribution that may be indistinguishable from that of ductal carcinoma *in situ.*

The three main types of ductal carcinoma *in situ* are comedocarcinoma, cribriform carcinoma, and micropapillary carcinoma. Comedocarcinoma is characterized by necrotic cellular debris in ductal and lobular spaces. The calcifications in comedocarcinoma are frequently elongated, rod-shaped, or branching and may appear to form casts of the ducts **(Option (C) is true).** Cribriform carcinoma is characterized histologically by a duct lumen filled with an almost solid growth of malignant cells, perforated by round spaces or by bridges of malignant cells forming a cartwheel appearance. Micropapillary carcinoma is distinguished by frondlike projections of cells within the lumen of a duct. The calcifications in cribriform and micropapillary carcinoma occur within cystic spaces or intraluminal papillary projections and are punctate or can have irregular shapes that present a "crushed stone" appearance. Since comedocarcinoma often coexists with cribriform and micropapillary carcinoma, mammography can often show both types of calcifications in the same location. Most cases of ductal carcinoma *in situ* are nonpalpable and are found by mammography alone. Ductal carcinoma *in situ* generally does not produce clinical signs or symptoms until after it evolves into invasive carcinoma. It is usually found among women older than 40 years.

Paget's disease of the nipple is a condition diagnosed clinically when *in situ* or invasive ductal carcinoma involves the nipple epidermis, producing an eczematoid lesion (Figure 17-5). Paget's cells, which are large

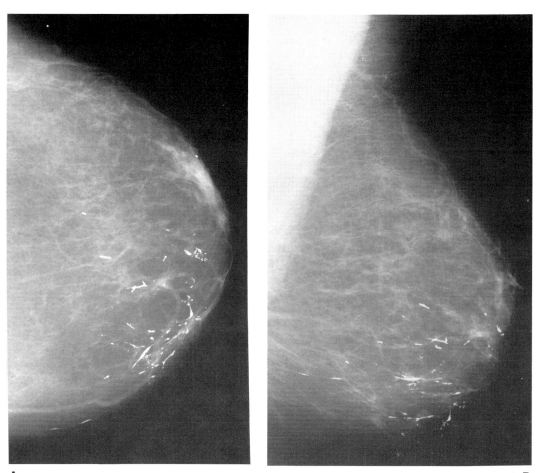

A

B

Figure 17-4. Benign duct ectasia. Secretory calcifications are much longer and wider than nearly all malignant microcalcifications. Their arclike distribution extending away from the retroareolar region is characteristic; it parallels the normal ductal anatomy of the breast on the CC (A) and MLO (B) views.

adenocarcinoma cells with clear cytoplasm, are seen within the skin. Microcalcifications in a ductal pattern can be seen on mammograms and are due to the underlying cancer (Figure 17-6) **(Option (D) is true).**

Adenosis represents benign epithelial proliferation and architectural alteration of the acini and terminal ductules of the lobules. Each lobule is a collection of acini, which are the blind-ending sacs at the end of the terminal ductules. Sclerosing adenosis is a type of adenosis characterized by fibrotic proliferation. Calcifications in adenosis are usually round, punctate, and scattered (see Case 18, Figures 18-1 and 18-2), not elon-

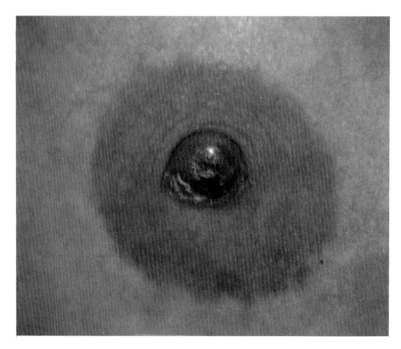

Figure 17-5. Paget's disease of the nipple. Note the involvement of the skin of the nipple. (Courtesy of Gordon F. Schwartz, M.D., Jefferson Medical College, Philadelphia, Pa.)

gated and clustered. These calcifications occur predominantly in the acini rather than in the ducts **(Option (E) is false).** As is the case with ductal hyperplasia, adenosis (lobular hyperplasia) does not produce symptoms unless it coexists with gross cysts.

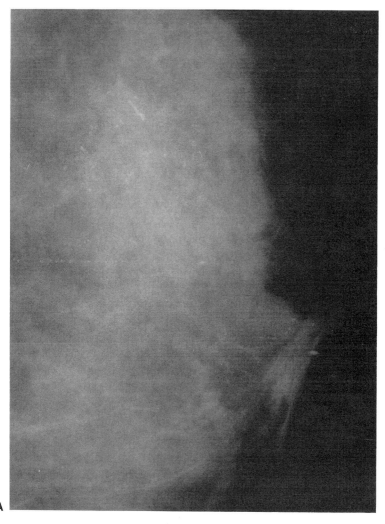

A

Figure 17-6. Paget's disease of the nipple. Note the retroareolar calcifications within the ducts, a finding suspicious for ductal carcinoma *in situ*. In this case, some calcifications can actually be seen within the nipple itself in the coned-down 90° mediolateral (A) and CC (B) views.

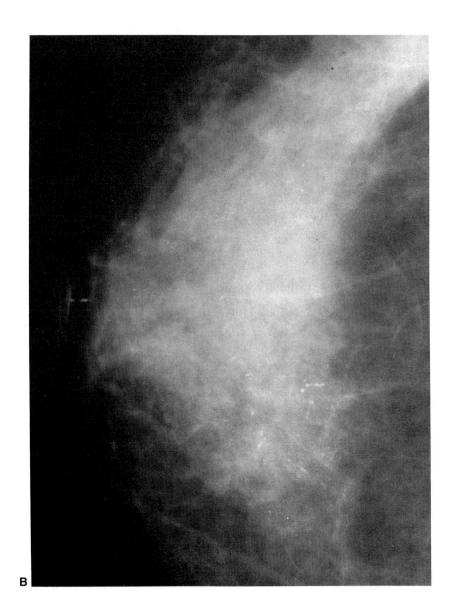

B

Question 79

Which *one* of the following types of calcifications is LEAST likely to be associated with carcinoma?

    (A) Linearly distributed
    (B) Branching
    (C) Casting
    (D) Solid round or oval
    (E) Ringlike

Calcifications that are linearly distributed (Option (A)), branching (Option (B)), or casting (Option (C)) suggest the presence of intraductal abnormalities. Since most invasive breast cancers arise in the ducts rather than in the lobules, intraductal calcifications are often associated with malignancy. Casting calcifications, also termed elongated or rod-shaped calcifications, form a cast of the duct lumen within which they occur (Figures 17-7 and 17-8). Ductal carcinoma *in situ* may also present as solid, round, or oval calcifications (Option (D)) in a linear array (Figure 17-9) or in a clustered distribution. Ringlike calcifications are almost never due to malignancy **(Option (E) is correct).** Very small ringlike calcifications, 1 mm in size, may be due to senile involution of the acini. Calcifications of this size and larger (Figure 17-10) may be due to fat

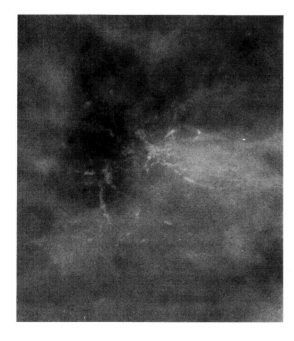

Figure 17-7. Comedo-carcinoma. The image shows casting calcifications, several of which are branching.

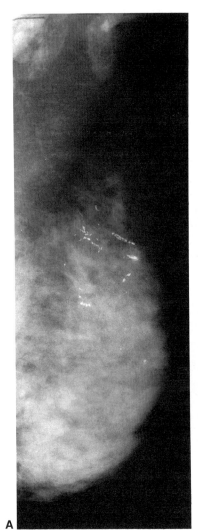

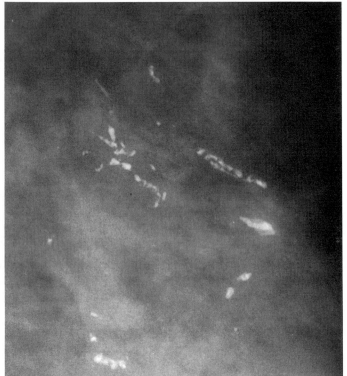

Figure 17-8. Comedocarcinoma with coarse casting calcifications. An MLO view (A) and a photographic enlargement of the MLO view (B) are shown.

A

B

necrosis. Rarely, larger ringlike calcifications are found in the walls of cysts.

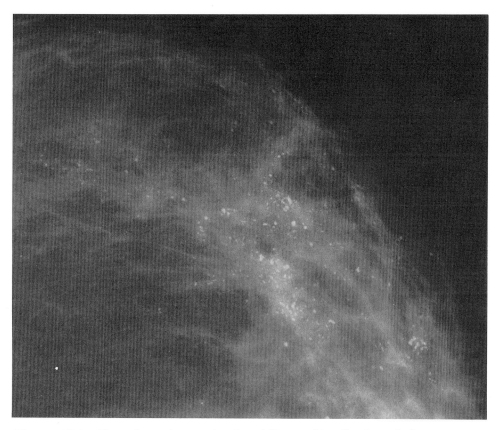

Figure 17-9. Ductal carcinoma *in situ*. A linear distribution of pleomorphic calcifications in ducts can be seen.

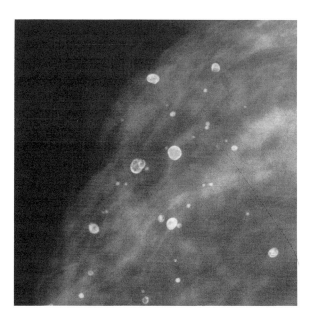

Figure 17-10 (left).
Fat necrosis with
round calcifications.
Lucent centers are ob-
vious in the larger cal-
cifications, whereas the
smallest calcifications
appear as solid
spheres.

Question 80

In the absence of calcifications elsewhere in the breast, biopsy of a solitary cluster of indeterminate microcalcifications should be considered if their number equals or exceeds:

    (A) $2/cm^2$
    (B) $5/cm^2$
    (C) $10/cm^2$
    (D) $15/cm^2$
    (E) $20/cm^2$

Several studies have shown a correlation between the number of calcifications in a solitary cluster and the likelihood of malignancy. It is generally agreed that a cluster containing fewer than five indeterminate calcifications/cm^2 need not be biopsied since such clusters are so common and since the chance of their being associated with malignancy is negligible. For calcifications of indeterminate shape and distribution, biopsy should be considered for solitary clusters of at least 5/cm^2 **(Option (B) is correct).** Restricting biopsy to isolated clusters of 10 or more calcific particles/cm^2 is inappropriate because this approach would forego biopsy of many early cases of ductal carcinoma *in situ*. It should be emphasized that calcification morphology and the relationship of calcifications to one another are more important criteria for suggesting biopsy than is the number of particles. For example, the presence of one or more rod-like calcifications in a cluster of four or fewer calcific particles or in a linear arrangement of four punctate calcifications is suspicious for malignancy. It must also be stressed that the rule of thumb that a cluster containing at least 5 calcifications/cm^2 should be biopsied applies only to a solitary cluster and not to the multiple clusters consistent with adenosis (see Case 18).

Stephen A. Feig, M.D.

SUGGESTED READINGS

DUCTAL CARCINOMA *IN SITU*

1. Bassett LW. Mammographic analysis of calcifications. Radiol Clin North Am 1992; 30:93–105
2. Ikeda DM, Helvie MA, Frank TS, Chapel KL, Andersson IT. Paget disease of the nipple: radiologic-pathologic correlation. Radiology 1993; 189:89–94

3. Lanyi M. Diagnosis and differential diagnosis of breast calcifications. New York: Springer-Verlag; 1986:81–139

4. Muir BB, Lamb J, Anderson TJ, Kirkpatrick AE. Microcalcification and its relationship to cancer of the breast: experience in a screening clinic. Clin Radiol 1983; 34:193–200

5. Page DL, Anderson TJ, Rogers LW. Carcinoma *in situ* (CIS). In: Page DL, Anderson TJ (eds), Diagnostic histopathology of the breast. New York: Churchill Livingstone; 1987:157–192

6. Rogers JV Jr, Powell RW. Mammographic indications for biopsy of clinically normal breasts: correlation with pathologic findings in 72 cases. AJR 1972; 115:794–800

7. Schnitt SJ, Silen W, Sadowsky NL, Connolly JL, Harris JR. Ductal carcinoma *in situ* (intraductal carcinoma) of the breast. N Engl J Med 1988; 318:898–903

8. Stomper PC, Connolly JL, Meyer JE, Harris JR. Clinically occult ductal carcinoma *in situ* detected with mammography: analysis of 100 cases with radiologic-pathologic correlation. Radiology 1989; 172:235–241

DUCTAL AND LOBULAR HYPERPLASIA

9. Bartow SA, Pathak DR, Mettler FA. Radiographic microcalcification and parenchymal patterns as indicators of histologic "high-risk" benign breast disease. Cancer 1990; 66:1721–1725

10. de Paredes E, Abbitt PL, Tabbarah S, Bickers MA, Smith DC. Mammographic and histologic correlations of microcalcifications. RadioGraphics 1990; 10:577–589

11. Page DL, Anderson TJ, Rogers LW. Epithelial hyperplasia. In: Page DL, Anderson TJ (eds), Diagnostic histopathology of the breast. New York: Churchill-Livingstone; 1987:120–156

12. Thomas DB, Whitehead J, Dorce C, et al. Mammographic calcifications and risk of subsequent breast cancer. J Natl Cancer Inst 1993; 85:230–235

DUCT ECTASIA

13. Haagensen CD. Diseases of the breast, 3rd ed. Philadelphia: WB Saunders; 1986:357–368

14. Hughes LE, Mansel RE, Webster DJT. Benign disorders and diseases of the breast. London: Balliere Tindall; 1989:107–132

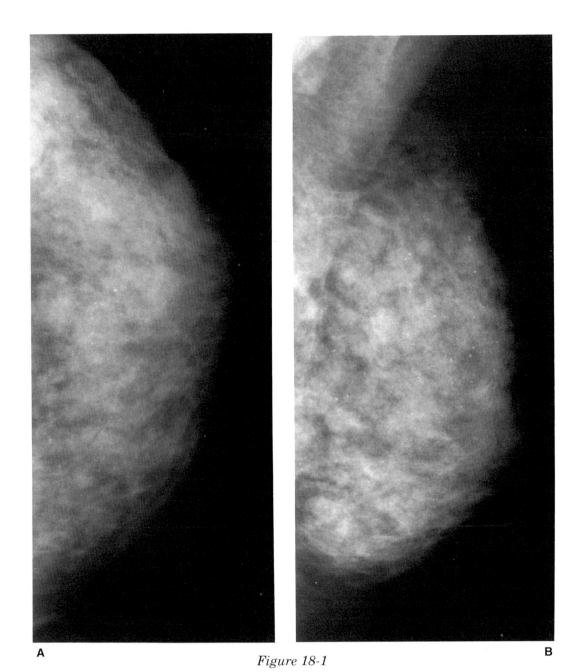

A

B

Figure 18-1

Figures 18-1 and 18-2. You are shown CC (A) and MLO (B) views of the left breast from the mammography examination of a 60-year-old asymptomatic woman who underwent right mastectomy 4 years ago (Figure 18-1). Corresponding spot-compression magnification views are also shown (Figure 18-2).

Case 18: Bilateral Benign Scattered Calcifications

Question 81

Which *one* of the following is the MOST likely cause of the calcifications?

    (A) Atypical hyperplasia
    (B) Sclerosing adenosis
    (C) Ductal carcinoma *in situ* (comedo)
    (D) Ductal carcinoma *in situ* (micropapillary)
    (E) Lobular neoplasia

General symmetry in the distribution of calcifications between the breasts is a highly useful, reliable sign of a benign process. However, evaluation of calcifications in the postmastectomy patient can be difficult if previous mammograms of the opposite breast are not available for comparison. In such cases, the radiologist can rely only on other signs, such as the morphology of the calcifications themselves and their distribution within the remaining breast, and on a comparison with previous studies of the same breast.

The calcifications seen in this case are most likely due to sclerosing adenosis **(Option (B) is correct).** The key finding leading to this conclusion is that the distribution of calcifications is fairly diffuse, even though most are confined to the upper-outer quadrant. Malignant calcifications, such as those seen in comedo or micropapillary ductal carcinoma *in situ* (DCIS) (Options (C) and (D)), would be more clustered. Although the calcifications seen in the test patient are not completely regularly distributed, i.e., some calcific particles are closer to nearby particles than others, the distribution is basically random. Groups consisting of 3 to 5 calcifications are in individual acini of single lobules, which are separated from other lobules by areas of fatty and fibrotic tissue containing few if any calcifications.

Sclerosing adenosis is characterized histologically by enlargement and distortion of the lobular units. There is an increase in the number of

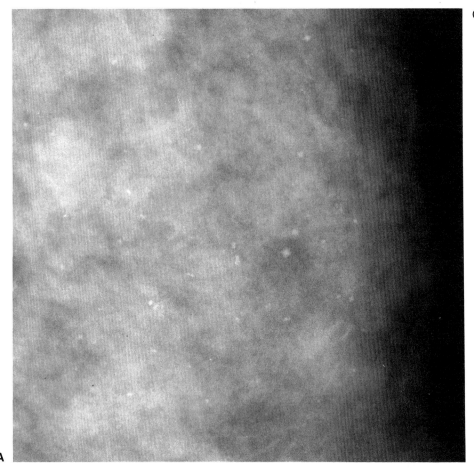

A

Figure 18-2

acini in each lobule, as well as fibrous alteration of the lobule, so that the acini are often compressed. However, the acini maintain the normal pattern of only-two-cell-thick layers central to the basement membrane.

As seen best in the spot-compression magnification views of the test patient (Figure 18-2), the benign calcifications of adenosis vary in size and shape. Such variation is frequent and should not be of concern. Although most of the calcifications are smooth, the calcifications of adenosis can at times have irregular or poorly defined margins. Indeed, some of the calcifications in the MLO view (Figure 18-2B) appear elongated, but these are generally parallel to the horizontal plane, indicating early milk-of-calcium formation (see Case 19), which frequently develops in the later stages of adenosis when acini dilate into microcysts.

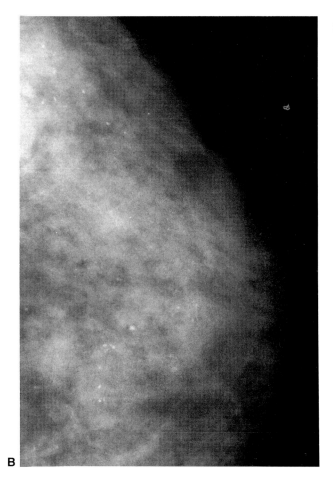

MLO

B

Lobular neoplasia (Option (E)), another type of lobular proliferation, is synonymous with lobular carcinoma *in situ*. Histologically, all acini in the lobule are filled by uniform cells having round or oval nuclei. Most of the acini in the lobule are distended. In most cases of lobular neoplasia undergoing biopsy because of mammographic microcalcifications, the calcifications are located in an area of benign disease rather than in the (contiguous) area of lobular neoplasia. The few calcifications associated with lobular neoplasia are probably associated with preexisting benign disease that was engulfed by the lobular neoplasia. There are no direct or indirect mammographic signs of lobular neoplasia. Lobular neoplasia detected following biopsy for calcifications should be considered an incidental pathologic finding.

Similarly, there are no specific mammographic findings for atypical hyperplasia (Option (A)). When suspicious microcalcifications are biopsied and found to be benign, the histologic diagnosis is usually due to some type of hyperplastic process, whether bland or with cellular atypia. There is nothing in the appearance of the calcifications in Figures 18-1 and 18-2 to suggest atypical hyperplasia rather than sclerosing adenosis. However, in contradistinction to lobular neoplasia, the area of mammographic calcifications for lesions representing atypical hyperplasia does generally correspond to the area of histologic abnormality.

Question 82

Calcifications in adenosis:

  (A) occur primarily in acini
  (B) are most often in the upper-outer quadrant
  (C) often have hollow centers
  (D) are often rod-shaped
  (E) are usually scattered in distribution

Calcifications in adenosis occur mainly in the acini **(Option (A) is true)**, which may have enlarged to the point of cystic dilatation. Although such microcystic adenosis is also termed blunt duct adenosis, the word "duct" in blunt duct adenosis is a misnomer because this lesion actually involves the acinus.

Although the calcifications of adenosis can be seen throughout the breast, they are most often found in the upper-outer quadrant since this region contains the most glandular tissue **(Option (B) is true)**.

The calcifications of adenosis are often round or oval but can have a triangular, irregular, or amorphous appearance when the calcification process is incomplete. Hollow spherical calcifications are an infrequent sequela of adenosis and are thought to result from spontaneous rupture of microcysts and consequent fat necrosis **(Option (C) is false)**.

Rod-shaped calcifications are seen infrequently in adenosis **(Option (D) is false)** and can be explained by concurrent epithelial ductal hyperplasia, DCIS, or stagnation of secretions in benign dilated ducts. Meniscus-shaped calcifications described by the term "milk of calcium" occur frequently in adenosis. Although at times these mimic rod-shaped calcifications, they can be correctly identified by means of their slightly concave upper surface, slightly convex lower surface, tapered ends, and horizontal orientation on the MLO view and their less well defined, often smudgy shapes on the CC view (see Case 19).

Since adenosis is a diffuse process, the distribution of calcifications is typically scattered. Even when confined to a single area of the breast, the calcifications are fairly dispersed **(Option (E) is true)**.

Question 83

Concerning ductal carcinoma *in situ*,

(A) it is synonymous with comedocarcinoma
(B) multicentricity describes tumors that involve more than one quadrant
(C) it is often multicentric
(D) an extensive intraductal component reduces the effectiveness of radiation therapy
(E) it is a precursor of invasive disease

DCIS is classified as either comedo type or noncomedo type. The latter consists of micropapillary, cribriform, and solid carcinoma **(Option (A) is false),** although mixtures of the various types are seen. The comedo subtype is more likely than the noncomedo subtypes to be associated with subsequent invasive disease. Page and DuPont have suggested that noncomedo DCIS should be regarded not as a frank cancer but as an indicator of extremely high risk of invasive cancer (8 to 10 times the normal risk).

The definition of cancer multicentricity is not universally accepted. Some researchers use the terms "multicentric" and "multifocal" interchangeably. However, multicentricity is generally defined as the presence of independent cancer foci remote from or in a quadrant different from that of the primary tumor **(Option (B) is true).** In contrast, multifocality refers to tumor foci in the vicinity of the main tumor. This distinction has therapeutic implications. Patchefsky and Schwartz have proposed that cribriform and solid DCIS lesions may be treated by local excision alone since they are rarely multicentric. In contradistinction, comedo and micropapillary DCIS lesions are frequently multicentric and require whole-breast treatment. Reviewing the results of numerous studies available on this topic, McDivitt concluded that the overall rate of multicentricity is in the range of 25 to 50% **(Option (C) is true).** A recent study of "multicentric" DCIS by Holland et al. utilizing serial slices and radiographs of whole-breast specimens indicates that much of what has traditionally been thought to be separate multicentric foci is actually contiguous growth along the ductal system.

An extensive intraductal component is defined as widespread DCIS associated with an invasive ductal carcinoma mass or as a large tumor composed primarily of DCIS with a small area of local invasion. Invasive cancers with moderate or extensive intraductal components are more likely to recur locally, whereas tumors without extensive intraductal components treated by limited resection and radiation therapy have a low risk of local recurrence. Tumors with extensive intraductal components must be widely excised because radiation therapy is relatively ineffective in achieving local tumor control **(Option (D) is true)**. The poorer prognosis of such tumors is limited to their propensity for local recurrence, not to an association with systemic metastasis or impaired breast cancer survival.

The mammographic appearance of a carcinoma can be used to predict its intraductal component. For cancers presenting as calcifications without a mass, Healey et al. found that there was a 73% likelihood that the tumor had an extensive intraductal component. For cancers appearing as a mass or architectural distortion without calcifications, there was a 92% likelihood that the lesion lacked an extensive intraductal component.

Although all invasive ductal carcinomas must arise from DCIS **(Option (E) is true),** there are data to suggest that not all cases of DCIS actually progress to invasive disease. One autopsy series from Denmark found DCIS in 15% of breasts of patients who died of diseases other than breast cancer. This suggests that the lesion can remain clinically unimportant for a long time, since far fewer than 15% of women ever develop invasive breast cancer. However, the diagnostic criteria for DCIS used in this study have been questioned. Two autopsy series performed in the United States demonstrated occult DCIS less frequently.

Question 84

Concerning lobular carcinoma *in situ*,

    (A) it has a poorer prognosis than lobular neoplasia
    (B) it occurs primarily in ducts
    (C) it is less aggressive than ductal carcinoma *in situ*
    (D) the mammographic findings are specific
    (E) it usually progresses to invasive disease

Since lobular carcinoma *in situ* (LCIS) is synonymous with lobular neoplasia, the prognosis is identical **(Option (A) is false)**. LCIS is confined to the acini of the lobules. There is no involvement of the ducts **(Option (B) is false).**

LCIS is considerably less aggressive than comedocarcinoma and even less aggressive than noncomedo DCIS **(Option (C) is true)**. The mammographic findings are nonspecific **(Option (D) is false)** and are usually located adjacent to rather than within the area of LCIS.

Follow-up of women with biopsy-proven lobular neoplasia has shown that only 20 to 30% develop invasive breast cancer over the next 15 to 20 years. Approximately half of these invasive breast cancers develop in the contralateral breast. Therefore, it appears that LCIS does not often progress to invasive carcinoma **(Option (E) is false).**

Stephen A. Feig, M.D.

SUGGESTED READINGS

SCLEROSING ADENOSIS

1. Helvie MA, Hessler C, Frank TS, Ikeda DM. Atypical hyperplasia of the breast: mammographic appearance and histologic correlation. Radiology 1991; 179:759–764
2. Lanyi M. Diagnosis and differential diagnosis of breast calcifications. New York: Springer Verlag; 1988:29–81, 157–173
3. MacErlean DP, Nathan BE. Calcification in sclerosing adenosis simulating malignant breast calcification. Br J Radiol 1972; 45:944–945

DUCTAL CARCINOMA *IN SITU*

4. Alpers CE, Wellings SR. The prevalence of carcinoma *in situ* in normal and cancer-associated breasts. Hum Pathol 1985; 16:796–807
5. Andersen J, Nielsen M, Christensen L. New aspects of the natural history of *in situ* and invasive carcinoma in the female breast. Results from autopsy investigations. Verh Dtsch Ges Pathol 1985; 69:88–95
6. Bartow SA, Pathak DR, Black WC, Key CR, Teaf SR. Prevalence of benign, atypical, and malignant breast lesions in populations at different risk for breast cancer. A forensic autopsy study. Cancer 1987; 60:2751–2760
7. Dutt PL, Page DL. Multicentricity of *in situ* and invasive carcinoma. In: Bland KI, Copeland EM (eds), The breast: comprehensive management of benign and malignant diseases. Philadelphia: WB Saunders; 1991: 299–308
8. Harris JR, Lippman ME, Veronesi U, Willett W. Breast cancer (2). N Engl J Med 1992; 327:390–398
9. Healey EA, Osteen RT, Schnitt SJ, et al. Can the clinical and mammographic findings at presentation predict the presence of an extensive intraductal component in early stage breast cancer? Int J Radiat Oncol Biol Phys 1989; 17:1217–1221
10. Holland R, Connolly JL, Gelman R, et al. The presence of an extensive intraductal component following a limited excision correlates with prominent residual disease in the remainder of the breast. J Clin Oncol 1990; 8:113–118
11. Holland R, Hendriks JH, Verbeek AL, Mravunac M, Schuurmans Stekhoven JH. Extent, distribution, and mammographic/histological correlations of breast ductal carcinoma *in situ*. Lancet 1990; 335:519–522
12. Jacquemier J, Kurtz JM, Amalric R, Brandone H, Ayme Y, Spitalier JM. An assessment of extensive intraductal component as a risk factor for local recurrence after breast-conserving therapy. Br J Cancer 1990; 61:873–876

13. McDivitt RW. Breast cancer multicentricity. In: McDivitt RW, Oberman HA, Ozello L, Kaufman N (eds), The breast. Baltimore: Williams & Wilkins; 1984:139–148

14. Page DL, DuPont WD. Anatomic markers of human premalignancy and risk of breast cancer. Cancer 1990; 66:1326–1335

15. Patchefsky AS, Schwartz GF, Finkelstein SD, et al. Heterogeneity of intraductal carcinoma of the breast. Cancer 1989; 63:731–741

16. Schwartz GF, Patchefsky AS, Finkelstein SD, et al. Nonpalpable *in situ* ductal carcinoma of the breast. Predictors of multicentricity and microinvasion and implications for treatment. Arch Surg 1989; 124:29–32

17. Stomper PC, Connolly JL. Mammographic features predicting an extensive intraductal component in early-stage infiltrating ductal carcinoma. AJR 1992; 158:269–272

LOBULAR CARCINOMA *IN SITU*

18. Beute BJ, Kalisher L, Hutter RV. Lobular carcinoma *in situ* of the breast: clinical, pathologic, and mammographic features. AJR 1991; 157:257–265

19. Haagensen CD, Lane N, Lattes R, Bodian C. Lobular neoplasia (so-called lobular carcinoma *in situ*) of the breast. Cancer 1978; 42:737–769

20. Hutter RV, Snyder RE, Lucas JC, Foote FW Jr, Farrow JH. Clinical and pathologic correlation with mammographic findings in lobular carcinoma *in situ*. Cancer 1969; 23:826–839

21. Page DL, Anderson TJ, Rogers LW. Carcinoma *in situ* (CIS). In: Page DL, Anderson TJ (eds), Diagnostic histopathology of the breast. New York: Churchill Livingstone; 1987:157–192

22. Rosen PP, Kosloff C, Lieberman PH, Adair F, Braun DW Jr. Lobular carcinoma *in situ* of the breast. Detailed analysis of 99 patients with average follow-up of 24 years. Am J Surg Pathol 1978; 2:225–251

23. Sonnenfeld MR, Frenna TH, Weidner N, Meyer JE. Lobular carcinoma *in situ*: mammographic-pathologic correlation of results of needle-directed biopsy. Radiology 1991; 181:363–367

Notes

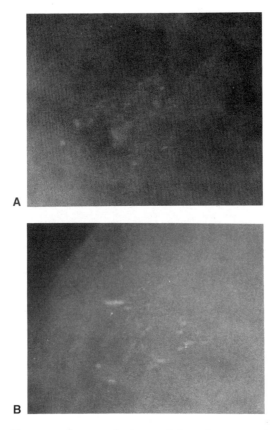

Figure 19-1. You are shown photographic enlargements of CC (A) and 90° mediolateral (B) spot-compression magnification views obtained following the first mammographic screening examination of a 50-year-old asymptomatic woman.

Case 19: Milk of Calcium in Tiny Benign Cysts

Question 85

Which *one* of the following is the MOST likely diagnosis?

(A) Fat necrosis
(B) Microcystic hyperplasia
(C) Ductal carcinoma *in situ*
(D) Lobular neoplasia
(E) Ductal ectasia

The cluster of approximately 30 microcalcifications seen in Figure 19-1 represents milk of calcium layering in the lower portions of the very tiny cysts that occur in microcystic hyperplasia **(Option (B) is correct).** This case illustrates several of the characteristic mammographic features that may be seen in this condition.

On the spot-compression magnification 90° mediolateral (ML) view (Figure 19-1B), some of the calcifications have meniscus shapes. Others appear as tiny linear densities. All are oriented in a parallel fashion along the horizontal axis. These features are usually harder to see on a nonmagnified 90° ML view (Figure 19-2) or on a magnified MLO view and are hardest to see on a nonmagnified MLO view (Figure 19-3).

Meniscus- and linear-shaped calcifications are not evident on the CC projection (Figure 19-1A) because this vertical-beam radiograph shows the calcifications as seen from above, thereby causing them to appear round, less dense, and often smudgy. This dramatic change in the appearance of the calcifications between CC and lateral projections is another feature characteristic of milk of calcium.

Although milk of calcium is frequently seen in multiple areas of the breast and is usually bilateral, it may be a diagnostic problem when present as a unilateral focus. If the condition is not correctly recognized, an unnecessary biopsy may be performed. When the diagnosis of milk of calcium is suspected on routine views, spot-compression magnification

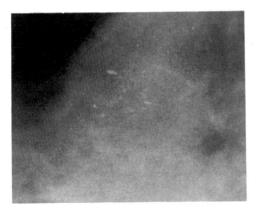

Figure 19-2 (left). Same patient as in Figure 19-1. Milk of calcium in tiny benign cysts. Photographic enlargement of the calcifications on a nonmagnified 90° ML view. Typical features of milk of calcium are less well demonstrated than on the comparable spot-compression magnification view (Figure 19-1B).

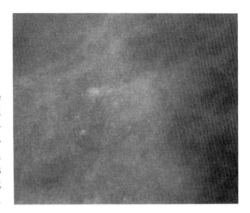

Figure 19-3 (right). Same patient as in Figures 19-1 and 19-2. Milk of calcium in tiny benign cysts. A photographic enlargement of the calcifications on a nonmagnified MLO view does not show any features to suggest milk of calcium.

views in 90° ML and CC projections should be obtained to elicit the characteristic features of this condition so that the calcifications are not mistaken for ductal carcinoma *in situ* (Option (C)) or lobular neoplasia (Option (D)).

The calcifications in fat necrosis (Option (A)) can be curvilinear. However, this represents calcification within the walls of lipoid cysts rather than calcific debris suspended in fluid. Since these calcifications do not sediment, there are no consistent differences between their appearances on vertical- and horizontal-beam projection mammograms.

The calcifications in ductal ectasia (Option (E)) are elongated rods of wide caliber, with a typical distribution (see Case 17). These calcifications should be readily distinguished from those seen with microcystic hyperplasia.

Question 86

Characteristics of calcifications in microcysts as seen on a lateral view include:

(A) crescent shape
(B) semilunar shape
(C) horizontal orientation
(D) upper margins better defined than lower margins
(E) appearance similar to that on the CC view

Milk of calcium represents calcified debris that has sedimented in the dependent portions of cystically dilated acini. These tiny cystic structures are one stage in a sequence of development that progresses to gross cysts. First, there is an increase in the number of acini in a lobule (adenosis), as a result of lobular hyperplasia (see Cases 17 and 18). The acini then dilate (blunt duct adenosis) and subsequently undergo further dilatation (microcystic adenosis), which eventually can extend beyond lobular boundaries to form larger microcysts and eventually gross cysts.

The milk of calcium within these tiny cysts can appear as curvilinear calcifications that measure 0.5 to 1.5 mm in length. The shapes of these calcifications have also been described as meniscus, crescent, teacup, and semilunar **(Options (A) and (B) are true).** All milk of calcium should have a convex lower margin on a 90° lateral view. Those calcifications that are curvilinear and have a concave upper surface are best described as meniscus- or crescent-shaped. Other calcifications that have a flat upper surface should be termed teacup- or semilunar-shaped.

The meniscus or crescent shape is best seen on an erect 90° lateral projection since the X-ray beam is horizontal and therefore tangential to the cyst fluid-calcium interface. This characteristic appearance may not be seen as well on a 45° MLO view (Figure 19-4). On the 90° lateral view, the tops of these calcifications will be oriented parallel to one another along the horizontal axis **(Option (C) is true).**

Another helpful distinguishing feature of the meniscus or crescent shape is that the upper convex border of the meniscus (where calcific debris and noncalcified cyst fluid gradually merge) is less distinct than the lower convex border where calcific debris is sharply bounded by the cyst wall **(Option (D) is false).**

The curvilinear shapes of sedimented calcium cannot be demonstrated on the CC projection since the X-ray beam is vertical and therefore perpendicular to the cyst fluid-calcium interface. Here, the calcifications are seen *en face*. They can appear as discrete punctate, clustered densities in the central (lowermost) portion of the cyst (Figure 19-5). However, since most sedimented material represents true milk of calcium (suspended calcific debris rather than discrete particles) and since

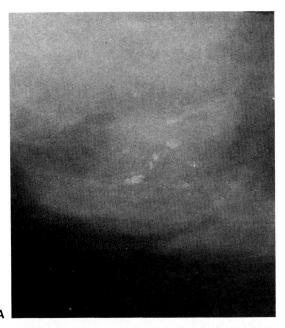

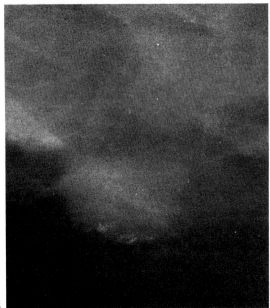

Figure 19-4. Milk of calcium in tiny benign cysts. (A) A spot-compression magnification MLO view of a 45-year-old woman demonstrates nonspecific calcifications in the lower breast. (B) A spot-compression magnification 90° lateral view of the same calcifications reveals that they have meniscus shapes and are located in the dependent portion of a 1-cm multiloculated mass.

the vertically oriented X-ray beam is transmitted through calcium of lesser thickness, the calcifications can also appear as poorly defined plaquelike smudges or even be so faint as to be invisible **(Option (E) is false).**

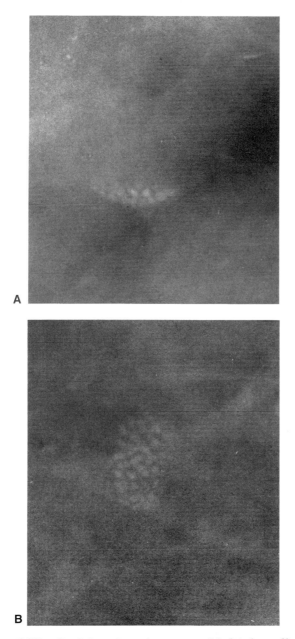

Figure 19-5. Milk of calcium in a 1-cm cyst. Multiple well-defined particles sediment in lowermost (central) portion of a large cyst to form a crescent pattern on the spot-compression magnification lateral view (A) and
an oval pattern on the spot-compression magnification CC view (B).

Question 87

In a solitary cluster of microcalcifications, the characteristic MOST suspicious for malignancy is:

(A) variation in density
(B) variation in size
(C) oval shape
(D) number of calcifications more than 10
(E) dot-dash appearance

Although certain types and patterns of calcifications are pathognomonic of a benign process and others provide a very strong indication of malignancy, many are indeterminate. A number of criteria have been used to estimate the likelihood of malignancy for an isolated cluster of microcalcifications in order to determine whether biopsy is indicated. Some criteria are more useful than others.

The mammographic feature most suspicious for malignancy is a dot-dash pattern **(Option (E) is correct).** This pattern contains two different features, either of which by itself would be highly suggestive of malignancy (see Figures 17-1 and 17-9). The "dash" component refers to the presence of a thin linear microcalcification (width, ≤1 mm; length, ≤3 mm). This has also been termed a "casting type" calcification since it forms a cast of that portion of the duct in which it occurs. Its presence indicates that an abnormal ductal process is causing production and subsequent calcification of necrotic debris within the duct. This type of calcification indicates a strong probability of malignancy, particularly comedo ductal carcinoma *in situ*.

The second feature of the dot-dash pattern is the linear arrangement of "dots" (nonlinear calcifications that can be irregular, oval, or round) and "dashes," also suggesting an intraductal process. This too is highly suspicious for ductal carcinoma *in situ*.

Management of clusters containing more than 10 calcifications (Option (D)) should be determined in part by the presence of other, similar-appearing calcifications in the same or opposite breast. If such a cluster does not appear significantly different from those seen in other areas, it is most likely due to a benign process such as adenosis and can be managed by follow-up alone (see Case 18). When such calcifications occur as an isolated cluster, spot-compression magnification mammography and other supplementary views will often be helpful in documenting either benign or malignant characteristics to determine whether biopsy is indicated (Figure 19-1).

The classic studies on microcalcifications, reported by Leborgne from 1949–1951, were the first to document that calcifications can be the sole mammographic manifestation of carcinoma. Although Leborgne described them as "tiny, dot-like, and resembling fine grains of salt," subsequent investigators have been unable to separate calcifications smaller than 2 mm into benign or malignant types simply on the basis of their size. Although some experts consider variation in size (Option (B)) as suggestive of malignancy, this criterion is often hard to apply due to the small size of the particles and the resolution limitations of mammography. Smooth, round particles of identical size, especially when they measure 2 mm or more, suggest a benign process. However, variation in the size of calcific particles is the rule rather than the exception and can be seen in both benign and malignant disease.

Oval calcifications (Option (C)) are more likely to be benign than are rod-shaped or irregular calcifications. However, smooth-bordered oval calcifications do not always indicate a benign process.

Although malignant calcifications have been described as typically dense, many experts believe there is no difference in radiologic density between benign and malignant particles. Variations in density among calcific particles (Option (A)) and within individual particles suggest malignancy to some investigators but not to others. Moreover, variation in density is hard to assess among particles that themselves vary in size.

Question 88

Characteristics of secretory calcifications include:

(A) location in the duct wall
(B) polarity toward the nipple
(C) smoothly tapered shape
(D) hollow, cylindrical shape
(E) unilaterality

On gross pathologic inspection, the ducts of patients with secretory disease will be filled with thick secretions (see Case 17). Distended ducts can burst, releasing their secretions into the surrounding tissues. An inflammatory reaction consisting of lipid-filled macrophages, plasma cells, and lymphocytes ensues. Periductal fibrosis, parenchymal scarring, nipple retraction, and calcifications represent late sequelae. Secretory disease has also been termed duct ectasia, plasma cell mastitis, and comedomastitis.

Calcifications in secretory disease can be located in the duct lumen or duct wall **(Option (A) is true),** or they can be periductal. Those in the duct lumen appear as long solid cores. Calcifications in the duct wall and periductal calcifications can be equally long but are usually much wider,

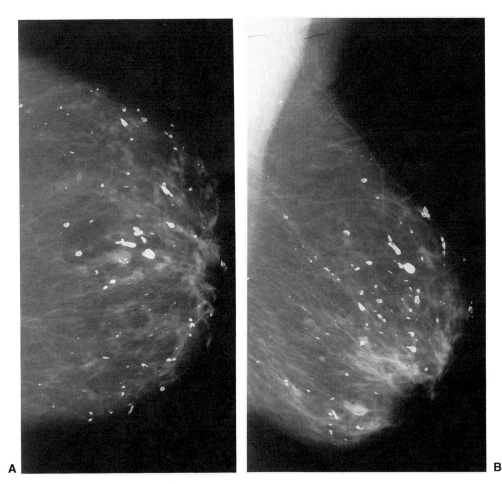

A   B

Figure 19-6. Secretory calcifications. Hollow cylindrical calcifications located in the walls of ectatic ducts in a patient with secretory disease can be seen on the CC (A) and MLO (B) views. The central lucency within each calcification represents the nonopacified duct lumen.

especially if the duct is distended (Figure 19-6). Since calcifications in the sides of a duct wall are projected tangentially, they appear denser than those projected *en face* and produce a hollow cylindrical appearance **(Option (D) is true).**

The distribution of secretory calcifications is orderly and dispersed, in contrast to the focal clustered distribution of malignant calcifications. The long axes of secretory calcifications follow the course of the ducts, branching out in a series of arcs that radiate from the retroareolar region, thereby assuming an overall polarity toward the nipple **(Option (B) is true).**

Another characteristic of secretory calcifications is that each one has a smoothly tapered shape **(Option (C) is true).** Individual calcifications usually have areas of increasing and decreasing caliber along their long axis, but these regions of widening and narrowing occur gradually. This appearance represents another distinguishing feature from malignant linear calcifications.

Secretory calcifications tend to be bilateral **(Option (E) is false),** still another feature that contributes to the relative ease with which they can be distinguished from malignancy. However, secretory calcifications that occur unilaterally, especially when confined to a localized area of the breast, provide a greater diagnostic challenge.

Stephen A. Feig, M.D.

SUGGESTED READINGS

MICROCYSTIC HYPERPLASIA

1. Homer MJ, Cooper AG, Pile-Spellman ER. Milk of calcium in breast microcysts: manifestation as a solitary focal disease. AJR 1988; 150:789–790
2. Lanyi M. Diagnosis and differential diagnosis of breast calcifications. New York: Springer-Verlag; 1988:29–81
3. Linden SS, Sickles EA. Sedimented calcium in benign breast cysts: the full spectrum of mammographic presentations. AJR 1989; 152:967–971
4. Sickles EA. Further experience with microfocal spot magnification mammography in assessment of clustered breast microcalcifications. Radiology 1980; 137:9–14
5. Sickles EA, Abele JS. Milk of calcium within tiny benign breast cysts. Radiology 1981; 141:655–658

FAT NECROSIS

6. Bassett LW, Gold RH, Cove HC. Mammographic spectrum of traumatic fat necrosis: the fallibility of "pathognomonic" signs of carcinoma. AJR 1978; 130:119–122
7. Lanyi M. Diagnosis and differential diagnosis of breast calcifications. New York: Springer-Verlag; 1988:157–173

BIOPSY CRITERIA FOR CALCIFICATIONS

8. Bjurstam NG. Radiology of the female breast and axilla. Acta Radiol 1978; Suppl 357:1–131
9. Egan RL, McSweeney MB, Sewell CW. Intramammary calcifications without an associated mass in benign and malignant diseases. Radiology 1980; 137:1–7

10. Leborgne R. Diagnosis of tumors of the breast by simple roentgenography: calcifications in carcinomas. AJR 1951; 65:1–11

11. Millis RR, Davis R, Stacey AJ. The detection and significance of calcifications in the breast: a radiological and pathological study. Br J Radiol 1976; 49:12–26

12. Moskowitz M. The predictive value of certain mammographic signs in screening for breast cancer. Cancer 1983; 51:1007–1011

13. Murphy WA, DeSchryver-Kecskemeti K. Isolated clustered microcalcifications in the breast: radiologic-pathologic correlation. Radiology 1978; 127:335–341

14. Sickles EA. Breast calcifications: mammographic evaluation. Radiology 1986; 160:289–293

15. Sigfüsson BF, Andersson I, Aspegren K, Janzon L, Linell F, Ljungberg O. Clustered breast calcifications. Acta Radiol [Diagn] (Stockh) 1983; 24:273–281

16. Wolfe JN. Xeroradiography of the breast, 2nd ed. Springfield, IL: Charles C Thomas; 1983:516–544

SECRETORY CALCIFICATIONS

17. Gershon-Cohen J, Ingleby H, Hermel MB. Calcifications in secretory disease of the breast. AJR 1956; 76:132–135

18. Ingleby H, Gershon-Cohen J. Comparative anatomy, pathology and roentgenology of the breast. Philadelphia: University of Pennsylvania; 1960:237–265

Notes

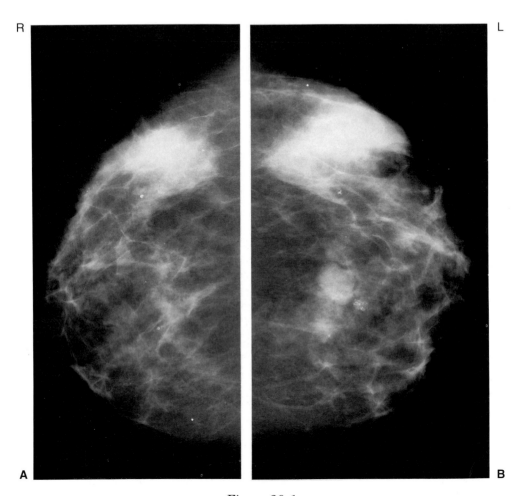

R   L

A   B

Figure 20-1

Figures 20-1 and 20-2. You are shown CC (A and B) and MLO (C and D) views of both breasts from the first screening examination of a 40-year-old asymptomatic woman with no breast cancer risk factors (Figure 20-1). Spot-compression magnification CC (A) and MLO (B) views of the left breast obtained following this screening examination are also shown (Figure 20-2).

Case 20: Calcification in a Circumscribed Mass

Question 89

The NEXT step should be:

(A) ultrasonography
(B) biopsy
(C) follow-up mammography in 6 months
(D) follow-up mammography in 1 year
(E) follow-up mammography in 2 years

A 0.8-cm circumscribed mass containing approximately 35 irregular calcifications is present in the upper inner quadrant of the left breast. The calcifications are irregular and vary in size, shape, and density. They are diffusely distributed throughout the central portion of the mass. No other similar calcifications can be seen in either breast. However, a circumscribed noncalcified lobulated 2.5-cm mass is adjacent to the calcified mass.

The calcific pattern indicates that the mass is solid and not a cyst. The appearance is consistent with either a calcified fibroadenoma or a circumscribed carcinoma. Ultrasonography (Option (A)) would not be useful since it cannot reliably distinguish benign from malignant solid masses. Moreover, microcalcifications frequently cannot be demonstrated on ultrasonography due to their small size and the difficulty in distinguishing them from other specular reflectors in the soft tissues. Ultrasonography does not provide relevant clinical information about microcalcifications.

Since the appearance of the calcified mass is moderately suspicious for carcinoma, follow-up in 6 months, 1 year, or 2 years (Options (C), (D), and (E)) would not be reasonable alternatives. Lack of change does not avert the need for biopsy. Malignant masses and calcifications can maintain a stable mammographic appearance for 3 years or longer. Proper

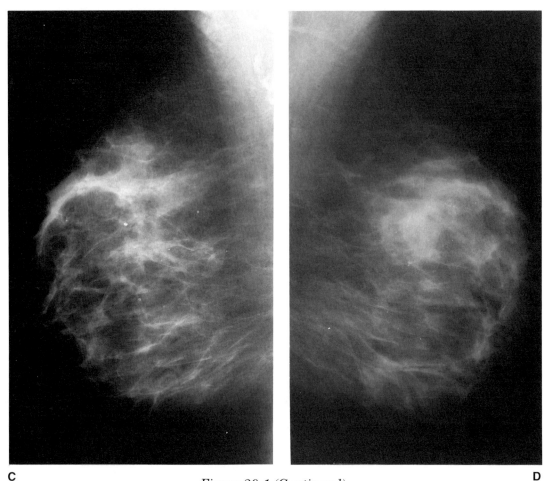

C

D

Figure 20-1 (Continued)

management involves biopsy to provide a tissue diagnosis **(Option (B) is correct).**

Excisional biopsy was performed in the test patient and demonstrated a partially calcified fibroadenoma. This case represents atypical calcification in a fibroadenoma, which is indistinguishable from malignant calcification.

Calcifications in a mass seen on mammography do not necessarily indicate the diagnosis of fibroadenoma unless they are either of the very large "popcorn" type or preferentially concentrated along the circumference of the mass. If calcifications are eccentric but not at the periphery of a mass, the lesion may still be malignant.

Although it is conceivable that follow-up in 1 or 2 years would have allowed the fibroadenoma to further calcify and present a more typical

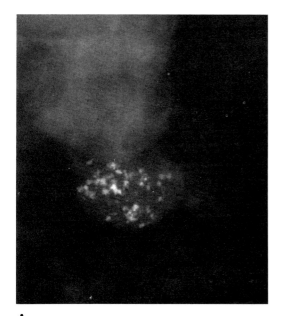
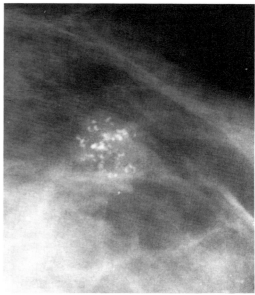

A   *Figure 20-2*   B

appearance, this is unlikely since fibroadenomatous calcifications usually develop slowly over many years. Deferring a biopsy would have risked progression of a possible malignancy, as well as loss of the patient to follow-up.

Question 90

Distributions of fine calcifications in a circumscribed mass indicating that it is benign include:

    (A) predominantly central
    (B) eccentric
    (C) diffuse
    (D) predominantly marginal
    (E) ringlike peripheral

Fine calcifications (<2 mm) can be found in either benign or malignant circumscribed masses. A benign diagnosis can be made with certainty only when such calcifications are concentrated more along or near the margin of a mass than in the central portion of the mass or when they form a complete ring around the periphery of the mass (Figure 20-3) **(Options (D) and (E) are true).** In the absence of a definite mass, it is

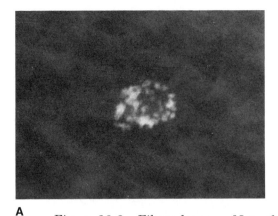
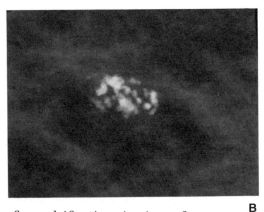

A

B

Figure 20-3. Fibroadenoma. Note the fine calcifications in circumferential distribution within a circumscribed mass in these spot-compression magnification CC (A) and MLO (B) views.

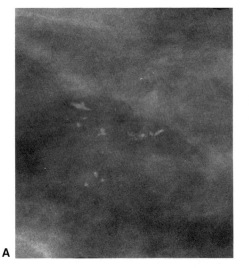
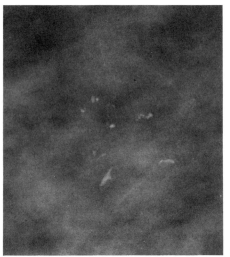

A

B

Figure 20-4. Ductal carcinoma *in situ*. Random distribution of irregular and linear calcifications in ductal carcinoma *in situ* should not be mistaken for the ringlike distribution of calcifications occasionally seen at the margins of a benign mass. In these spot-compression CC (A) and MLO (B) projection images, no mass is seen.

important not to mistake a random distribution of suspicious microcalcifications for a benign ringlike distribution (Figure 20-4).

Fine calcifications with a predominantly central, eccentric (Figure 20-5), or diffuse (Figure 20-6) distribution in a circumscribed mass can

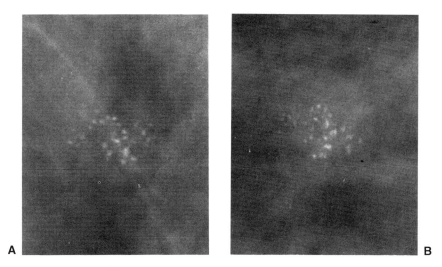

Figure 20-5. Ductal carcinoma *in situ*. Eccentric distribution of fine calcifications in a mass shown on spot-compression magnification views in CC (A) and MLO (B) projections.

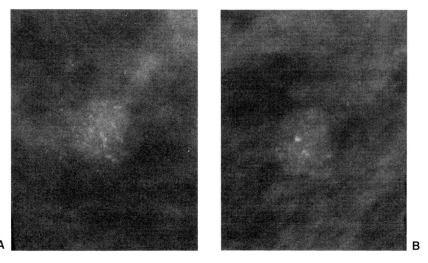

Figure 20-6. Ductal carcinoma *in situ*. Diffuse distribution of fine calcifications in a circumscribed mass can be seen in spot-compression magnification CC (A) and MLO (B) views.

represent ductal carcinoma *in situ* **(Options (A), (B), and (C) are false),** although fibroadenoma is still a major differential diagnostic possibility. Mitnick et al. reported the empiric observation that some lesions with this type of appearance were found to be malignant on biopsy. However, the relative frequency of carcinoma versus fibroadenoma for these types of calcifications is not known since no biopsy data from a series of benign and malignant lesions with this appearance have yet been published.

Question 91

Distributions of coarse calcifications in a circumscribed mass indicating the need for biopsy include:

(A) predominantly central
(B) eccentric
(C) diffuse
(D) predominantly marginal

A circumscribed mass with coarse calcifications ($\geq$2 mm) is more likely to be benign than is one with fine calcifications. Nevertheless, coarse calcifications in a predominantly central, eccentric (Figure 20-7), or diffuse distribution do not necessarily indicate that a mass is benign, and biopsy may be necessary in some cases **(Options (A), (B), and (C) are true).** Only when coarse calcifications are predominantly distributed along the margins of a mass (Figure 20-8) is a benign diagnosis of fibroadenoma assured **(Option (D) is false).**

Carcinoma arising within a fibroadenoma is rare. Since fibroadenomas that harbor cancer can be indistinguishable from the usual benign fibroadenomas, biopsy of a circumscribed indeterminate mass is usually not indicated unless the mass is solid and large or has such features as indistinct margins, suspicious calcifications, or increasing size. In addition, unless the mammographic features suggest invasive cancer, the cancer within a fibroadenoma is likely to represent *in situ* disease. In one report by Baker et al. of 24 cancers arising within fibroadenomas, only one was invasive. All of the other lesions were lobular carcinoma *in situ* or ductal carcinoma *in situ*.

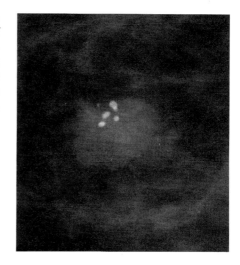

Figure 20-7 (right). Fibroadenoma. Eccentric distribution of coarse calcifications in a circumscribed mass. Biopsy was performed since this appearance could also be compatible with a carcinoma.

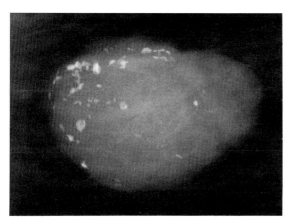

A

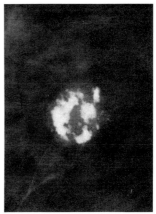

B

C

Figure 20-8 (above and left). Peripheral calcifications in three fibroadenomas. (A) Predominantly peripheral distribution of coarse calcifications in a circumscribed mass. (B) Peripheral distribution of coarse calcifications in a circumscribed mass. (C) Peripheral distribution of two coarse calcifications in a circumscribed mass.

Question 92

Types of calcifications in a circumscribed mass indicating that it is benign include:

(A) irregular shape, ringlike distribution
(B) thick, curvilinear, peripheral distribution
(C) thin, curvilinear distribution
(D) plaquelike
(E) popcornlike

Regardless of their size or shape, calcifications distributed in a ring-like fashion around the periphery of a mass indicate that it is benign **(Option (A) is true).** The differential diagnosis includes fibroadenoma, calcified cyst, lipoid cyst, and fat necrosis (see Figure 17-10).

Curvilinear calcifications along the periphery of a mass are always indicative of benign disease whether or not the calcifications extend around the entire circumference of the mass and whether or not they are thick or thin and eggshell-like (Figure 20-9) **(Options (B) and (C) are true).**

Thin curvilinear calcifications extending across a sufficient area on the surface of a circumscribed mass that are projected *en face* appear as plaquelike calcifications (Figure 20-10A). These lesions are always benign **(Option (D) is true).**

Popcornlike calcifications (Figure 20-10B) are very large, coarse, and amorphous. Regardless of their location in a circumscribed mass, they indicate that the mass represents a fibroadenoma **(Option (E) is true).**

Stephen A. Feig, M.D.

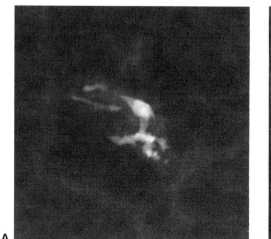
A

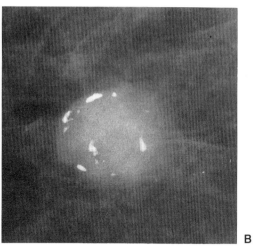
B

Figure 20-9. Curvilinear calcifications in two fibroadenomas. Thick (A) and thin (B) curvilinear calcifications are seen at the margins of these circumscribed masses.

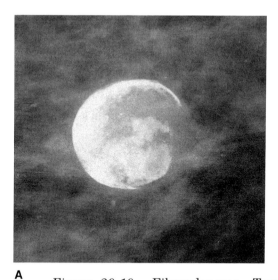
A

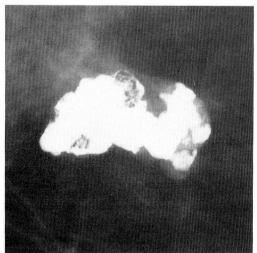
B

Figure 20-10. Fibroadenoma. Two examples of fibroadenoma show plaquelike (A) and popcornlike (B) calcifications.

SUGGESTED READINGS

CALCIFICATIONS IN FIBROADENOMA

1. Baker KS, Monsees BS, Diaz NM, Destouet JM, McDivitt RW. Carcinoma within fibroadenomas: mammographic features. Radiology 1990; 176:371–374
2. Cole-Beuglet C, Soriano RZ, Kurtz AB, Goldberg BB. Fibroadenoma of the breast: sonomammography correlated with pathology in 122 patients. AJR 1983; 140:369–375
3. Jackson VP, Rothschild PA, Kreipke DL, Mail JT, Holden RW. The spectrum of sonographic findings of fibroadenoma of the breast. Invest Radiol 1986; 21:34–40
4. Lanyi M. Diagnosis and differential diagnosis of breast calcifications. New York: Springer-Verlag; 1988:145–156
5. Meyer JE, Frenna TH, Polger M, Sonnenfeld MR, Shaffer K. Enlarging occult fibroadenomas. Radiology 1992; 183:639–641

CALCIFICATIONS IN CIRCUMSCRIBED CARCINOMA

6. Mitnick JS, Roses DF, Harris MN, Feiner HD. Circumscribed intraductal carcinoma of the breast. Radiology 1989; 170:423–425

Notes

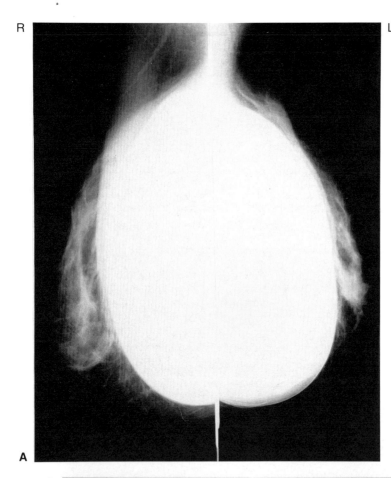

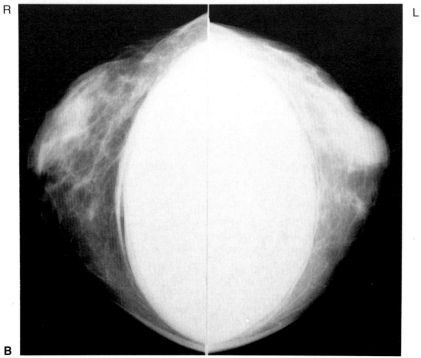

Figure 21-1. You are shown standard MLO (A) and CC (B) mammograms of augmented breasts.

Case 21: Mammography of the Augmented Breast

Question 93

The mammograms demonstrate:

    (A) double-lumen implants
    (B) subpectoral implants
    (C) leakage of silicone
    (D) capsular contracture
    (E) capsular calcification

Augmentation implants are available as single-lumen devices containing either silicone or saline and as double-lumen devices containing silicone in the inner envelope and saline in the outer envelope or saline in the inner envelope and silicone in the outer envelope. The test images (Figure 21-1) demonstrate implants consisting of a higher-density silicone-filled inner envelope and a lower-density saline-filled outer envelope (Figure 21-2A) **(Option (A) is true).** Implants can be placed under the glandular tissue of the breast, directly anterior to the pectoral fascia (subglandular or intramammary), or they can be placed under the pectoral muscle (subpectoral or submuscular). The layer of pectoral muscle over the implant may be so thin that it cannot be seen mammographically. Usually, however, as in the test patient, the pectoral muscle can be identified on the MLO view reflecting over the upper contour of the implant (Figure 21-2A) **(Option (B) is true).** Only occasionally, the pectoral muscle can be identified on the CC view (Figure 21-2B). With subglandular (intramammary) placement of the implant, the anterior margin of the pectoral muscle shows no anterior reflection but is directed behind the implant (Figure 21-3).

There are no radiographic findings to suggest silicone leakage **(Option (C) is false).** Implant rupture and leakage are discussed below (See Question 97).

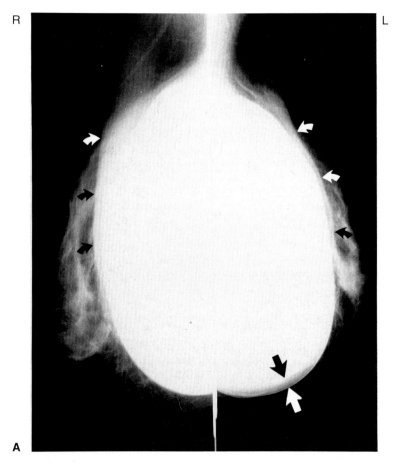

R

L

A

Figure 21-2 (Same as Figure 21-1). Mammographic appearance of subpectoral, double-lumen implants. Note the pectoral muscles (curved
arrows) over and in front of the implants, indicating subpectoral placement. The lower-density area between the straight arrows over the inferior aspect of the implant on the left breast MLO view (Figure 21-2A)
indicates a small rim of the saline-filled outer envelope of the double-
lumen implant. The more radiodense inner lumen is filled with silicone.

Fibrous capsular contracture around an implant is a common physio-
logical response, representing an attempt to wall off a foreign body; it
occurs most commonly in the first 6 months after surgery. The reported
frequency varies widely, from 0 to 75%. Contracture can occur bilaterally
or in only one breast, leaving the contralateral breast unaffected. The
contracting capsule deforms the contour of the implant, changing the
normal teardrop shape into a ball-like appearance, especially as seen in
the MLO projection. The process of capsular contracture may not be uniform. Occasionally, constriction bands form, creating deforming bulges in

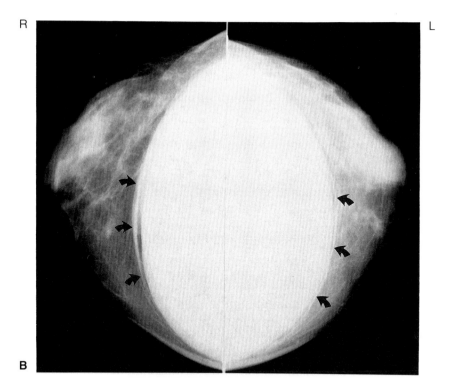

the implant contour (Figure 21-4) (See Question 96). However, none of the mammographic signs of encapsulation are present in the test images **(Option (D) is false)**.

There are no visible calcifications surrounding the implant in the test images **(Option (E) is false)**. Calcification can be very difficult to detect without overexposed images (Figure 21-4).

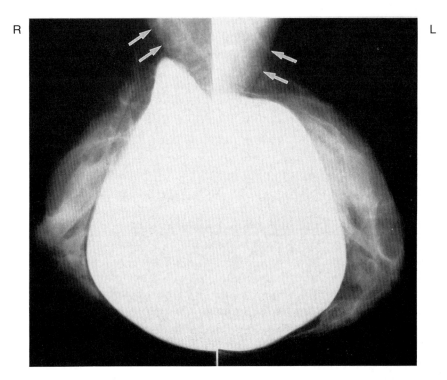

Figure 21-3. Mammographic appearance of subglandular implants. Standard MLO mammograms of a patient with bilateral augmentation implants confirm the subglandular placement of these implants by the appearance of the pectoral muscles extending posteriorly behind the implants (arrows). Compare this appearance with that of Figure 21-2, which illustrates subpectoral implants. Also, in this figure the "bulge" of silicone density toward the axilla on the right is a "reducible" herniation of the implant through the fibrous capsule, and not a perforation.

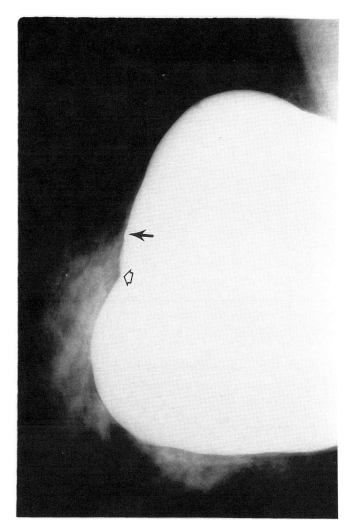

Figure 21-4.
Mammographic
appearance of
nonuniform cap-
sular contracture
around an im-
plant. A standard
MLO view of right
breast shows an
encapsulated
subglandular im-
plant with a fi-
brous constric-
tion band (open
arrow). A plaque
of calcium in the
fibrous capsule is
barely percepti-
ble (solid arrow).
Calcifications in
the capsule are
better seen on
overexposed
films taken with
higher kVp.

Question 94

The NEXT step should be:

    (A) ultrasonography
    (B) modified compression mammography
    (C) axillary mammographic view
    (D) CT scan
    (E) MRI

Ultrasonography (Option (A)) is not beneficial as a routine imaging
procedure and should be used as a problem-solving tool in the evaluation

of palpable or mammographically detected masses, just as for nonaugmented breasts. Ultrasonography also can be useful in the evaluation of suspected pockets of extra-luminal silicone or in the evaluation of intracapsular implant rupture.

Standard CC and MLO projection mammograms are important for visualizing both the most posterior tissues surrounding the implant and the implant itself. However, with the implant included in the field of view, the native breast tissue that is superimposed on the image of the implant will be obscured. In addition, compression is severely limited by the presence of an implant, so that native tissue surrounding the periphery of the implant remains relatively uncompressed. When the full implant is included in the field of compression, only sufficient compression to immobilize the breast is necessary. Excessive compression on the implant itself risks damage to the implant and does nothing to improve visualization of native breast tissue. Our imaging goal for all patients, including those with implants, remains optimal visualization of as much breast tissue as possible, with proper compression.

To maximize visualization of native breast tissue and achieve proper compression, the implant must be excluded from the field of compression. Several factors influence the degree to which this goal can be achieved: (1) the relative compressibility of the implant (lack of encapsulation), (2) the relative mobility of the implant, (3) the size of the implant in relation to the amount of residual native breast tissue (implant/native-tissue ratio) and (4) the location of the implant (subglandular versus subpectoral). If there has been no firm fibrous encapsulation and the implant is not so large that skin and native tissue are tightly stretched over the implant surface (simulating capsular contracture), the implant may be soft enough to flatten against the chest wall. Indeed, in the absence of firm encapsulation, many implants are sufficiently mobile on the chest wall that they can be moved out of the field of compression. Subpectoral implants, which are less prone to firm encapsulation, have the effect of projecting the entire breast and the underlying pectoral fascia anteriorly.

Depending on the degree to which these various factors are present, the implant can be moved out of the field of compression or else flattened against the chest wall and the native breast tissue can be pulled over and in front of the implant, enabling compression to be limited to native breast tissue alone (Figure 21-5). This modified compression technique, now called the implant-displaced (ID) view, enables visualization of more and better-compressed native breast tissue in most patients and should be included routinely in mammographic imaging of patients with implants **(Option (B) is correct)** (Figure 21-6). If an implant is firmly encapsulated, it is usually relatively immobile and cannot be flattened against the chest wall. In this circumstance, the only modified technique

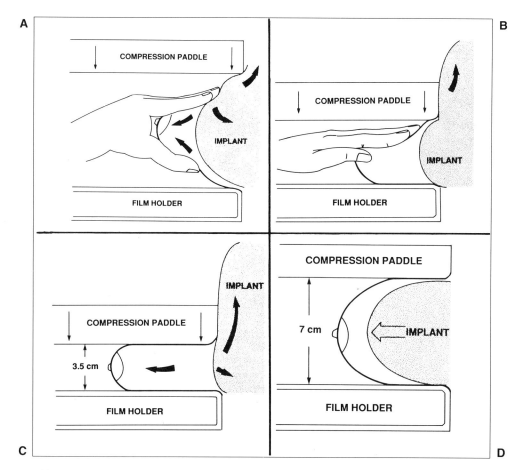

Figure 21-5. Illustrations demonstrating the modified compression technique for implant-displaced views. (A) Breast tissue is being pulled over and in front of the implant while the implant is pushed back against the chest wall. (B) As compression is applied and the compression paddle engages the convex contour of the implant, the paddle forces the implant back posteriorly, keeping the implant out of the field of view, flattened against the chest wall. (C) If the implant is soft and compressible and the native breast tissue is not tightly stretched over the implant, significantly more native tissue can be visualized anterior to the implant when little or no implant remains in the field. With standard compression images, which include the implant in the field of view, it is important to understand that the native tissue visualized is the tissue surrounding the implant and that this tissue will be poorly compressed because of the limitation on compression imposed by the implant. (D) Compression directly on the implant causes the implant to expand circumferentially, moving the outer wall of the silicone envelope toward the skin. This has the effect of making the surrounding breast tissue more "compact" and appear more dense due to the limited compression. The only purpose of compression with the standard views, which include the implant, is to immobilize the breast.

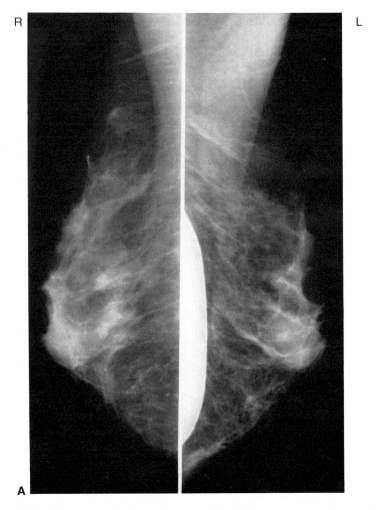

Figure 21-6. Implant-displaced views. Modified compression technique used in MLO (A) and CC (B) projections of the test patient shows that most of the native breast tissue is visualized and effectively compressed without the implants remaining in the field of view (compare with Figure 21-1). A small portion of implant is seen on the left MLO view, and a trace of implant is seen on the posterior edge of the left CC image (arrowhead). The arrows mark the anterior margins of the pectoral muscles seen on both CC views.

available for achieving good compression is to pull as much breast tissue as possible over and in front of the implant, limiting compression to the tissue anterior to the implant. Although some breast tissue is inevitably excluded from view under such circumstances, more native breast tissue can be visualized than when only standard views (which include the implant) are used.

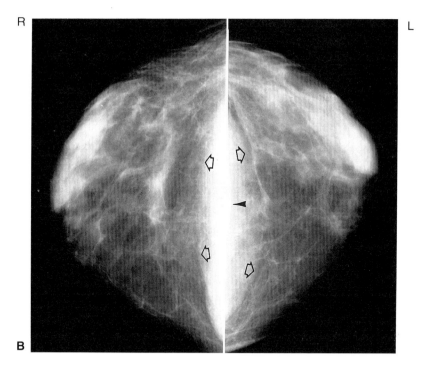

Axillary views (Option (C)) are appropriate only if there is concern about clinical axillary findings or for evaluation of axillary densities that are incompletely imaged by standard and ID CC or MLO views.

CT scanning and MRI (Options (D) and (E)) have the advantage of being able to visualize the entire circumference of the implant and therefore can be useful in evaluation of suspected implant rupture. MRI seems to have the greatest sensitivity and specificity. However, cost considerations certainly will limit routine use of CT scanning or MRI.

Question 95

Concerning mammography of the augmented breast,

(A) detection of lesions is easier in patients with saline-filled implants than in those with silicone-filled implants
(B) phototiming should not be used for implant-displaced views
(C) by including implant-displaced views, the augmented breast is imaged as completely as the breast without an implant
(D) it is essential to use a high-kVp technique

Saline is less radiodense than silicone, but both provide sufficient density to obscure superimposed breast parenchyma and early signs of breast cancer. Therefore, saline offers no significant advantage over silicone in mammographic imaging **(Option (A) is false)**.

With standard CC and MLO views, the photocell is positioned partially or completely under the implant, resulting in very high levels of exposure and "burn out" of the surrounding native breast tissue when phototiming technique is used. Whenever the photocell is positioned to "see" areas that are too dense (implants) or much more radiolucent (air) than breast tissue, manual technique should be used to achieve appropriate exposure of the surrounding parenchyma. However, ID views are also part of the routine imaging of women with implants. Phototimed technique should be used for the ID views, because the implant will not overlie the photocell **(Option (B) is false)**.

In some patients virtually all of the breast parenchyma can be visualized free of the implant with modified compression technique. However, in most patients with augmentation implants, some breast tissue will be obscured, even with the added benefits of ID views. It is a mistake to suggest to patients or referring physicians that the augmented breast can be imaged as completely as the nonaugmented breast **(Option (C) is false)**.

High-kVp technique is required only to penetrate very dense glandular tissue; it serves no purpose in imaging the augmented breast, since the proper imaging goal is not to see through the implant **(Option (D) is false)**. Manual technique is used for the standard views that include the implants in the field, and 25 or 26 kVp (when combined with extended developer processing) is usually quite adequate for such exposures, keeping in mind that it is the native breast tissue that must be properly visualized.

Question 96

Concerning encapsulation of an implant,

    (A) it is the result of fibrosis developing around the implant wall

    (B) it occurs more often in patients with subglandular implants than in those with subpectoral implants

    (C) it is suggested by the shape of the implant on mammography

    (D) mammography is the most reliable method for its detection

    (E) calcium deposition occurs on the surface of the implant wall

    (F) firm encapsulation is a contraindication to mammography

The relatively common process of encapsulation involves the development of a sheet of fibrosis around the outer envelope or wall of the implant **(Option (A) is true)**. This phenomenon, which seems to be a host response to a foreign object, appears less commonly in patients with subpectoral implants than in those with subglandular implants **(Option (B) is true)**.

The process of encapsulation tends to mold the implant into a spherical or ball-like shape, causing it to lose the teardrop contour typical of soft, nonencapsulated implants on the MLO view **(Option (C) is true)**. Although the spherical shape of the implant on the MLO view is strongly suggestive of fibrous encapsulation, the lack of compressibility of the implant on physical examination is the most reliable method for identifying fibrous encapsulation **(Option (D) is false)**.

Calcium deposition around the implant is common, but calcium is deposited in the fibrous capsule, not on the implant wall itself **(Option (E) is false)**. Underexposed films may not reveal calcifications, whereas overexposed films may reveal more calcifications than do films ideally exposed for evaluation of native breast tissue. However, there is seldom any need to evaluate the extent of capsular calcification, which is regarded as an incidental finding of no great pathological significance. The presence of extensive calcification in the capsule can result in increased firmness of an encapsulated implant. Calcification is rarely seen without firm fibrous encapsulation, but firm fibrous encapsulation is common with no mammographic evidence of calcification.

Women with encapsulated implants are at no less risk for the development of breast cancer than are women without implants. Mammography remains the only reliable method for detection of clinically occult breast cancer; therefore, women with encapsulated implants should not be discouraged from participation in mammographic screening programs. Fibrous encapsulation may mean that less tissue can be visualized mammographically. As a result, additional views may be required to increase the amount of tissue seen. Patients with encapsulation also may not tolerate compression as well as those with soft implants; however, encapsulation is not a contraindication to mammography **(Option (F) is false).**

Question 97

Concerning implant rupture or leakage,

  (A) a soft, palpable bulge in the side of an implant is most likely a pocket of free silicone
  (B) peri-implant calcification is an important mammographic sign of silicone leakage
  (C) dense lymph nodes with loss of fatty hila suggest lymphatic sequestration of silicone
  (D) a closed capsulotomy occasionally results from compression during mammography
  (E) saline-filled implants are less prone to decompression than are silicone-filled implants

Collagen vascular diseases have been suggested, but not proven, to be related to the presence of free or extra-luminal silicone in breast-augmented patients. Scleroderma, systemic lupus, rheumatoid arthritis, Raynaud's disease, fibromyalgia, and psoriatic arthritis are a few of the conditions that have been implicated. Human leukocyte antigen has shown elevation in symptomatic patients with breast implants. Auto-antibodies also have been demonstrated in as many as 50% of symptomatic patients, probably in response to some component of silicone gel or the silicone envelope. However, these manifestations of immune response do not prove a connection between free silicone and autoimmune diseases. This subject has been, and continues to be, the target of several investigations, all of which have failed to show any definite association.

The recent media attention to possible adverse side effects from "free" silicone has caused the detection of extraluminal silicone to become a major concern of women with implants, who want to know if their implants are intact every time they undergo mammography. Because of the fear of rupture or leakage, soft bulges in the wall of an implant will often bring a patient to her doctor's office. The most common cause of this finding is a herniation of the outer implant wall through a weakened area in the fibrous capsule **(Option (A) is false).** Clinically, such a herniation presents as a soft bulge on palpation, usually "reducible" (Figure 21-7). Occasionally, pockets of extra-luminal silicone do present in this manner.

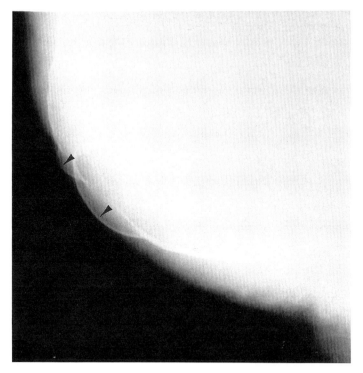

Figure 21-7. Mammographic appearance of implant herniation through its fibrous capsule. Bulges (arrowheads) seen along the outer margin of this subglandular saline implant were clinically palpable and raised concern about possible implant rupture. However, they represent herniations of the implant through areas of weakness in the surrounding fibrous capsule. They can be easily "reduced" with the tip of a finger, which can also palpate the defect in the fibrous capsule.

The presence of extra-luminal silicone can be suspected if small globules or islands of silicone density appear adjacent to the outer contour of the implant (Figure 21-8). The presence of calcification in the capsule bears no relationship to the presence of extraluminal silicone and should not be confused with free silicone **(Option (B) is false).** Silicone can be picked up by the lymphatics and carried to regional nodes, resulting in increased density of the nodes with "filling in" of the fatty hila. Unusually dense axillary nodes, especially with loss of the fatty hila, should raise the possibility of nodal sequestration of free silicone **(Option (C) is true).**

Again, because of media attention, undue anxiety about the risk of damage to implants during mammography has raised many questions in the minds of patients and their referring physicians. Rupture of the

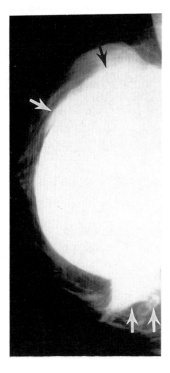

Figure 21-8. Mammographic appearance of free intramammary silicone. The implant has ruptured, and pockets of extraluminal silicone are visible adjacent to the implant envelope (arrows).

fibrous capsule surrounding the implant (closed capsulotomy) can occur but is a very uncommon complication of mammographic compression with standard MLO and CC views **(Option (D) is true).** Actual rupture of the implant during mammographic compression is extremely rare. It is important to understand that only minimal compression is required for the standard MLO and CC views, since immobilization of the breast is the primary purpose of compression when the implant is included in the field of view. Therefore, the risk of implant rupture as a result of compression is remote. With ID views, in which the implant is flattened against the chest wall or moved out of the field of view, the compression paddle is being applied to breast tissue anterior to the implant.

All implants can rupture as a result of direct trauma, such as seat belt injuries in auto accidents. Implants also have been known to decompress or leak spontaneously; however, spontaneous decompression appears to be more commonly associated with saline implants rather than with silicone implants **(Option (E) is false).**

G. W. Eklund, M.D.

SUGGESTED READINGS

1. Argenta LC. Migration of silicone gel into breast parenchyma following mammary breast prosthesis rupture. Anesthetic Plast Surg 1983; 7:253–254

2. Berg WA, Caskey CI, Hamper UM, et al. Diagnosing breast implant rupture with MR imaging, US, and mammography. RadioGraphics 1993; 1323–1336

3. Biggs TM, Yarish RS. Augmentation mammoplasty: retropectoral versus retromammary implantation. Clin Plast Surg 1988; 15:549–555

4. Burkhardt BR. Capsular contracture: hard breasts, soft data. Clin Plast Surg 1988; 15:521–532

5. DeBruhl ND, Gorczyca DP, Ahn CY, Shaw WW, Bassett LW. Silicone breast implants: US evaluation. Radiology 1993; 189:95–98

6. Destouet JM, Monsees BS, Oser RF, Nemecek JR, Young VL, Pilgram TK. Screening mammography in 350 women with breast implants: prevalence and findings of implant complications. AJR 1992; 159:973–978; discussion 979–981

7. Eklund GW. Diagnostic breast imaging in plastic surgery of the breast. In: Noone RB (ed), Plastic and reconstructive surgery of the breast. St. Louis: Mosby-Year Book; 1991:48–69

8. Eklund GW, Busby RC, Miller SM, Job JS. Improved imaging of the augmented breast. AJR 1988; 151:469–473

9. Fock KM, Feng PM, Tey BH. Autoimmune disease developing after augmentation mammoplasty: report of 3 cases. J Rheumatol 1984; 11:98–100

10. Ganott MA, Harris KM, Ilkhanipour ZS, Costa-Greco MA. Augmentation mammoplasty: normal and abnormal findings with mammography and US. RadioGraphics 1992; 12:281–295

11. Gorczyca DP, Sinha S, Ahn CY, et al. Silicone breast implants *in vivo*: MR imaging. Radiology 1992; 185:407–410

12. Grace GT, Roberts C, Cohen IK. The role of mammography in detecting breast cancer in augmented breasts. Ann Plast Surg 1990; 25:119–123

13. Harris KM, Ganott MA, Shestak KC, Losken HW, Tobon H. Silicone implant rupture: detection with US. Radiology 1993; 187:761–768

14. Liebman AJ, Kruse B. Breast cancer: mammographic and sonographic findings after augmentation mammoplasty. Radiology 1990; 174:195–198

15. Mendelson EB. Silicone implants present mammographic challenge. Diagn Imaging 1992; 14(9):70–76

16. Mund DF, Farria DM, Gorczyca DP, et al. MR imaging of the breast in patients with silicone-gel implants: spectrum of findings. AJR 1993; 161: 773–778

17. Rosculet KA, Ikeda DM, Forrest ME, et al. Ruptured gel-filled silicone breast implants: sonographic findings in 19 cases. AJR 1992; 159:711–716

18. Sahn EE, Garen PD, Silver RM, Maize JC. Scleroderma following augmentation mammoplasty. Report of a case and review of the literature. Arch Dermatol 1990; 126:1198–1202

19. Steinbach BG, Hardt NS, Abbitt PL. Mammography: breast implants—types, complications, and adjacent breast pathology. Curr Probl Diagn Radiol 1993; 22:39–86

20. Thomsen JL, et al. Histological changes and silicone concentrations in human breast tissue surrounding silicone breast prostheses. Plast Recon Surg 1990; 85:38

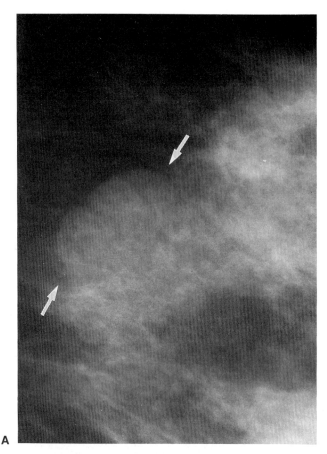

Figure 22-1. A new circumscribed, 8-mm bilobed mass (arrows) was found on MLO (A) and CC (B) mammograms in this 44-year-old woman. The lesion was not palpable. Ultrasonography (not shown) demonstrated a hypoechoic mass with low-level internal echoes.

A

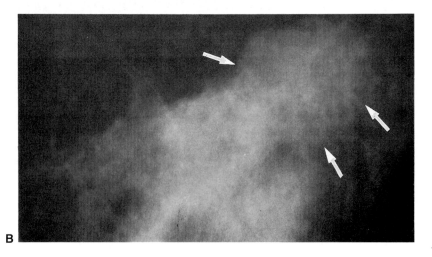

B

Case 22: Needle Aspiration of the Circumscribed Noncalcified Mass

Question 98

A reasonable next step would be:

- (A) sonographic fine-needle aspiration
- (B) stereotactic fine-needle aspiration
- (C) freehand needle localization
- (D) grid coordinate needle placement
- (E) follow-up mammography in 6 months
- (F) follow-up ultrasonography in 6 months

The clinical management of probably benign breast lesions has received considerable attention in the mammography literature. With the onset of large-scale mammography screening, radiologists commonly encounter case scenarios such as that illustrated by the test patient (Figure 22-1). The mammographic evaluation of a nonpalpable neodensity should begin with spot-compression magnification views. If the lesion has irregular margins or is a spiculated mass, cytologic or histologic analysis is warranted to determine whether it is benign or malignant.

When the lesion is a circumscribed mass, as in the test patient, ultrasonography is used next to determine whether the mass is cystic or solid. However, for a lesion less than 1 cm in diameter, particularly if the lesion is deep in a large breast or if the breast is primarily fatty replaced, it may be difficult to establish with confidence that it is cystic. A reasonable next step would be sonographically guided fine-needle aspiration **(Option (A) is true).** If the lesion is truly solid, aspirated cellular material should be submitted for cytologic analysis. After one becomes adept with this procedure, sonographically guided fine-needle aspiration can be performed quickly and with little patient morbidity.

Stereotactic fine-needle aspiration is also a reasonable next step **(Option (B) is true).** However, this procedure requires specially designed equipment and, in most hands, takes longer to perform than sonographically guided aspiration. Recent advances in digital imaging in conjunction with stereotactically guided procedures should result in a shortened procedure time.

Before the development of stereotactic devices, use of a perforated compression plate marked with alphanumeric grid coordinates was the only method available for consistently accurate needle placement. This method is still an option since the equipment is less expensive and readily available in nearly all radiology facilities and the procedure time is shorter than with stereotactically guided procedures **(Option (D) is true).** After a scout film is taken by using the alphanumeric-grid compression paddle, the x and y coordinates indicate where the needle should be placed. The depth or z coordinate is calculated from the location of the lesion on an orthogonal (right-angle) projection. This distance is decreased by approximately 20% to compensate for compression and magnification. Precise needle placement within a cyst is necessary to aspirate fluid from it successfully. If the needle is not placed accurately and fluid is not obtained, this will incorrectly suggest that the mass is solid and can result in unnecessary open surgical biopsy. As a result, freehand needle localization is not a reasonable next step **(Option (C) is false),** because this procedure does not consistently ensure accurate needle placement. In some cases, multiple freehand passes must be performed to place a needle within the lesion.

Several investigators have published results of mammographic follow-up of nonpalpable, probably benign lesions. In a recent series of 21,855 cases by Varas et al., 9 of 535 patients who underwent follow-up (1.7%) were found to have cancer. Sickles reported that of 3,184 nonpalpable probably benign lesions monitored by mammography, only 0.5% were cancer. However, before any lesion can be placed in the probably benign category and relegated to periodic mammographic follow-up, it must meet all accepted imaging criteria. Most authorities require demonstration that at least 75% of the margins of a mass are well defined, on magnification views, before designating a mass as "probably benign." These criteria are not met in the test patient. The medial and anterior margins of the lesion are obscured by adjacent glandular tissue. In addition, the presence of low-level internal echoes is not compatible with the sonographic diagnosis of a simple cyst. Given the mammographic appearance and the sonographic characteristics of this lesion, the differential diagnosis includes a complex cyst, a benign solid mass such as a fibroadenoma, and a circumscribed malignancy. Therefore, follow-up imaging in 6 months is inappropriate because the mass does not qualify as a probably benign lesion **(Options (E) and (F) are false).**

Question 99

Concerning aspiration of cystic lesions,

  (A) it is indicated if a mural nodule is seen on ultrasonography
  (B) bloody aspirates should be sent for cytologic testing
  (C) postaspiration mammography is essential
  (D) multiloculated cysts should be aspirated
  (E) an associated cancer is usually adjacent to a cyst rather than within the wall

As a general rule, a simple cyst is aspirated only when it is painful and troublesome to the patient, enlarges over time, or is equivocal in sonographic appearance or when there is a substantial discrepancy in lesion size as seen at mammography and ultrasonography (Figure 22-2).

A circumscribed anechoic mass with posterior acoustic enhancement and a well-defined back wall requires no further intervention. On the other hand, when a cystic lesion contains a mural nodule, aspiration is indicated **(Option (A) is true).**

After aspiration of a complicated or equivocal cyst, pneumocystography can be performed to delineate further the inner wall of the cyst and to exclude the presence of an intracystic mass (Figure 22-3). This simple procedure involves replacing 75% of the cyst fluid volume with air. After filling the cyst with air, CC and 90° lateral views are obtained. Overdistension of the cyst will result in rupture of the cyst wall and in pneumocystograms that show air within the breast parenchyma.

In the report by Tabar and Pentek of 20 patients with intracystic tumors among 132 patients who underwent pneumocystography, 11 intracystic carcinomas and 9 benign intracystic growths were found. However, cytologic testing of the aspirated fluid led to the diagnosis of malignant cells for only 2 of the 11 cancers. Ciatto et al. have suggested that the yield of malignant cells from cytologic analysis of straw-colored, clear, or greenish cyst fluid is too low to justify the routine submission of these types of fluid for cytologic testing. However, most authorities agree that bloody aspirates should be sent for cytologic testing **(Option (B) is true).** In some cases a serosanguineous aspirate is the result of a traumatic procedure instead of an indication of blood within the cyst.

For an uncomplicated simple cyst, postaspiration mammography is not essential **(Option (C) is false).** This would involve additional radiation exposure to the patient, increased procedure time, and increased cost and is unnecessary for diagnosis. However, if a patient is scheduled

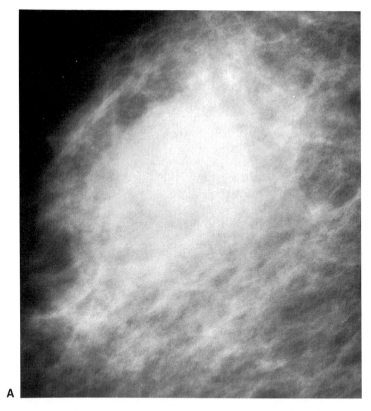

A

Figure 22-2. Simple benign cyst surrounded by dense tissue. (A) A spot-compression MLO view of a 42-year-old woman with a painful mass shows an ill-defined 3-cm density in the upper aspect of the right breast. (B) Pneumocystography was performed because the cyst measured only 1 cm on sonography. The dense tissue that surrounds the cyst may represent an inflammatory reaction from fluid leaking through the cyst wall.

for open surgical biopsy and the lesion proves to be a simple cyst during the needle localization procedure, pneumocystography followed by postaspiration mammography can be performed to provide convincing evidence that the lesion in question was a cyst (Figure 22-4).

Occasionally, a multiloculated cyst seen on ultrasonography appears to contain a mural nodule. This is usually due to a septum presenting as a thickened area where it attaches to the cyst wall (Figures 22-3 and 22-5). However, by scanning in different projections, the diagnosis of a multiloculated cyst can frequently be made without aspiration **(Option (D) is false).** The presence of multiloculation does not connote an increased frequency of associated neoplasm, since a cancer found in the vicinity of a cyst is usually adjacent to the cyst rather than within the cyst wall

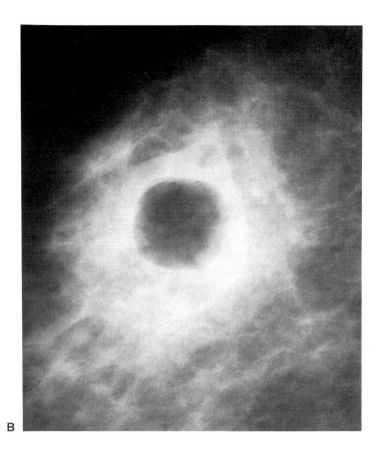

B

(Option (E) is true). Coincident breast carcinoma is found in fewer than 1% of cyst biopsy specimens and is virtually always a serendipitous finding during histologic evaluation. Reaccumulation of fluid in a cyst that has been drained more than three times is suspicious for an associated neoplasm and is an indication for surgical removal. Thickening or irregularity of a cyst wall on mammography or ultrasonography and the presence of a hypoechoic mass adjacent to a cyst on ultrasonography are suspicious findings that warrant biopsy.

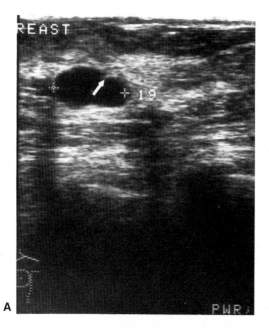

A

Figure 22-3. Septated cyst. (A) A longitudinal sonogram shows a 19-mm dumbbell-shaped anechoic mass. There is focal thickening of the superior wall (arrow). (B) A pneumocystogram shows that a thin, incomplete septum (arrowhead) in the midportion of the cyst accounts for the apparent wall thickening seen on ultrasonography.

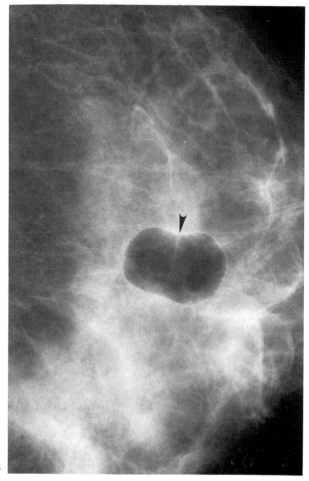

B

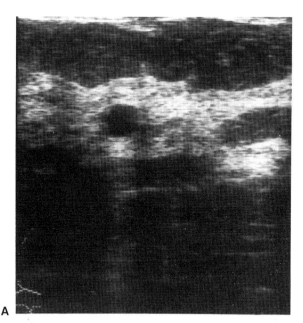

A

Figure 22-4. Simple benign cyst identified during needle localization. (A) A transverse sonogram of a 52-year-old woman referred for needle localization and breast biopsy shows a 7-mm hypoechoic (but not anechoic) circumscribed mass with acoustic enhancement, suggestive but not diagnostic of a cyst. (B) A pneumocystogram following aspiration of fluid with stereotactic guidance confirmed that the lesion was a simple cyst.

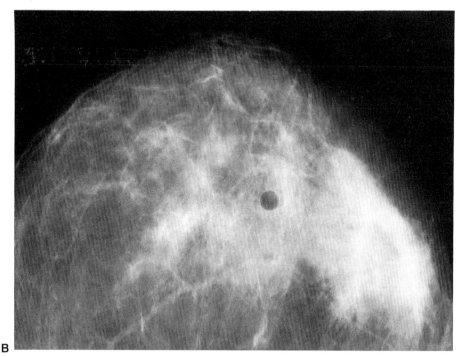

B

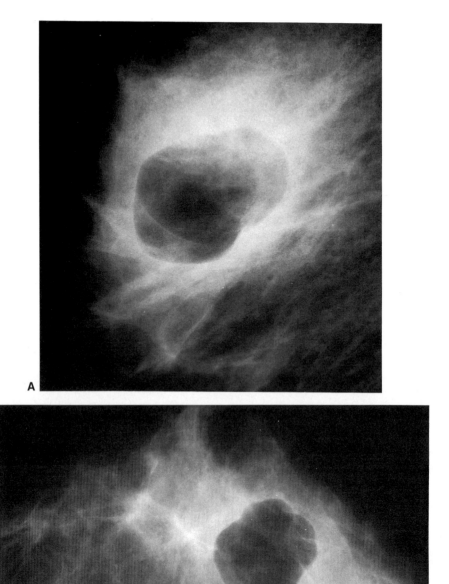

Figure 22-5. Multiloculated cyst. Mediolateral (A) and CC (B) views following pneumocystography show a multiloculated, thin-walled cyst in a
patient who presented with a rock-hard 5-cm palpable mass.

Question 100

Intracystic papillary lesions:

(A) are usually found in women under age 50
(B) when malignant, are usually *in situ*
(C) usually present with bloody nipple discharge
(D) usually appear as circumscribed masses
(E) usually contain microcalcifications

The incidence of intracystic papillary lesions is unknown, but experience with breast ultrasonography and pneumocystography suggests these lesions are rare. In the series of Tabar et al., involving 434 pneumocystograms in 338 women, 26 (6%) intracystic lesions were detected. Of these intracystic tumors, 13 (50%) were malignant.

Intracystic cancers make up 0.5 to 1.5% of all malignant breast tumors. On gross inspection, these tumors are encapsulated or cystic, fleshy or firm, and frequently hemorrhagic. Microscopically, they are circumscribed and are located in one or a few connected large cysts or ducts. They all have a papillary pattern. Pure intracystic papillary carcinoma is rare and is a noninvasive lesion. This term has been used synonymously with *in situ* carcinoma by McDivitt et al.**(Option (B) is true).**

The study by Carter et al. of 41 patients with intracystic papillary carcinoma revealed no instance of lymph node metastasis. However, intracystic papillary carcinoma can be associated with a variable amount of invasive ductal carcinoma, and the clinical outcome depends on the most aggressive part of the neoplasm.

In the series of Tabar and Pentek, 60% of women with malignant intracystic tumors were age 50 and older **(Option (A) is false).** There are no specific clinical signs for the diagnosis of intracystic carcinoma, since these lesions are usually slow growing. Of the 41 patients with intracystic papillary carcinoma studied by Carter et al., 85% had a palpable mass for an average of 16 months prior to diagnosis. However, intracystic papillary carcinoma can also present as a rapidly enlarging palpable mass as a result of hemorrhage.

Only 22% of the patients studied by Carter et al. had a history of nipple discharge **(Option (C) is false).** Of the intracystic carcinomas, 12% were described either clinically or pathologically as subareolar. The others were scattered throughout the four quadrants of the breast. In the series of Tabar and Pentek, of 20 patients with intracystic lesions, only 3 presented with bloody nipple discharge. In this series, nine benign intracystic papillomas were relatively small and were mainly subareolar. The location of the malignant intracystic tumors was not specified.

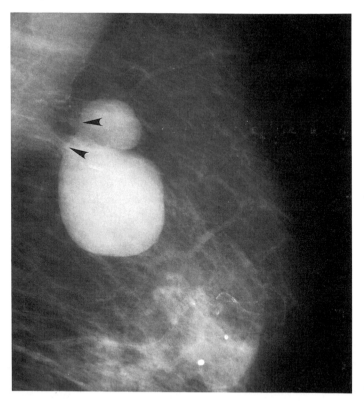

Figure 22-6. Intracystic carcinoma. An MLO mammogram shows a lobulated, fairly well circumscribed dense mass in the upper portion of the
breast in a 75-year-old woman. Note that the posterior border of this
intracystic papillary carcinoma has a "comet-tail" sign (arrowheads)
where the mass abuts adjacent fatty tissue.

These lesions have no pathognomonic mammographic appearance,
but intracystic carcinoma commonly presents as a very dense, solitary,
circumscribed nodule (Figure 22-6) **(Option (D) is true)**. Rarely, a
"comet-tail" sign is present (Figure 22-6), suggesting invasive carcinoma.
Even more rare is the presence of microcalcifications in intracystic
tumors **(Option (E) is false)**.

Ultrasonography plays a key role in the diagnosis of intracystic lesions, particularly when the lesions are nonpalpable. An intracystic tumor can present as a mass, mural nodule, focal thickening of a cyst wall,
or a fluid level within the cyst indicating intracystic hemorrhage (Figure
22-7). Sonographically guided aspiration of cyst fluid or cellular material
from the solid tumor may yield the correct diagnosis of malignancy. However, sonographic demonstration of an atypical or complex mass war-

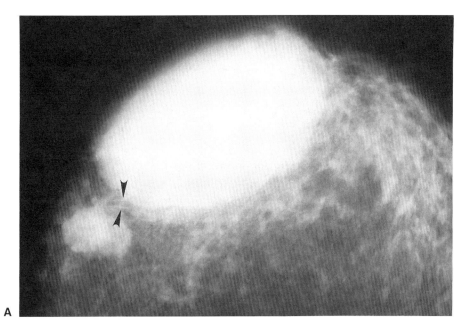

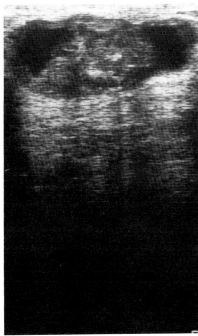

Figure 22-7. Intracystic papillary carcinoma. (A) A CC mammogram in a patient with a palpable subareolar mass shows a large, dense, slightly irregular mass with a small satellite lesion posteriorly. Subtle branching microcalcifications (arrowheads) are noted at the posteromedial aspect of this large intracystic papillary carcinoma. (B) A transverse sonogram shows a large echogenic intracystic mass that corresponds to the *in situ* papillary carcinoma.

rants biopsy despite a benign cytologic diagnosis. Cytologic analysis of aspirated fluid led to the detection of malignant cells in only 2 of 11 intracystic cancers in the series of Tabar and Pentek. Ciatto et al. recommend that cytology be used only when bloodstained fluid is aspirated. In a series of cytologic examinations of 6,782 consecutive breast cyst fluid aspirates from 4,105 women, intraductal papilloma was correctly identified in only 2 of 5 patients, although all 5 had bloodstained fluid.

Question 101

Concerning sonographically guided aspiration of breast masses,

  (A) it requires the use of a needle-guide attachment
  (B) visualization of the needle tip requires the use of a burnished needle
  (C) the use of a sector transducer rather than a linear-array transducer is preferred
  (D) it should not be attempted for lesions ≤1 cm in diameter

Sonographically guided fine-needle aspiration and core biopsy have been reported to be accurate methods for managing some indeterminate breast masses. The equipment required to perform these interventional procedures can be found in any modern radiology department. No special equipment is needed **(Option (A) is false).** A hand-held high-frequency transducer (7.5 MHz) should be used.

Although the use of a needle with a roughened (and therefore more echogenic) tip is preferable, this is not required for visualization of the needle tip within a lesion **(Option (B) is false).** If the needle is aligned along the long axis of the transducer, the entire needle can be visualized as it passes into a lesion.

Most sonographically guided interventional procedures are performed with linear-array transducers, particularly when a freehand technique is used. High-resolution sector scanners produce similar high-quality images, but without the assistance of a needle guide they are difficult to use for interventional procedures **(Option (C) is false).**

Fornage et al. reported 92% sensitivity and 93% specificity in the cytologic diagnosis of malignancy with sonographically guided fine-needle aspiration. The carcinomas ranged in size from 8 to 35 mm in greatest dimension. D'Orsi and Mendelson also report the sampling of lesions as small as 8 mm **(Option (D) is false).** However, regardless of lesion size, one must develop expertise with this procedure before relying on its results to determine the management of indeterminate breast masses.

Judy M. Destouet, M.D.

SUGGESTED READINGS

PROBABLY BENIGN BREAST MASS

1. Destouet JM, Monsees BS. Differential diagnosis of breast lesions on mammography. Curr Imaging 1989; 1:91–99

2. Helvie MA, Pennes DR, Rebner M, Adler DD. Mammographic follow-up of low-suspicion lesions: compliance rate and diagnostic yield. Radiology 1991; 178:155–158

3. Sickles EA. Periodic mammographic follow-up of probably benign lesions: results in 3,184 consecutive cases. Radiology 1991; 179:463–468

4. Varas X, Leborgne F, Leborgne JH. Nonpalpable, probably benign lesions: role of follow-up mammography. Radiology 1992; 184:409–414

SONOGRAPHICALLY GUIDED INTERVENTIONAL PROCEDURES

5. Adler DD. Ultrasound of benign breast conditions. Semin US CT MR 1989; 10:106–118

6. D'Orsi CJ, Mendelson EB. Interventional breast ultrasonography. Semin US CT MR 1989; 10:132–138

7. Fornage BD, Faroux MJ, Simatos A. Breast masses: US-guided fine-needle aspiration biopsy. Radiology 1987; 162:409–414

8. Fornage BD, Sneige N, Faroux MJ, Andry E. Sonographic appearance and ultrasound-guided fine-needle aspiration biopsy of breast carcinomas smaller than 1 cm^3. J Ultrasound Med 1990; 9:559–568

9. Parker SH, Jobe WE, Dennis MA, et al. US-guided automated large-core breast biopsy. Radiology 1993; 187:507–511

10. Svensson WE, Tohno E, Cosgrove DO, Powles TJ, al Murrani B, Jones AL. Effects of fine-needle aspiration on the US appearance of the breast. Radiology 1992; 185:709–711

INTRACYSTIC PAPILLARY BREAST LESIONS

11. Carter D, Orr SL, Merino MJ. Intracystic papillary carcinoma of the breast. After mastectomy, radiotherapy or excisional biopsy alone. Cancer 1983; 52:14–19

12. Ciatto S, Cariaggi P, Bulgaresi P. The value of routine cytologic examination of breast cyst fluids. Acta Cytol 1987; 31:301–304

13. Corkill ME, Sneige N, Fanning T, el-Naggar A. Fine-needle aspiration cytology and flow cytometry of intracystic papillary carcinoma of breast. Am J Clin Pathol 1990; 94:673–680

14. Knight DC, Lowell DM, Heimann A, Dunn E. Aspiration of the breast and nipple discharge cytology. Surg Gynecol Obstet 1986; 163:415–420

15. McDivitt RW, Stewart FW, Berg JW. Tumors of the breast. In: Atlas of tumor pathology, series II, fasc 2. Washington, DC: Armed Forces Institute of Pathology; 1968:22

16. Mitnick JS, Vazquez MF, Harris MN, Schechter S, Roses DF. Invasive papillary carcinoma of the breast: mammographic appearance. Radiology 1990; 177:803–806

17. Sanders TJ, Morris DM, Cederbom G, Gonzalez E. Pneumocystography as an aid in the diagnosis of cystic lesions of the breast. J Surg Oncol 1986; 31:210–213

18. Tabar L, Pentek Z. Pneumocystography of benign and malignant intracystic growths of the female breast. Acta Radiol [Diagn] (Stockh) 1976; 17:829–837

19. Tabar L, Pentek Z, Dean PB. The diagnostic and therapeutic value of breast cyst puncture and pneumocystography. Radiology 1981; 141:659–663

Notes

R L

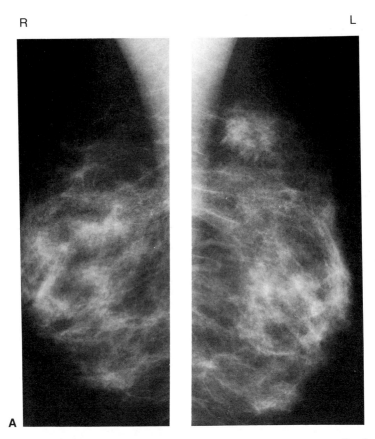

Figure 23-1. This 43-year-old woman was referred for needle localization of a nonpalpable lesion in the left breast. You are shown MLO (A) and CC (B) mammograms of both breasts.

Case 23: Proper Indications for Mammographic Needle Localization

Question 102

The NEXT step should be:

    (A) needle localization
    (B) ultrasonography
    (C) spot-compression mammogram
    (D) tangential mammogram
    (E) follow-up mammography in 6 months

The MLO mammograms (Figure 23-1A) demonstrate an asymmetric density in the upper left breast near the pectoralis muscle (Figure 23-2). The borders of the lesion are not well defined, but there is evidence of fat interspersed within the density. The CC views (Figure 23-1B) demonstrate no abnormality in either breast. Further radiographic evaluation of this asymmetric density is indicated prior to needle localization (Option (A)), because it must first be seen on at least two different projections to establish its existence and location.

The next step in the mammographic workup of the density seen in the test image should be a spot-compression view, in MLO projection, to establish or exclude the diagnosis of superimposed but asymmetric benign fibroglandular tissue **(Option (C) is correct).** A spot-compression magnification mammogram would probably be even more effective than a spot-compression mammogram alone, since the increased resolution and reduced noise produced by magnification imaging would probably portray the marginal characteristics of the asymmetric density with greater clarity. If spot-compression mammography excludes superimposition of glandular tissue as the basis for the density, confirmation of the existence of a mass still requires that the lesion must be seen on at least

R   L

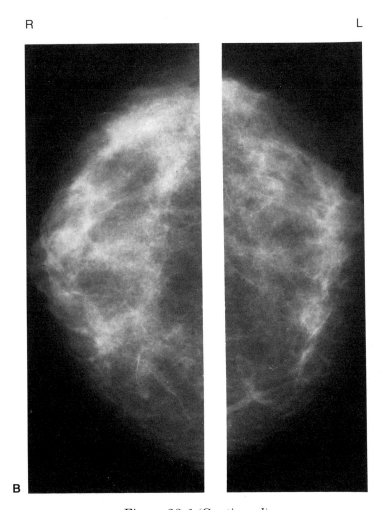

B

Figure 23-1 (Continued)

two different projections, preferably on two orthogonal views (e.g., CC and 90° lateral) to determine its exact location in the breast.

Ultrasonography (Option (B)) would be indicated if a mass had a mammographic appearance suggesting a breast cyst. However, ultrasonography is indicated only after the mammographic evaluation is complete and the existence of a mass has been confirmed.

Tangential views (Option (D)) of the breast are most helpful for evaluating possible skin lesions or palpable masses. These views are performed by placing a radiopaque marker on the skin precisely overlying the area of concern. The breast is then positioned such that the marker lies tangential to the X-ray beam. The area immediately underneath the marker can then be evaluated for a possible abnormality. This approach is very helpful in evaluating superficial or palpable lesions, but it was

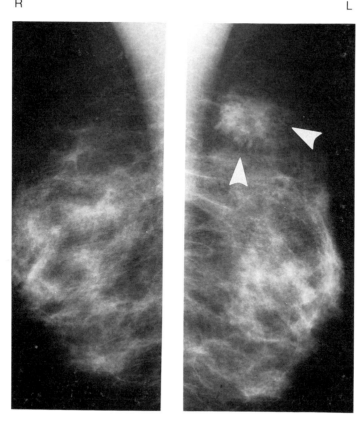

Figure 23-2 (Same as Figure 23-1A). The MLO mammogram shows a 3-cm asymmetric density in the upper portion of the left breast (arrowheads).

not indicated in the test patient, whose finding was nonpalpable and without suggestion of skin involvement.

Only after the mammographic evaluation is complete and indicates that no suspicious lesion exists should the option of a 6-month follow-up (Option (E)) be considered. If spot-compression magnification views had demonstrated a probably benign mass that was solid on ultrasonography, a 6-month follow-up would be a reasonable alternative to biopsy. Previous mammograms are invaluable in assessing the stability of a probably benign mass and may render short-term follow-up unnecessary. In fact, obtaining old mammograms and comparing them with the current ones should precede all other steps in the work-up of a possible mammographic abnormality. This simple maneuver may save time, money, and patient morbidity.

A spot-compression magnification view of the asymmetric density in the test patient was obtained (Figure 23-3); it demonstrated focal fibro-

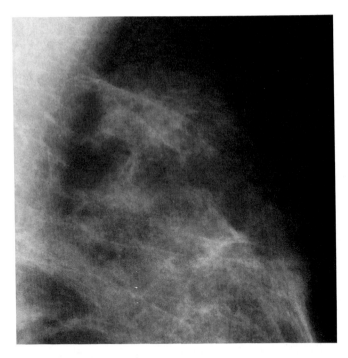

Figure 23-3. Same patient as in Figures 23-1 and 23-2. Ectopic fibro-glandular tissue producing asymmetric density. An MLO spot-compres-sion magnification mammogram shows normal fibroglandular tissue and no discrete mass in the region where the asymmetric density was seen previously.

glandular tissue without evidence of a mass. This mammographic find-ing probably represents ectopic fibroglandular tissue, which is indeed found more commonly in the upper outer quadrant than in either the lower or inner breast. Ectopic fibroglandular tissue is also frequently asymmetric in distribution.

Question 103

Reasonable explanations for asymmetric density seen on a mammogram include:

(A) invasive lobular carcinoma
(B) exogenous estrogen therapy
(C) mastitis
(D) prior surgery
(E) congestive heart failure

Proliferation of glandular elements in the breast results in mammographically visible increased density in approximately 17 to 24% of postmenopausal women undergoing hormonal replacement therapy. This change in density is asymmetric in approximately 14% of patients **(Option (B) is true)** (Figure 23-4). Hormone replacement therapy also results in new cyst formation in approximately 6% of women. A careful history can be very helpful in discerning the etiology of changing breast density, but this is not limited to exogenous estrogen or progesterone therapy. A history of breast pain, erythema, and fever raises the possibility of mastitis. Mastitis commonly presents mammographically as asymmetric density with skin edema in a location that correlates with the area of clinical symptoms **(Option (C) is true).**

Prior surgery is also a common cause of mammographic asymmetry **(Option (D) is true),** and some radiologists find it helpful to mark surgical scars with radiopaque markers (Figure 23-5). Scarring can also result in parenchymal distortion and skin retraction. Tangential views and shallow oblique views help distinguish scar tissue from a true mass. Most mammographic changes secondary to surgery become less obvious with time. However, an asymmetric density is occasionally seen in the contralateral breast, representing remaining normal fibroglandular tissue that appears asymmetric because of the tissue deficit in the breast that has undergone surgery (Figure 23-6).

Edema for any reason, localized or systemic, can result in increased density in the breast, and this can be asymmetric **(Option (E) is true)** (Figure 23-7). A history of congestive heart failure, hypoproteinemia, or other causes of edema will provide helpful clinical correlation. Asymmetry can be secondary to dependent edema if a patient was recently lying on one side more than the other.

Inflammatory carcinoma of the breast is an invasive cancer that has infiltrated the dermal lymphatics. Inflammatory carcinoma results in asymmetry in breast tissue density secondary to obstruction of lymphatic drainage and an edematous breast.

Unilateral edema is also found in patients who have undergone lumpectomy and radiotherapy for treatment of breast cancer. After

R   L

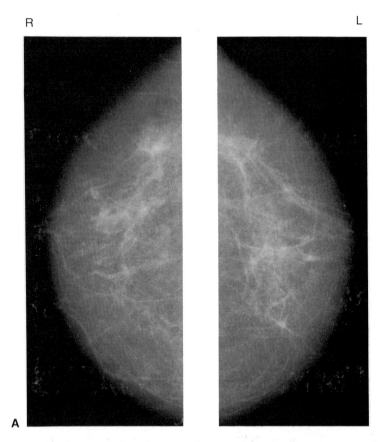

A

Figure 23-4. Asymmetric density due to exogenous estrogen therapy. (A) Baseline CC mammograms show fatty replacement in the breasts of this postmenopausal woman. (B) Following exogenous estrogen therapy, CC mammograms show marked asymmetric density in the outer half of the right breast. A biopsy of the palpable thickened tissue in this area revealed normal fibroglandular tissue.

breast conservation therapy, mammographic findings of edema and skin thickening should gradually decrease and then stabilize after approximately 2 years. Any area of increasing density should be thoroughly evaluated, including possible biopsy, to rule out tumor recurrence.

Invasive lobular carcinoma sometimes presents as an asymmetric density or focal parenchymal distortion in the breast **(Option (A) is true)**. Invasive lobular carcinoma is discussed in greater detail subsequently.

R

L

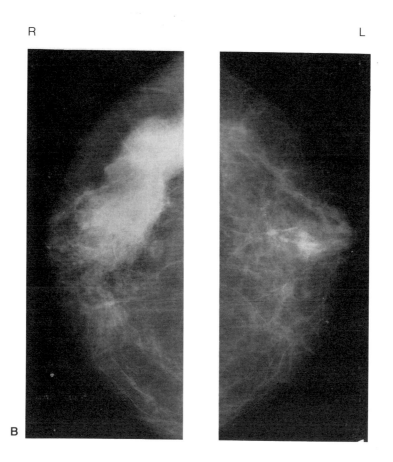

B

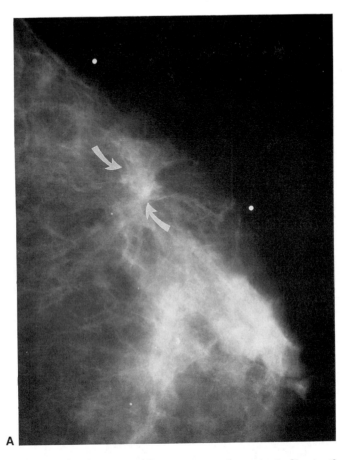

A

Figure 23-5. Value of using radiopaque markers to indicate the location of a postoperative scar. (A) A CC mammogram of a patient with a postoperative scar indicated by radiopaque markers shows a 3-cm focal parenchymal distortion (arrows) just below the skin surface. (B) An MLO view shows that the spiculated mass (arrows), which represents an invasive ductal cancer, is distant from the scar.

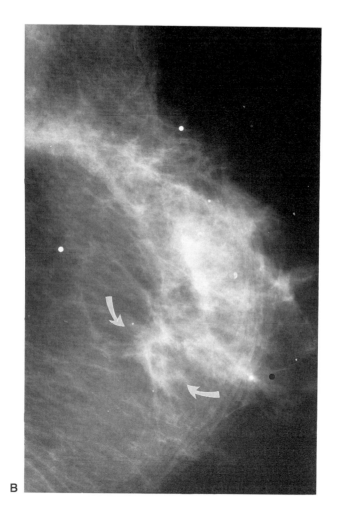

R   L

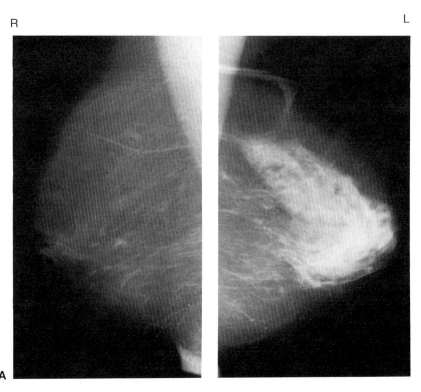

A

Figure 23-6. Asymmetric density due to removal of dense tissue from
the contralateral breast. MLO (A) and CC (B) mammograms show
marked asymmetric density in the left breast as a result of extensive surgery performed on the right breast.

R

L

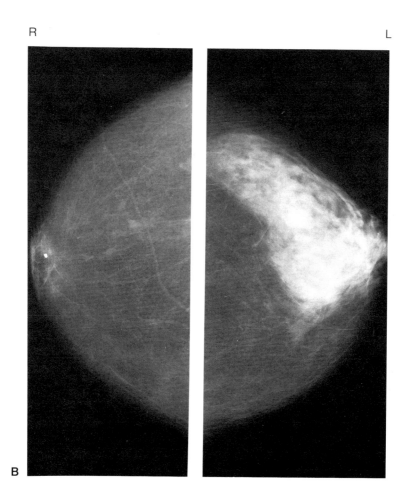

B

R 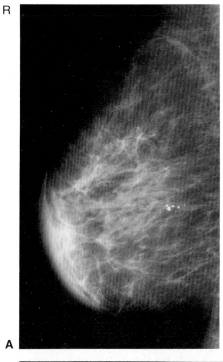 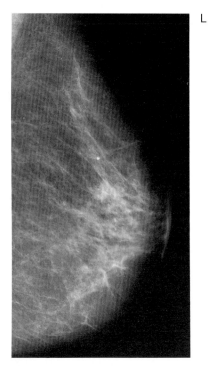 L

A

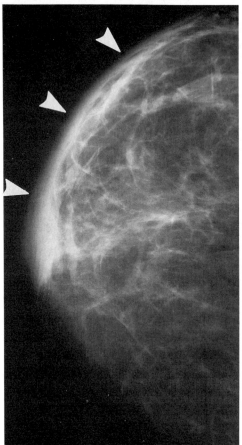

B

Figure 23-7. Asymmetric density due to breast edema. (A) 90° lateral views of both breasts show marked periareolar skin thickening and increased density in the anterior portion of the right breast. (B) A CC view of the right breast shows that edema is confined to the lateral half of the breast (arrowheads) because the patient was lying on her right side.

312

Question 104

Concerning acute mastitis,

    (A) calcifications are frequently present
    (B) fluid collections identifiable by sonography are present in most patients
    (C) purulent discharge from the nipple is a frequent presenting complaint
    (D) an associated abscess is usually subareolar
    (E) no organism is cultured on aspirates in more than 50% of cases

Acute mastitis is an infectious process involving the breast and is seen most commonly in the postpartum period during lactation, affecting 1 to 3% of nursing mothers. It is usually secondary to bacterial entry through a cracked nipple. The etiology is less clear in nonlactating women. The affected breast is typically warm, erythematous, and exquisitely tender to palpation. Treatment of mastitis includes a course of broad-spectrum antibiotics, with clinical follow-up to confirm resolution of symptoms. Differentiation from inflammatory carcinoma is important, and mammography is indicated if symptoms persist after antibiotic therapy. Punch biopsy of the skin is sometimes performed to exclude inflammatory carcinoma, if clinical suspicion warrants, even before antibiotic therapy has ended.

Calcifications are not a frequent finding in acute mastitis **(Option (A) is false)**. The mammographic appearance typically demonstrates an ill-defined, asymmetric density correlating with the area of clinical findings (Figure 23-8).

Fluid collections and purulent nipple discharge are occasionally present but are not common findings in mastitis **(Options (B) and (C) are false)**. A fluid collection indicative of abscess formation is usually subareolar in location **(Option (D) is true)** but can be found anywhere in the breast. The usual sonographic appearance of an abscess is that of a hypoechoic mass with areas of mixed echogenicity and irregular walls. Treatment of an abscess requires percutaneous aspiration or surgical drainage in addition to antibiotic therapy. Pretreatment aspirates are negative on culture at least 50% of the time; in one series, no organism was recovered from 12 of 19 patients **(Option (E) is true)**. When an organism is cultured, it is usually *Staphylococcus aureus*.

R

L

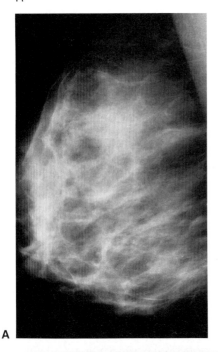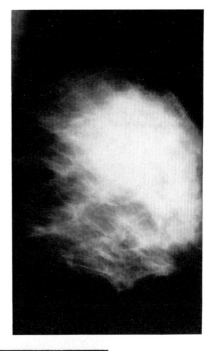

A

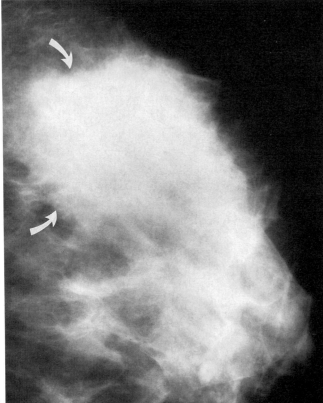

B

Figure 23-8. Asymmetric density due to mastitis. (A) MLO mammograms of both breasts show a large asymmetric density in the upper half of the left breast, which corresponded to clinically evident mastitis. (B) An MLO spot-compression magnification view of the left breast shows that the asymmetric density has irregular margins (arrows).

Question 105

Concerning invasive lobular carcinoma,

    (A) presenting physical findings are subtle or nonspecific in most patients

    (B) presenting mammographic findings are subtle or nonspecific in most patients

    (C) it constitutes 30% of invasive breast carcinoma

    (D) it often contains round, punctate calcifications

    (E) it is often more conspicuous on the CC view than on the MLO view

The pathogenesis of invasive lobular carcinoma is somewhat controversial. The cells of this tumor resemble those of the lobule and, although lobular carcinoma *in situ* can be found in association, its presence is not required for the diagnosis of invasive lobular carcinoma. The incidence of bilaterality is higher in invasive lobular carcinoma than in invasive ductal carcinoma, and it is felt to carry a worse prognosis by some investigators.

Both the physical and mammographic findings in patients presenting with invasive lobular carcinoma are often subtle or nonspecific **(Options (A) and (B) are true).** Depending on the series, palpable abnormalities have been identified in 64 to 89% of patients. When present, these range from an ill-defined thickening to a focal mass. Mammographic findings frequently include asymmetric density, subtle parenchymal distortion, or normal-appearing breast parenchyma (Figure 23-9). The most common mammographic pattern of invasive lobular carcinoma in the series by Mendelson et al. was a poorly defined asymmetric density with architectural distortion. The common histologic infiltrative pattern of invasive lobular carcinoma (it usually insinuates itself throughout the breast parenchyma without forming a discrete mass) helps to explain its subtle mammographic and physical findings.

Less than 10% of invasive breast carcinomas are lobular **(Option (C) is false);** the great majority (approximately 90%) are ductal in origin. Other malignancies, not representing carcinomas, include sarcomas, lymphomas, and metastases from cancers arising outside the breast.

Calcifications are associated with invasive lobular carcinoma only infrequently **(Option (D) is false).** When calcifications are visible, they are usually nonspecific in appearance. Many times they are an incidental finding and are adjacent to rather than within an area of invasive lobular carcinoma.

Mammographic findings of invasive lobular carcinoma are often best seen on the CC view **(Option (E) is true).** The compression of the breast obtained in the CC view is usually better than that obtained in the MLO view. This results in superior visualization of subtle architectural distor-

R   L

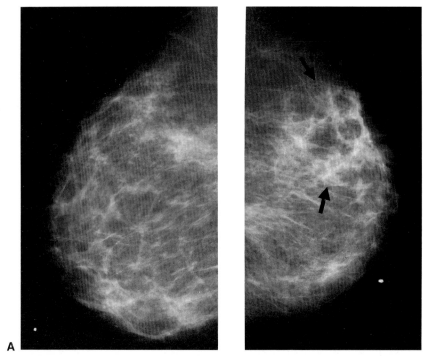

A

Figure 23-9. Parenchymal distortion due to invasive lobular carcinoma. Mediolateral (A) and CC (B) mammograms show a 5-cm area of focal parenchymal distortion (arrows) in the left upper inner quadrant in this patient with a palpable infiltrating lobular carcinoma.

tion, which is especially important in the detection of invasive lobular carcinoma.

Correlation with physical findings is essential in the timely identification of invasive lobular carcinoma. If a patient presents with a new palpable mass or thickening and there is no mammographic correlate, then biopsy should be strongly considered, primarily on the basis of the physical examination. Approximately 10% of breast cancers are mammographically occult.

Tracy L. Roberts, M.D.
Judy M. Destouet, M.D.

R   L

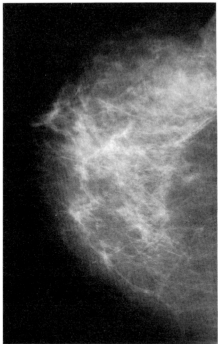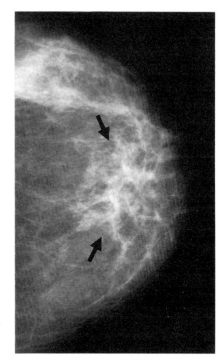

B

SUGGESTED READINGS

EVALUATION OF NONPALPABLE BREAST LESIONS

1. Adler DD. Ultrasound of benign breast conditions. Semin US CT MR 1989; 10:106–118

2. Bassett LW, Kimme-Smith C. Breast sonography. AJR 1991; 156:449–455

3. Berkowitz JE, Gatewood OM, Gayler BW. Equivocal mammographic findings: evaluation with spot compression. Radiology 1989; 171:369–371

4. Brenner RJ, Sickles EA. Acceptability of periodic follow-up as an alternative to biopsy for mammographically detected lesions interpreted as probably benign. Radiology 1989; 171:645–646

5. Hall FM. Magnification spot compression of the breast. (Letter to the editor). Radiology 1989; 173:284

6. Helvie MA, Pennes DR, Rebner M, Adler DD. Mammographic follow-up of low-suspicion lesions: compliance rate and diagnostic yield. Radiology 1991; 178:155–158

7. Jackson VP. The role of US in breast imaging. Radiology 1990; 177:305–311

8. Meyer JE, Sonnenfeld MR, Greenes RA, Stomper PC. Cancellation of preoperative breast localization procedure: analysis of 53 cases. Radiology 1988; 169:629–630

9. Pamilo M, Soiva M, Anttinen I, Roiha M, Suramo I. Ultrasonography of breast lesions detected in mammography screening. Acta Radiol 1991; 32:220–225

10. Sickles EA. Practical solutions to common mammographic problems: tailoring the examination. AJR 1988; 151:31–39

11. Sickles EA. Combining spot compression and other special views to maximize mammographic information. (Letter to the editor). Radiology 1989; 173:571

12. Sickles EA. Periodic mammographic follow-up of probably benign lesions: results in 3,184 consecutive cases. Radiology 1991; 179:463–468

13. Varas X, Leborgne F, Leborgne JH. Nonpalpable, probably benign lesions: role of follow-up mammography. Radiology 1992; 184:409–414

ASYMMETRIC DENSITY

14. Adler DD, Rebner M, Pennes DR. Accessory breast tissue in the axilla: mammographic appearance. Radiology 1987; 163:709–711

15. Berkowitz JE, Gatewood OM, Goldblum LE, Gayler BW. Hormonal replacement therapy: mammographic manifestations. Radiology 1990; 174:199–201

16. Destouet JM. Mammography of the altered breast. Curr Opin Radiol 1990; 2:734–740

17. Henderson MA, McBride CM. Secondary inflammatory breast cancer: treatment options. South Med J 1988; 81:1512–1517

18. Kaufman Z, Garstin WI, Hayes R, Michell MJ, Baum M. The mammographic parenchymal patterns of women on hormonal replacement therapy. Clin Radiol 1991; 43:389–392

19. Kopans DB, Swann CA, White G, et al. Asymmetric breast tissue. Radiology 1989; 171:639–643

20. Mendelson EB. Imaging the post-surgical breast. Semin US CT MR 1989; 10:154–170

21. Mitnick J, Roses DF, Harris MN. Differentiation of postsurgical changes from carcinoma of the breast. Surg Gynecol Obstet 1988; 166:549–550

22. Stomper PC, Van Voorhis BJ, Ravnikar VA, Meyer JE. Mammographic changes associated with postmenopausal hormone replacement therapy: a longitudinal study. Radiology 1990; 174:487–490

MASTITIS

23. Destouet JM, Monsees BS. Differential diagnosis of breast lesions on mammography. Curr Imaging 1989; 1:91–99

24. Karstrup S, Nolsøe C, Brabrand K, Nielsen KR. Ultrasonically guided percutaneous drainage of breast abscesses. Acta Radiol 1990; 31:157–159

INVASIVE LOBULAR CARCINOMA

25. Helvie MA, Paramagul C, Oberman HA, Adler DD. Invasive lobular carcinoma. Imaging features and clinical detection. Invest Radiol 1993; 28:202–207

26. Hilleren DJ, Andersson IT, Lindholm K, Linnell FS. Invasive lobular carcinoma: mammographic findings in a 10-year experience. Radiology 1991; 78:149–154

27. Mendelson EB, Harris KM, Doshi N, Tobon H. Infiltrating lobular carcinoma: mammographic patterns with pathologic correlation. AJR 1989; 153:265–271

28. Sickles EA. The subtle and atypical mammographic features of invasive lobular carcinoma. Radiology 1991; 178:25–26

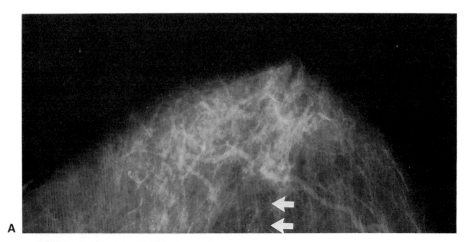

Figure 24-1

Figures 24-1 and 24-2. This
84-year-old woman was re-
ferred for needle localization
of microcalcifications associated with an area of in-
creased density in the right
breast. You are shown CC (A)
and 90° lateral (B) mammograms (Figure 24-1) and a
photographic enlargement of
the 90° lateral view (Figure
24-2). The microcalcifications
and density are indicated by
arrows. This lesion was not
present on mammograms
taken 14 months previously.

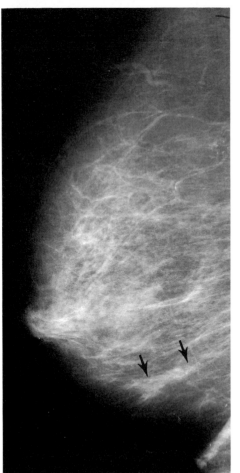

B

Case 24: Mammographic Needle Localization Techniques

Question 106

Which *one* of the following would be the BEST approach to localize this lesion?

(A) Mediolateral
(B) Superior (CC)
(C) Lateromedial
(D) Inferior (caudocranial)
(E) Periareolar

Needle localization of nonpalpable breast lesions is an essential procedure in the treatment of mammographically detected abnormalities. Several principles guide the correct placement of the localization needle. Most important, the needle must pass through or be immediately adjacent to the lesion. The surgeon then simply excises tissue along the shaft of the localization needle or wire until the tip of the needle or wire is reached. Excision will be much less precise if the surgeon must compensate for inaccurate placement. If placement is shallow, the surgeon must judge the direction in which to extend the dissection into a breast, a difficult decision because the orientation of the supine-positioned breast in the operating room is far different from the orientation of the breast in the mammography suite.

Selection of the localization path is not always clear-cut. A simple guiding principle is to choose the needle approach that provides the surgeon with the shortest path to the lesion. This is best assessed with CC and 90° lateral mammograms. There are instances, discussed below, when other approaches could be considered.

The approach to the lesion in the test patient is technically challenging because it is in the lower part of the breast at approximately the 6 o'clock position (Figures 24-1 and 24-2). Its location relatively close to the chest wall increases the chance of pneumothorax as a complication.

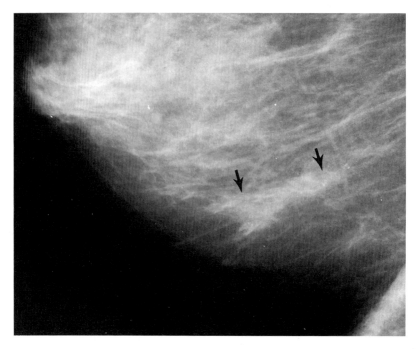

Figure 24-2

Therefore, the safest and most direct needle path to the lesion is an inferior (caudocranial) approach **(Option (D) is correct).**

For the lesion in the test patient, alternative anatomic approaches would not be as advantageous as an inferior approach. A mediolateral approach (Option (A)) would not be the shortest path to the lesion. For the same reason, superior (CC) and lateromedial approaches (Options (B) and (C)) would traverse too much normal breast tissue. In fact, a CC localization would require inserting the needle through almost the entire thickness of the breast to reach the lesion.

Several techniques of needle localization are used, especially the parallel-to-chest-wall and freehand methods. The parallel-to-chest-wall technique, coupled with the use of a perforated compression plate, is the easiest and safest to master. When properly performed, there is no risk of pneumothorax (Figure 24-3). For an inferiorly located lesion the localization grid is positioned over the lower aspect of the breast. This results in an awkward posture for the radiologist at the time of needle placement but is otherwise no different from approaches from the CC, medial, or lateral aspect of the breast.

Some radiologists use ultrasonographic guidance to place localization needles when lesions are unequivocally demonstrated by ultrasonog-

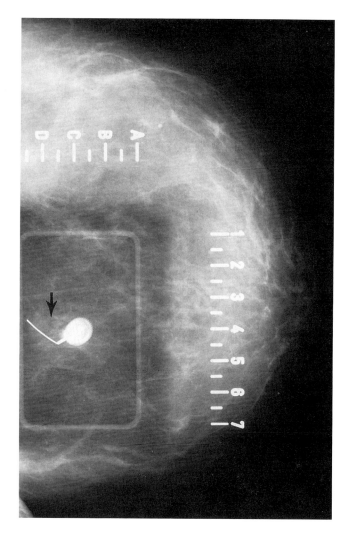

Figure 24-3. Rectangular-grid localization (not the test patient). When using a rectangular grid, placement of a needle aimed at, into, or passing through the lesion (arrow) is confirmed immediately after needle insertion. A second radiograph, obtained in an orthogonal plane, will then determine the appropriate needle depth.

raphy. This approach may be faster in selected cases. However, ultrasonography often fails to visualize small (<0.8-cm) solid masses and rarely images lesions that present as clustered microcalcifications. Furthermore, ultrasonographic guidance may not readily permit parallel-to-chest-wall needle insertion, therefore creating a slight risk of pneumothorax.

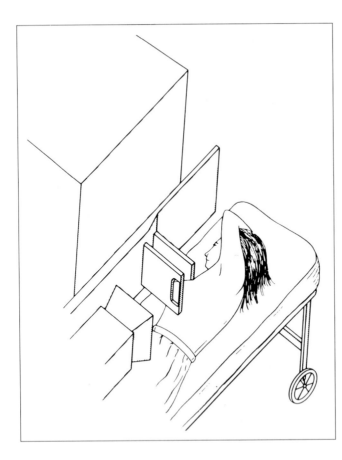

Figure 24-4. Inferior localization with a perforated compression plate. The patient is positioned on a stretcher during preoperative localization of a lesion situated inferiorly in the breast. (Reprinted with permission from Pisano and Hall [4].)

With some mammographic equipment, a limitation in gantry rotation means that inferior-approach needle placement cannot be done through a perforated compression plate if the patient is seated. For these units, two inferior-approach methods are available: use of a perforated compression plate with the patient lying on a stretcher, and a freehand approach from below with the patient seated. For the former method, the patient lies on her side and her breast is positioned with the compression applied in the horizontal plane (Figure 24-4). For the inferior freehand approach (used with the test patient), metal markers are placed at the inferior aspect of the breast over the approximate location of the lesion and a CC projection mammogram is obtained (Figure 24-5). An entry point under the lesion is determined relative to these markers, and the needle is inserted. Then two orthogonal views are taken to confirm accurate needle placement (Figure 24-6). Figure 24-7 is an enlargement of Figure 24-6B, showing the positioning of the needle and wire with respect to the lesion.

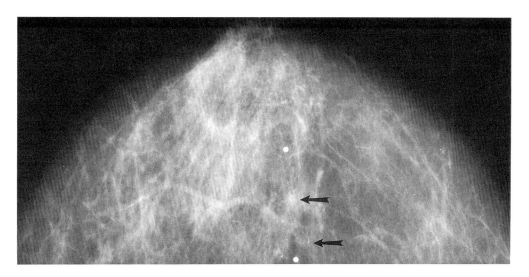

Figure 24-5

Figures 24-5 through 24-7. Inferior localization by the freehand technique. A scout CC mammogram (Figure 24-5), with metal markers placed under the approximate location of the lesion (arrows), is taken to determine the proper skin entry point relative to the location of the skin markers. After insertion of the localization needle and deployment of the J-wire, CC (Figure 24-6A) and 90° lateral (Figure 24-6B) mammograms are taken to verify satisfactory needle and wire placement. Figure 24-7 is a photographic enlargement of Figure 24-6B, showing the position of the localization needle and wire along the inferior aspect of the lesion (arrows).

Some surgeons prefer to approach all localized lesions via a circumareolar incision to produce a more cosmetically acceptable surgical scar. This usually requires that the radiologist perform freehand needle placement. Some radiologists have become proficient at the freehand technique. However, a potential complication of freehand localization is pneumothorax, caused when an inexperienced radiologist inadvertently places the localization needle into the pleural cavity. Radiologists who are not skilled at freehand localization are also likely to cause increased patient morbidity, since multiple needle passes may be needed to achieve the required accuracy. In the test patient, periareolar needle placement (Option (E)) would require the needle to traverse an extended path to reach the lesion. As discussed above, a freehand approach from the inferior aspect of the breast would be acceptable because it involves a shorter needle path.

The cosmetic consequences of needle placement should be considered when a lesion can be reached by either a lateral or a CC approach with

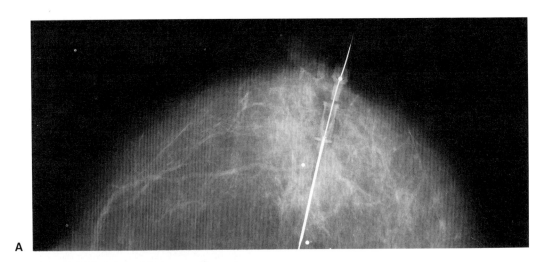

A

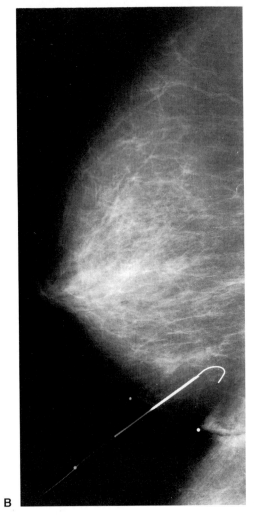

B

Figure 24-6

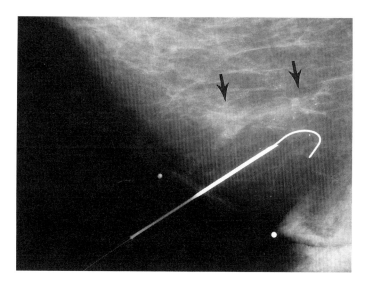

Figure 24-7

no significant difference in the length of the needle path. When this occurs, the lateral approach is usually preferred, because a lateral scar is cosmetically more acceptable than a scar on the superior aspect of the breast. These considerations do not apply for surgeons who routinely perform periareolar incisions.

Most manufacturers of mammography units provide a localization accessory for their equipment. These usually fall into two general categories: compression plates with a single rectangular perforation and those with multiple circular perforations (Figure 24-8). Some radiologists routinely use a stereotactic device for their localization procedures, but such a device is not required for accurate prebiopsy needle placement.

The choice of localization needle system should be based on both the radiologist's and the surgeon's preferences. Currently available systems designed specifically for breast lesion localization involve (1) hook wire systems in which a needle is used to introduce a hook wire, with subsequent removal of the needle, leaving the hook wire fixed in place, or (2) those that place a needle and a retractable wire, leaving both in the breast (Figure 24-9). Several authors have described methods in which dye markers, such as methylene blue or carbon black particles, are injected through the localization needle to make the area of interest more readily visible intraoperatively. These dye-marking methods, which can be used in addition to or in place of localization wires, are used more widely in Europe than in the United States.

Hook wire and retractable-wire systems both have inherent strengths and limitations. Hook wire systems have the advantage that

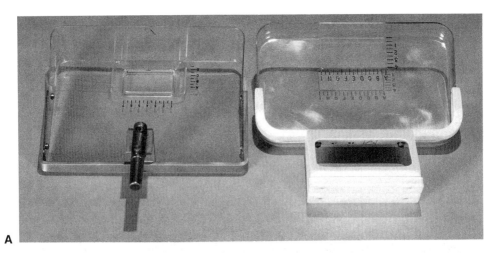

A

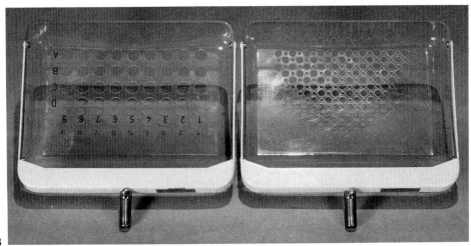

B

Figure 24-8. Preoperative compression plate devices. A variety of compression plates are available to assist with preoperative localization of nonpalpable lesions. These compression plates have either a single rectangular perforation (A) or an ordered set of circular perforations (B). The skin entry site is determined relative to alphanumeric grid coordinates or to the perforation that most closely overlies the lesion.

the barb of the wire usually stays anchored firmly in the breast both before and during surgery, even with incidental surgical retraction. This is also one of its disadvantages, because once a hook wire is deployed out of the needle it cannot be repositioned. Therefore, during the localization procedure, it is essential to confirm needle placement through and slightly beyond the lesion before the hook wire is deployed. Another consideration with hook wire systems is to select a long enough needle and

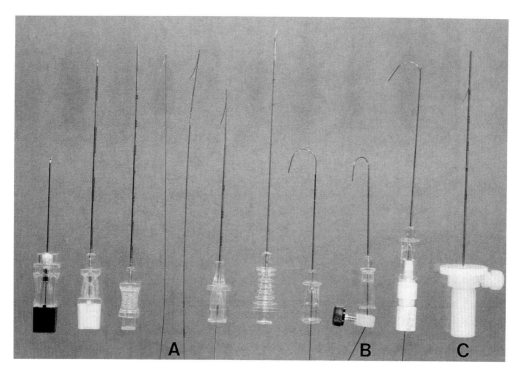

Figure 24-9. Localization needles. This is a representative sample of localization needle systems designed specifically for preoperative breast localization. These systems generally involve variations on either hook wire (A) or retractable-wire (B) design. Needles containing a retractable hook wire are also available (C).

wire. Use of too short a needle will not permit the wire to reach the lesion. Use of too short a wire (or the ill-advised practice of cutting away the excess length of exposed wire) can cause the external end of the wire to disappear beneath the skin when breast compression is released. This may compromise the ability of the surgeon to locate the wire, especially if a relatively thin wire is used.

Hook wires of various designs are available. Several systems have thick wire segments just proximal to the hook. These increase intraoperative palpability and minimize the likelihood of transection. Stiffening cannulas of various lengths are supplied with some systems to pass over the localization wire after deployment, serving to protect the hook wire from transection (similar to retractable-wire systems). A less expensive wire protection alternative would be to pass a standard needle over the hook wire. However, this should be done with caution, since it is possible for the sharp needle tip to shear the wire. Additional features of some hook wire systems include distinctive wire or needle markings, such as burnished areas or small embedded beads, to indicate 1-cm lengths along the shaft of the wire and needle. These markings can help the radiologist judge the depth of needle insertion during localization and can help the surgeon determine the depth of the needle or wire relative to the lesion during surgery.

Retractable-wire systems typically involve a curved or J-shaped wire that can be extended from the tip of the needle but can also be safely retracted to adjust the wire position during localization. This is an advantage over hook wire systems, in which wires cannot be retracted and relocated after suboptimal positioning or accidental wire deployment. Another advantage of retractable-wire systems is their durability during surgery; inadvertent wire transection is highly unlikely because of the protection provided by the outer needle shaft. A disadvantage of J-shaped retractable wires is that they do not anchor the breast tissue as firmly as hook wires do, thus slightly increasing the likelihood of wire displacement and the concomitant possibility of a failed biopsy, requiring repeat localization.

Question 107

Concerning specimen radiography,

   (A) it confirms excision of the lesion
   (B) it is not necessary for a lesion palpated in the specimen
   (C) it is essential only for assessment of lesions containing calcifications
   (D) a magnification technique should be used routinely
   (E) it facilitates detection of tumor extending to the margin of resection
   (F) radiographs of tissue blocks should be performed if resected calcifications are not seen on histologic sections

Specimen radiography is a mandatory procedure in the diagnosis of clinically occult breast carcinoma. The specimen radiograph confirms the excision of a suspicious mammographic lesion **(Option (A) is true)** and provides medicolegal documentation that a localized lesion has been excised. In the unusual circumstance when the lesion is not visible on specimen radiographs, some advocate taking a wider excision at the biopsy site. Others suggest immediately returning the patient to the mammography suite for relocalization of the lesion. If excision of a mammographic lesion ultimately cannot be confirmed by specimen radiography, the radiologist must recommend that the patient return for repeat mammography approximately 4 to 6 weeks after biopsy to reassess for removal of the lesion. Any patient with a failed needle localization, confirmed on follow-up mammography, should promptly undergo repeat localization and biopsy. This practice should ensure removal of all mammographically suspicious lesions within 6 to 8 weeks of the initial biopsy.

Some may question the need for specimen radiography when the surgeon palpates a mass within the specimen. However, it is prudent even in this situation to document that the mammographic lesion corresponds to the palpable findings and to confirm that the mammographic lesion has indeed been excised **(Option (B) is false)**.

Others may question the need for a specimen radiograph when the mammographic lesion does not contain calcifications, because of a presumed inability to visualize a noncalcified mass or area of architectural distortion. However, with the proper radiographic technique (including uniform specimen compression), all lesions seen on preoperative mammograms can also be identified on specimen radiographs **(Option (C) is false)**.

The preferred method of performing specimen radiography involves compressing the specimen to uniform thickness and taking a magnification exposure (Figure 24-10). Just as routine breast compression improves the mammographic detection of *in vivo* lesions, so does compression of the biopsy specimen. The use of a magnification technique during specimen radiography increases resolution and reduces system noise, thereby improving the conspicuity of both calcified and noncalcified lesions. For these reasons, a magnification technique should be used routinely **(Option (D) is true)**. Some radiologists also obtain a nonmagnified specimen radiograph to indicate the true size of the mammographic lesion. This occasionally proves helpful in staging a breast cancer when the pathologist fails to provide precise measurement of tumor size.

Dedicated specimen radiography units are used primarily within pathology departments. Unfortunately, these units do not conveniently permit either compression or magnification. High-quality specimen radiographs are best obtained with a full-feature dedicated mammography unit located in the radiology department. To minimize operating room delays, the radiology department should institute procedures to allow for specimen radiography immediately on receipt of biopsy material.

Specimen radiography can also help to indicate how close a mammographic lesion is to the margin of resection. Extension of microcalcifications, spiculations, or the border of a mass to the edge of a specimen should alert the pathologist to assess these areas for spread of cancer to the margin of resection **(Option (E) is true)**.

The specimen radiograph should serve not only as a means of confirming lesion excision but also as the initial step in quality assurance for pathologic analysis. Most mammographically detected abnormalities are not identified by the pathologist on gross examination of biopsy material;

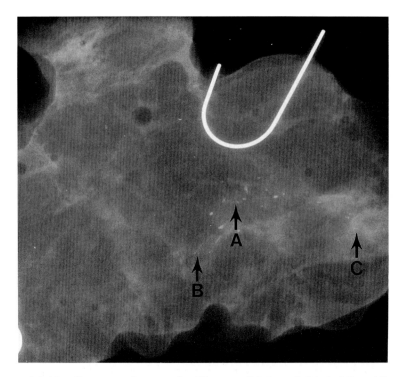

Figure 24-10. Same patient as in Figures 24-1 and 24-2. Magnification specimen radiograph. This specimen radiograph demonstrates the microcalcifications and density within the lower right aspect of the specimen, confirming successful excision of the lesion. The center arrow (A) indicates the lesion itself, and the outer arrows (B and C) indicate extension of calcifications. Note that it is generally inadvisable for the surgeon to cut the localization wire prior to specimen radiography. An intact wire lessens the possibility that a wire fragment will remain in the breast after surgery.

therefore, the specimen radiograph should direct the initial sectioning of the specimen by the pathologist. This applies to all mammographic lesions, whether or not they contain calcifications. However, specimen radiography is effective in guiding the pathologist to the site of the lesion only if the orientation of the specimen does not change during transport from the radiology department to the pathology department.

Several simple methods have been developed to assist in specimen radiography and maintenance of specimen orientation. For instance, some radiologists simply place a needle within the specimen prior to radiography and note the position of the needle relative to the lesion on a copy of the specimen radiograph sent to the pathologist. Other radiologists document the orientation of the specimen during radiography by

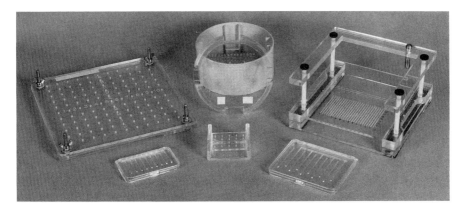

Figure 24-11. Specimen localization devices. Several breast specimen localization devices are commercially available to assist with biopsy specimen processing.

sandwiching the specimen between sheets of clear x-ray film and tracing the outline of the specimen contour on the film. The location of the lesion as seen on radiographs of the sandwiched specimen is then drawn on the overlying sheet of clear film. Both reusable and disposable specialized commercial devices are also available to facilitate specimen radiography. These usually provide for compression of the specimen by a perforated plate, through which the lesion is marked and held in place by a pin or needle (Figures 24-11 and 24-12). The known spacing of perforations on the compression plate can be used to measure lesion size by extrapolation.

The need to limit the contact of medical personnel with potentially infectious body tissues means that every breast specimen should be transported to the radiology department within a sealed plastic bag or other similarly sealed container. The method used for specimen radiography should minimize direct contact with the specimen by radiology personnel.

Tissue block radiography should be regarded as an adjunctive rather than a primary method of lesion identification. It is mandatory when the biopsy specimen contains microcalcifications that are not identified by the pathologist during routine histologic evaluation **(Option (F) is true)** (Figure 24-13). This ensures that the area of mammographic interest will be analyzed by the pathologist. One reported method of tissue block radiography involves imaging the tissue blocks in orthogonal projections to determine not only which tissue blocks actually contain the microcalcifications but also the depth of the calcifications within these selected tissue blocks.

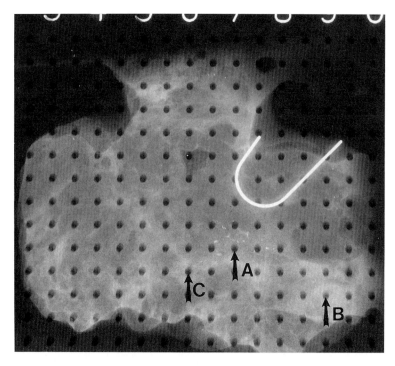

Figure 24-12. Same specimen as shown in Figure 24-10. Specimen radiography with a localization grid. The main area of calcification underlies the perforation labeled with arrow A, and calcifications extend to underlie the perforations labeled B and C. Marker pins are then inserted into the specimen through these perforations. Calcification and invasive ductal carcinoma were identified at position A. Calcification and ductal carcinoma *in situ* were identified at positions B and C. The pathologist measured the main lesion to be 1.5 cm. A similar measurement can be extrapolated from this specimen radiograph, because the grid perforations are spaced at 4-mm intervals.

In our experience with specimen localization and directed specimen sectioning, tissue block radiography is rarely required. There is cause for concern if tissue block radiography is routinely needed to identify microcalcifications that were not discovered on the initial microscopic analysis. Furthermore, although tissue block radiography works well for lesions that contain microcalcifications, it is unsuccessful for noncalcified lesions. Therefore, great care should be taken to optimize the specimen radiography technique. It is more efficient and cost effective to identify lesions prospectively without resorting to tissue block imaging. This will also minimize the possibility of a false-negative pathology interpretation.

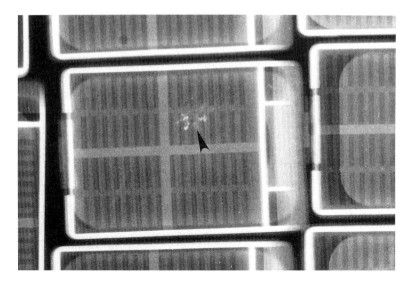

Figure 24-13. Tissue block radiograph. This patient had mammographically suspicious microcalcifications that were seen on a specimen radiograph (not shown) but not identified on the initial histologic evaluation. Specimen-radiography-directed specimen sectioning had not been done. This radiograph demonstrates the suspicious microcalcifications in only one of many tissue blocks (arrowhead). Additional sections were taken from this tissue block, and the pathologist then identified the microcalcifications, which were associated with a focus of atypical hyperplasia.

Question 108

Concerning microcalcifications seen on specimen radiographs,

(A) they nearly always correspond to the location of histologically demonstrated carcinoma

(B) if distant from the resected mass, they generally indicate intraductal extension of tumor

(C) those composed of calcium oxalate are better seen histologically with polarized light than on hematoxylin-and-eosin-stained sections

(D) they are a common manifestation of lobular neoplasia (lobular carcinoma *in situ*)

The strong association of microcalcifications with breast carcinoma is well known. Indeed, the presence of clustered microcalcifications is often an indication for breast biopsy. As mentioned above, it is essential for the pathologist to identify calcifications on histologic analysis of a specimen if biopsy was performed to evaluate suspicious calcifications. This step ensures that the pathologist has examined the lesion of mammographic concern. However, studies correlating the location of calcifications with the location of pathologically demonstrated carcinoma indicate that calcifications are not always present at the site of a carcinoma but can be adjacent to it or even as far as 1 cm away **(Option (A) is false).** Therefore, pathologists must thoroughly examine not only the exact location of mammographic calcifications but also the immediately adjacent tissues.

Once a carcinoma is identified, attention should be directed to determining the extent of the lesion within the biopsy specimen. The presence of extensive calcification within the specimen, distant from the excised lesion, generally indicates intraductal spread of carcinoma **(Option (B) is true).** Therefore, if specimen radiography indicates that calcifications extend away from the primary tumor site, the pathologist must direct histologic analysis to these areas as well.

Investigators have noted that even when examining sections from tissue blocks of some radiographically visible calcifications, the pathologist may not be able to identify calcifications. One such circumstance involves the presence of calcium oxalate crystals. These are radiopaque on mammography but usually imperceptible on routine histologic evaluation, unlike (the much more common) calcium phosphate crystals, which exhibit a characteristic blue tint on standard hematoxylin-and-eosin-stained sections. To demonstrate calcium oxalate crystals, polarized light microscopy is needed **(Option (C) is true).**

The mammographic features of lobular neoplasia (lobular carcinoma *in situ* [LCIS)]) are nonspecific; most often, no findings at all are seen. Microcalcification is not typically associated with LCIS **(Option (D) is false).** The discovery of LCIS is usually serendipitous when it is identified because of mammographic calcification. In these cases the calcification is typically found nearby but not within the area of LCIS.

Kevin W. McEnery, M.D.
Judy M. Destouet, M.D.

SUGGESTED READINGS

NEEDLE LOCALIZATION TECHNIQUES

1. Homer MJ. Preoperative needle localization of lesions in the lower half of the breast: needle entry from below. AJR 1987; 149:43–45
2. Homer MJ, Smith TJ, Safaii H. Prebiopsy needle localization. Methods, problems, and expected results. Radiol Clin North Am 1992; 30:139–153
3. Kopans DB, Swann CA. Preoperative imaging-guided needle placement and localization of clinically occult breast lesions. AJR 1989; 152:1–9

4. Pisano ED, Hall FM. Preoperative localization of inferior breast lesions. AJR 1989; 153:272

BREAST SPECIMEN RADIOGRAPHY

5. Bauermeister DE, Hall MH. Specimen radiography—a mandatory adjunct to mammography. Am J Clin Pathol 1973; 59:782–789
6. Cardenosa G, Eklund GW. Paraffin block radiography following breast biopsies: use of orthogonal views. Radiology 1991; 180:873–874
7. Rebner M, Pennes DR, Baker DE, Adler DD, Boyd P. Two-view specimen radiography in surgical biopsy of nonpalpable breast masses. AJR 1987; 149:283–285
8. Stomper PC, Davis SP, Sonnenfeld MR, Meyer JE, Greenes RA, Eberlein TJ. Efficacy of specimen radiography of clinically occult noncalcified breast lesions. AJR 1988; 151:43–47

MICROCALCIFICATION IDENTIFICATION

9. D'Orsi CJ, Reale FR, Davis MA, Brown VJ. Breast specimen microcalcifications: radiographic validation and pathologic-radiologic correlation. Radiology 1991; 180:397–401
10. Owings DV, Hann L, Schnitt SJ. How thoroughly should needle localization breast biopsies be sampled for microscopic examination? A prospective mammographic/pathologic correlative study. Am J Surg Pathol 1990; 14:578–583
11. Rebner M, Helvie MA, Pennes DR, Oberman HA, Ikeda DM, Adler DD. Paraffin tissue block radiography: adjunct to breast specimen radiography. Radiology 1989; 173:695–696
12. Stein MA, Karlan MS. Calcifications in breast biopsy specimens: discrepancies in radiologic-pathologic identification. Radiology 1991; 179:111–114
13. Surratt JT, Monsees BS, Mazoujian G. Calcium oxalate microcalcifications in the breast. Radiology 1991; 181:141–142
14. Tornos C, Silva E, el-Naggar A, Pritzker KP. Calcium oxalate crystals in breast biopsies. The missing microcalcifications. Am J Surg Pathol 1990; 14:961–968

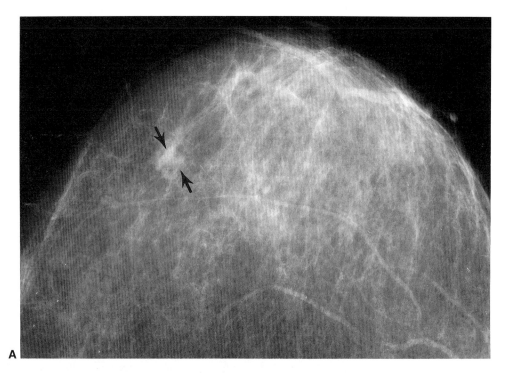

Figure 25-1

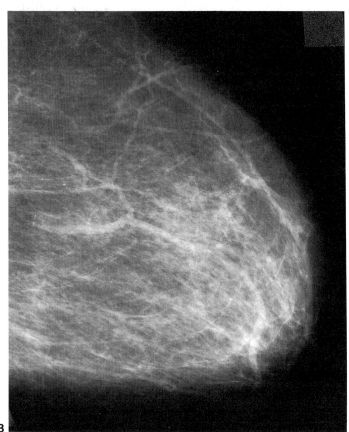

Figures 25-1 and 25-2. This 70-year-old woman underwent mammographic screening. You are shown CC (A) and MLO (B) views (Figure 25-1). A 6-mm density (arrows) not present 1 year ago was detected on the CC view. You are also shown CC (A) and 90° lateral (B) spot-compression magnification views (Figure 25-2). Spiculated margins are seen clearly on the CC view but are barely visible on the 90° lateral view (arrows). The patient is a poor operative risk.

Case 25: Stereotactic Localization of the Nonpalpable Breast Lesion

Question 109

The NEXT step should be:

(A) follow-up mammography in 6 months
(B) sonographically guided fine-needle aspiration cytology or core biopsy
(C) stereotactic fine-needle aspiration or core biopsy
(D) grid coordinate needle localization

Short-term mammographic follow-up of a solid mass (Option (A)) should be performed only when the mass fulfills all accepted imaging criteria for a probably benign lesion. Most authorities require demonstration that at least 75% of the margins of a mass are well defined on magnification views before assigning it "probably benign" status. These criteria are not met in the test images (Figures 25-1 and 25-2).

Furthermore, the development of a neodensity, particularly in a postmenopausal woman, raises the possibility of carcinoma. The evaluation of such an abnormality has changed dramatically over the past 5 years. Formerly, these patients routinely underwent needle localization followed by open surgical biopsy. However, technical improvements in alphanumeric grid localization systems and sonographic equipment, as well as the development of stereotactic devices and automated biopsy guns, now enable us to obtain tissue from nonpalpable lesions without open surgical biopsy.

With the development of high-frequency (7.5- and 10-MHz) ultrasound transducers, it is now possible to visualize and characterize small breast lesions. However, it remains difficult to differentiate a cyst from a solid mass when the lesion is smaller than 1 cm, especially in a large breast or one replaced with fat. The small size (6 mm) of the lesion in the test patient makes it unlikely that it would be seen on ultrasonography. As a general rule, ultrasonography of irregular masses is useful only if there is a possibility that an underlying cyst with surrounding inflamma-

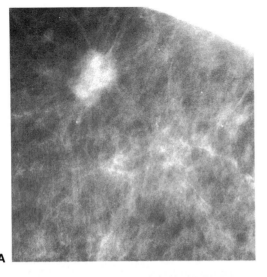

A

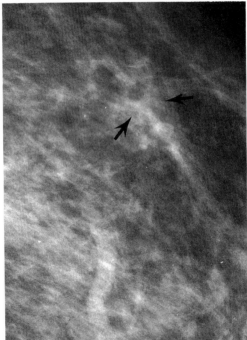

B

Figure 25-2

tory reaction is present. In such a situation aspiration of fluid from the cyst and pneumocystography would be indicated.

Some investigators have reported considerable success in fine-needle aspiration and core biopsy of nonpalpable lesions with sonographic guidance (Option (B)), but one must develop expertise with this procedure before relying on its results to determine the management of indeterminate breast masses. In 1987, Fornage et al. reported a 92% sensitivity and a 93% specificity in the cytologic diagnosis of malignancy, for lesions that ranged in size from 8 to 35 mm in greatest dimension. D'Orsi and Mendelson also report fine-needle aspiration of lesions as small as 8 mm. However, for most radiologists, sonographically guided fine-needle aspiration or core biopsy of a 6-mm lesion is fraught with enough difficulty to make this option unacceptable in the test patient.

Parker et al. (1993) combined sonographic guidance with the use of an automated gun and a 14-gauge needle to obtain core biopsies. This technique allows for continuous observation of the needle and lesion and permits one to approach the lesion at virtually any angle, even parallel to the chest wall. However, this is a freehand technique and hence requires greater skill and experience than are needed for procedures involving a biopsy needle guide. Biopsy guides are widely available for 3.5- and 5.0-MHz transducers, but they are not routinely available for 7.5-MHz transducers. A biopsy guide permits visualization of the needle as it traverses the lesion; however, it can be cumbersome to use, and it limits the angle at which the lesion can be approached. Indeed, use of a needle guide may preclude the use of the best pathway to sample the lesion while avoiding the chest wall. It can also be difficult to maintain sterility during multiple passes through a needle guide.

The fact that the test patient is a poor surgical risk means that grid coordinate needle localization followed by open surgical biopsy (Option (D)) is not the preferred procedure for establishing a diagnosis. In some centers, breast biopsies are still performed under general anesthesia. Furthermore, the lesion in the test patient was barely visible on orthogonal views, and even then was seen only on the spot-compression magnification view (Figure 25-2B). This would have substantially limited the likelihood of success with conventional grid coordinate needle localization. On the other hand, stereotactic devices are far more accurate in localizing suspicious lesions that cannot be seen readily on the orthogonal projection **(Option (C) is correct).**

Stereotactic fine-needle aspiration biopsy (SFNB) was developed in Sweden and has been in use at the Karolinska Hospital since 1976. This procedure is now enthusiastically embraced by the Swedish radiology community, in no small part because of the success reported by Azavedo et al. in the evaluation of 2,594 mammographically detected nonpalpable lesions, 2,005 (77.3%) of which were so characteristically benign by SFNB that surgical biopsy was averted. Only 1 of these 2,005 lesions turned out to be a cancer, 14 months later. Of the 567 patients who did undergo surgery, 429 (75.7%) had breast cancer, with lesions ranging in size from 3 to 30 mm. In 49 (8.6%) of the 567 patients who underwent surgery, there was insufficient or inadequate material from SFNB to establish a cytomorphologic diagnosis.

However, investigators in the United States have not been able to reproduce these highly successful results. The reported insufficient or inadequate rates for SFNB range up to 54%. One major source of difficulty is the paucity of pathologists trained in the interpretation of breast cytology. With the introduction of large-gauge (20- to 14-gauge) cutting needles, which produce tissue cores ranging in length from 10 to 17 mm, many of the difficulties encountered with SFNB were overcome. The pathologist can now perform histologic instead of cytologic analysis of breast specimens. In addition, large-gauge needles can be used in conjunction with automated biopsy guns, which provide a range of 15 to 23 mm forward needle excursion into the breast. Such long excursions eliminate the need for the pinpoint accuracy that is required with fine-needle aspiration cytology, in which the sampling needle may traverse 10 mm or less of breast tissue.

Parker et al. (1991) report 96% agreement between the histologic results from stereotactically guided automated-gun core biopsy and surgical biopsy specimens in 102 cases. One of 23 carcinomas and one benign lesion were missed with the automated large-core biopsy gun. On the other hand, two sclerotic fibroadenomas diagnosed by automated large-core biopsy were missed at open surgical biopsy.

For radiologists who do not have a stereotactic device, fine-needle aspiration can be performed by using standard, widely available, coordinate-grid localization equipment. Evans and Cade report comparable results in performing fine-needle aspiration between standard grid localization and stereotactic localization, with sensitivities of 71 and 80%, respectively. However, as discussed below, the precision of standard-grid localization is limited since the depth of the lesion is estimated from mammograms taken prior to localization and is not precisely known during the aspiration procedure.

Question 110

Concerning stereotactic procedures,

(A) they require expensive, specialized equipment
(B) they are highly operator dependent
(C) they require a cooperative patient
(D) they permit more precise wire localization

The principle behind the operation of all stereotactic equipment is basically the same. Two images of a lesion are obtained by angling the mammography tube 15° in one direction and then 15° in the other direction away from a reference projection, i.e., +15° and −15°. From these images a computer calculates the three-dimensional location of the lesion along the x, y, and z axes. The resulting x, y, and z coordinates are then either dialed in manually or automatically transferred from the computer to the stereotactic device, which aligns its needle holder directly over the lesion. After the skin is aseptically cleansed and infiltrated with local anesthetic, a small incision is made in the skin. Separation of the subcutaneous tissues with a "mosquito" clamp allows the needle to move freely through the breast toward the lesion. If the needle meets resistance as it passes through the skin and subcutaneous tissues, there will be interference with its excursion deeper into the breast, which may result in incomplete sampling of the lesion and discomfort to the patient because a pulling sensation is created at the skin. Once the needle has been advanced to the designated depth in the breast, repeat stereotactic views are obtained to determine the accuracy of needle placement. Before tissue sampling, the needle is retracted approximately 5 mm, to withdraw the needle tip from the center of the lesion. This maneuver is done so that sampling of the lesion begins at its anterior edge rather than at its center. After the specimen is obtained, by either fine-needle aspiration or core biopsy, the x, y, and z coordinates are adjusted to sample nearby areas within the lesion. Most radiologists perform at least five separate passes through a lesion to overcome sampling error (Figure 25-3).

For needle localization of a nonpalpable lesion, it is advisable to advance the z axis or depth coordinate by 10 mm to ensure that the localizing wire traverses a portion of the lesion before the breast is released from compression (Figure 25-4). If the localizing needle is not advanced deeper into the breast before the wire is deployed, the wire may end up being superficial to the lesion (Figure 25-5).

Stereotactic localization requires specialized equipment; two types of devices are commercially available for stereotactic localization: a stand-alone prone table and an add-on unit that can be attached to a standard mammography machine. As discussed below, each system has features that must be considered before such a purchase is made. The prone table is more expensive than the add-on unit, with current prices of over $100,000 and over $35,000, respectively **(Option (A) is true)**.

Stereotactic procedures are relatively easy to perform, but the learning curve is steep. These procedures require meticulous operator technique and an understanding of three-dimensional relationships **(Option (B) is true)**. Stereotactic biopsy procedures also require a cooperative patient who can remain motionless (Figure 25-6) **(Option (C) is true)**.

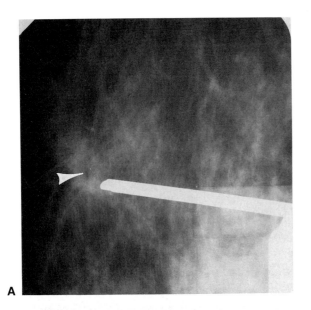

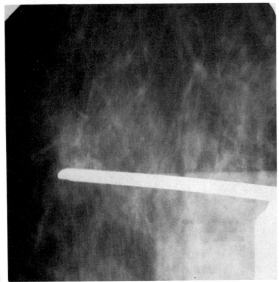

Figure 25-3. Stereotactically guided core biopsy, multiple passes. Stereotactic views before (A) and after (B) fire of the biopsy gun, showing the full excursion of a 22-mm throw, 14-gauge needle into an invasive ductal carcinoma. The small radiolucent defect in the center of the spiculated mass (arrowhead in panel A) indicates the site of a previous needle pass.

This is particularly important with use of an add-on stereotactic unit, since the patient sits upright for the procedure.

An advantage of stereotactically guided wire localization is the precise placement of the needle within a lesion since the x, y, and z axes are calculated by a computer and are not estimated from mammograms taken before the localization procedure (**Option (D) is true**). As mentioned above, the z or depth coordinate should be advanced 10 mm to

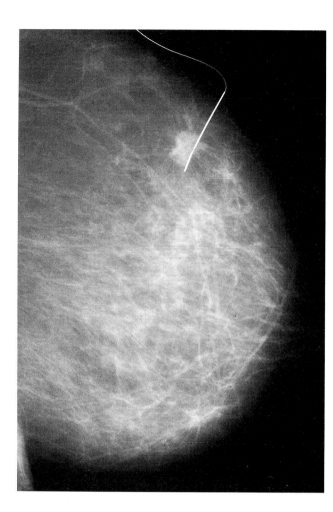

Figure 25-4. Stereotactically guided needle localization, proper wire placement. Mediolateral view following a stereotactic core biopsy and needle localization, prior to surgical excision of an invasive ductal carcinoma, shows optimal placement of the hook wire just inferior to the mass.

ensure that the needle traverses the entire lesion and does not lie superficial to it when the breast is released from compression.

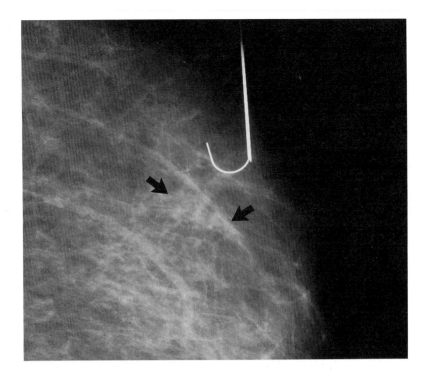

Figure 25-5. Stereotactically guided needle localization, improper wire placement. Mediolateral view following stereotactic needle localization shows a suboptimal position of the hook wire with respect to the mass (arrows). The needle should have been advanced 10 mm before the hook wire was engaged.

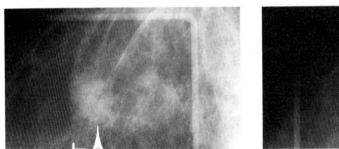
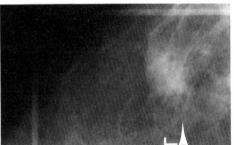

A　　　　　　　　　　　　　　　　　　　　　　　　　　　　　B

Figure 25-6. Stereotactically guided lesion localization complicated by patient motion. (A and B) Stereotactic CC views show movement of the spiculated mass along the *y* axis (arrowheads) (vertical displacement), which is due to patient motion between exposures. The mammography tube travels only along the *x* axis (lateral displacement), so any other movement is an indication for restarting the localization procedure. (C) Mediolateral view following wire deployment demonstates how incorrect the *z* axis or depth can be if motion occurs at any point during the localization procedure. The J-wire tip is 7 cm inferior to the cancer.

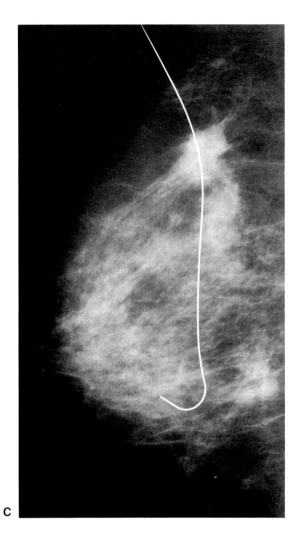

C

Question 111

Stereotactically guided procedures are preferable to the use of a grid coordinate system for:

    (A) biopsy of loosely grouped calcifications
    (B) biopsy of a mass smaller than 1 cm
    (C) biopsy of a deep lesion in a large breast
    (D) aspiration of a cyst smaller than 1 cm

    To calculate the coordinates for stereotactic biopsy, the center of the lesion must be indicated on two stereotactic images. For tightly grouped calcifications or a small, dense mass, it is relatively easy to determine the lesion center. However, for loosely grouped calcifications it can be difficult to mark the center of the lesion with precision **(Option (A) is false)**. In general, scattered or loosely grouped calcifications indicate a benign process, and unless they are pleomorphic or branching, they do not warrant biopsy. When percutaneous sampling of this type of large-area lesion is indicated, multiple sites may be subjected to biopsy or aspirated by using a grid coordinate system.

In a series involving grid coordinate-directed fine-needle aspiration of 61 nonpalpable breast lesions, Arishita et al. reported that 18 (30%) of the aspirates were inadequate for diagnosis, and 12 of 14 carcinomas were accurately diagnosed. Unfortunately, the lesion size was not specified. Helvie et al. reported that only 46% of 215 nonpalpable breast lesions that underwent grid coordinate aspiration provided sufficient specimens for diagnosis. Inaccurate needle placement in masses smaller than 1 cm and microcalcifications were the major source of sampling errors. Hann et al. concurred that fine-needle aspiration with a standard mammographic grid coordinate device has limitations for small lesions (<5 mm) or for firm masses, which can deflect the needle. For these reasons, the use of stereotactic guidance is generally preferred, especially for lesions smaller than 1 cm **(Option (B) is true)**.

Lofgren et al. reported that needle deviation was a major source of error in all localization procedures and that the deeper the lesion, the more difficult it was to place the needle tip accurately within the abnormality. This problem can be reduced by rotating the needle while advancing it. Such a maneuver also helps to minimize the likelihood of pushing the lesion aside or in front of the needle. In a large breast with a deep lesion, the superior accuracy of stereotactically guided needle placement is especially important to minimize the confounding effects of needle deviation **(Option (C) is true)**.

As discussed above, in some cases it is difficult to be sure that a mass smaller than 1 cm is truly cystic on ultrasonography, and aspiration of fluid from such a lesion is definitive for diagnosis. This procedure can be performed under ultrasonographic, grid coordinate, or stereotactic guidance, but stereotactic guidance is the most reliable method for aspiration of fluid from cysts smaller than 1 cm **(Option (D) is true)**. An initial attempt to aspirate fluid usually is made with sonographic guidance, and if this procedure is unsuccessful, stereotactic guidance is the next step.

Question 112

Concerning stereotactic devices,

(A) prone systems facilitate procedures in less cooperative patients
(B) prone systems facilitate sampling of lesions adjacent to the chest wall
(C) upright systems are designed to obtain cytological samples only
(D) each upright system works only with the mammography unit(s) of that manufacturer
(E) upright systems cost less than prone systems

Stereotactic technology is now several years old, but there continue to be a few technical problems associated with the units. The patient who is unstable or uncooperative should not undergo a stereotactically guided procedure, particularly if the available unit is an upright add-on device **(Option (A) is true).** Any breast motion incurred during the procedure will probably result in inaccurate needle placement and an incorrect diagnosis (Figure 25-6).

The use of prone systems is associated with a marked decrease, if not total elimination, of vasovagal reactions. However, some patients do complain of neck or arm discomfort when they lie on a prone table for an extended period. Prone systems do not appear to be any more effective in permitting the sampling of lesions adjacent to the chest wall **(Option (B) is false).** The one carcinoma missed by Parker et al. (1991), who used a prone unit, was a small cluster of microcalcifications that gradually retracted out of the field of view because it was so close to the chest wall.

Upright systems are designed to obtain both histologic and cytologic samples **(Option (C) is false).** However, some upright systems have a limited amount of working room between the breast and the mammography tube head, which makes it difficult to connect a syringe directly to an aspiration needle. A short length of tubing can be attached to the aspiration needle and syringe to overcome this problem. Similarly, it is difficult to use an automated biopsy gun with some upright units. However, several disposable automated biopsy guns have been shortened to be suitable for use with these upright units.

Each add-on or upright system works only with the mammography unit(s) of that specific manufacturer **(Option (D) is true).** However, most mammography equipment manufacturers provide an upright stereotactic biopsy device as an option, costing $35,000 or more. Currently only two manufacturers make free-standing prone systems, which cost $100,000 or more **(Option (E) is true).** Optional features, such as digital image processing and computerized storage of multiple coordinates for up to eight different needle positions, are available for an additional cost. One disadvantage of a prone-table unit is that it occupies a room that must then be used only to perform stereotactic biopsies, an expense that may be difficult to justify unless many stereotactic procedures are done each day. Multipurpose use of the room can be preserved by wiring the same generator to supply both a mammography unit and the stereotactic system, although a substantially larger room will be needed to accommodate the stereotactic table.

Questions 113 through 117

For each numbered statement listed below (Questions 113 through 117), indicate whether it is MORE closely associated with core biopsy (A) or fine-needle aspiration cytology (B), equally associated with both procedures (C), or associated with neither (D). Each lettered option may be used once, more than once, or not at all.

113. The pathologist needs special training for interpretation of the specimen
114. Invasive carcinoma is reliably differentiated from *in situ* carcinoma
115. Sclerosing duct hyperplasia (radial scar) is reliably diagnosed
116. Only one specimen is required for diagnosis
117. Fibroadenoma is reliably diagnosed

    (A)   Core biopsy
    (B)   Fine-needle aspiration cytology
    (C)   Both
    (D)   Neither

Proficiency in the cytologic diagnosis of breast disease is a prerequisite for interpretation of fine-needle aspirates of breast tissue. In the United States, fine-needle aspiration for the diagnosis of benign and malignant breast lesions has not been widely used, in part because of the lack of trained cytopathologists. Some radiologists have recently adopted the use of 20- to 14-gauge needles to obtain core biopsy specimens, which are suitable for conventional histologic analysis, since this does not require specialized training of the pathologist **(Option (B) is the correct answer to Question 113).**

Large-gauge core biopsy is evaluated by histologic rather than cytologic analysis; therefore, it reliably differentiates invasive carcinoma from *in situ* carcinoma **(Option (A) is the correct answer to Question 114).** However, neither fine-needle aspiration cytology (FNAC) nor core biopsy is recommended to diagnose sclerosing duct hyperplasia (radial scar) **(Option (D) is the correct answer to Question 115).** This lesion is also difficult to distinguish from invasive carcinoma at mammography, and because there is a possibility that radial scar is a risk marker for subsequent development of tubular carcinoma, some investigators believe that radial scars should be completely excised anyway.

Multiple tissue samples should be collected from all lesions to minimize the likelihood of sampling error. This rationale applies to core biopsy as well as to FNAC **(Option (D) is the correct answer to Question 116).** Neither procedure will yield accurate data if only one sample is obtained. Some investigators recommend having a cytotechnologist available to analyze specimen adequacy after each needle pass during a fine-needle aspiration procedure, in an attempt to decrease procedure time by reducing the number of passes. For core biopsy procedures, most radiologists routinely perform five (and sometimes more) passes through different sites in a lesion. With multiple core biopsy specimens, it can often be determined whether an *in situ* component coexists with invasive cancer.

FNAC often yields typical cells that allow the cytopathologist to diagnose a fibroadenoma, but usually it simply provides a nonspecific benign diagnosis. Core biopsy much more frequently provides sufficient tissue to make the confident diagnosis of fibroadenoma **(Option (A) is the correct answer to Question 117).** However, for the fibroadenoma that is large enough to prompt mammographic work-up, there is a very infrequent (perhaps 1%) association of *in situ* carcinoma located either within or immediately adjacent to the fibroadenoma. For this reason and because both FNAC and core biopsy techniques do not sample all of a targeted lesion, radiologists may recommend periodic mammographic surveillance when the tissue-sampling diagnosis is fibroadenoma, an approach similar to that used for "probably benign" lesions (which also carry an approximately 1% likelihood of malignancy).

Surprisingly, few complications have been reported with the use of either FNAC or core biopsy. Patients sometimes experience mild breast pain during or after the procedures. Hematomas may develop in the breast, apparently more frequently after core biopsy, but they are rarely a serious complication; in fact, there is only one reported case that required surgical drainage. More disturbing is the report of seeding of the needle track during large-core biopsy of a mucinous carcinoma. The risk of track seeding for large-core biopsy yielding breast cancer is approximately 1%. Incorporation of the core biopsy track within the resected specimen during definitive breast cancer surgery is one method to eliminate the possibility of track seeding.

Stereotactic FNAC and core biopsy promise to result in less costly work-up of mammographically detected nonpalpable lesions, primarily because the procedure may allow for a significant reduction in the number of open surgical biopsies of benign lesions. In addition, by establishing the diagnosis of carcinoma less invasively than open biopsy, stereotactic biopsy may eliminate some cases of two-stage breast cancer surgery, i.e., open surgery to establish the diagnosis and reexcision (when necessary) to achieve negative tumor margins. Once a definitive diagnosis of carcinoma is made by stereotactic biopsy, a one-step surgical approach will usually succeed.

However, the cost of stereotactic equipment is high, and currently third-party payers are reluctant to reimburse for the procedure because most authorities still consider stereotactic biopsy an experimental test. The National Cancer Institute is in the process of conducting a large-scale multi-institutional trial to determine the proper clinical role of stereotactic breast biopsy. Results of this trial may well provide the scientific support needed to gain widespread acceptance of the procedure in the United States.

Judy M. Destouet, M.D.

SUGGESTED READINGS

ULTRASONOGRAPHY

1. Adler DD. Ultrasound of benign breast conditions. Semin US CT MR 1989; 10:106–118
2. D'Orsi CJ, Mendelson EB. Interventional breast ultrasonography. Semin US CT MR 1989; 10:132–138
3. Fornage BD, Faroux MJ, Simatos A. Breast masses: US-guided fine-needle aspiration biopsy. Radiology 1987; 162:409–414
4. Fornage BD, Sneige N, Faroux MJ, Andry E. Sonographic appearance and ultrasound-guided fine-needle aspiration biopsy of breast carcinomas smaller than 1 cm^3. J Ultrasound Med 1990; 9:559–568
5. Hogg JP, Harris KM, Skolnick ML. The role of ultrasound-guided needle aspiration of breast masses. Ultrasound Med Biol 1988; 14(Suppl 1):13–21
6. Jackson VP. Sonography of malignant breast disease. Semin US CT MR 1989; 10:119–131
7. Parker SH, Jobe WE, Dennis MA, et al. US-guided automated large-core breast biopsy. Radiology 1993; 184:507–511
8. Rizzatto G, Solbiati L, Croce F, Derchi LE. Aspiration biopsy of superficial lesions: ultrasonic guidance with a linear-array probe. AJR 1987; 148:623–625
9. Svensson WE, Tohno E, Cosgrove DO, Powles TJ, al Murrani B, Jones AL. Effects of fine-needle aspiration on the US appearance of the breast. Radiology 1992; 185:709–711

FINE-NEEDLE ASPIRATION CYTOLOGY

10. Arishita GI, Cruz BK, Harding CT, Arbutina DR. Mammogram-directed fine-needle aspiration of nonpalpable breast lesions. J Surg Oncol 1991; 48:153–157

11. Evans WP, Cade SH. Needle localization and fine-needle aspiration biopsy of nonpalpable breast lesions with use of standard and stereotactic equipment. Radiology 1989; 173:53–56

12. Hann L, Ducatman BS, Wang HH, Fein V, McIntire JM. Nonpalpable breast lesions: evaluation by means of fine-needle aspiration cytology. Radiology 1989; 171:373–376

13. Helvie MA, Baker DE, Adler DD, Andersson I, Naylor B, Buckwalter KA. Radiographically guided fine-needle aspiration of nonpalpable breast lesions. Radiology 1990; 174:657–661

14. Kreula J. Effect of sampling technique on specimen size in fine needle aspiration biopsy. Invest Radiol 1990; 25:1294–1299

15. Lamb J, Anderson TJ. Influence of cancer histology on the success of fine needle aspiration of the breast. J Clin Pathol 1989; 42:733–735

16. Orel SG, Evers K, Yeh IT, Troupin RH. Radial scar with microcalcifications: radiologic-pathologic correlation. Radiology 1992; 183:479–482

STEREOTACTICALLY GUIDED BIOPSY

17. Azavedo E, Svane G, Auer G. Stereotactic fine-needle biopsy in 2594 mammographically detected non-palpable lesions. Lancet 1989; 1:1033–1036

18. Ciatto S, Rosselli Del Turco M, Bravetti P. Nonpalpable breast lesions: stereotaxic fine-needle aspiration cytology. Radiology 1989; 173:57–59

19. Dowlatshahi K, Gent HJ, Schmidt R, Jokich PM, Bibbo M, Sprenger E. Nonpalpable breast tumors: diagnosis with stereotaxic localization and fine-needle aspiration. Radiology 1989; 170:427–433

20. Dowlatshahi K, Yaremko ML, Kluskens LF, Jokich PM. Nonpalpable breast lesions: findings of stereotaxic needle-core biopsy and fine-needle aspiration cytology. Radiology 1991; 181:745 750

21. Fajardo LL, Davis JR, Wiens JL, Trego DC. Mammography-guided stereotactic fine-needle aspiration cytology of nonpalpable breast lesions: prospective comparison with surgical biopsy results. AJR 1990; 155:977–981

22. Harter LP, Curtis JS, Ponto G, Craig PH. Malignant seeding of the needle track during stereotaxic core needle breast biopsy. Radiology 1992; 185:713–714

23. Jackson VP, Bassett LW. Stereotactic fine-needle aspiration biopsy for nonpalpable breast lesions. AJR 1990; 154:1196–1197

24. Jackson VP, Reynolds HE. Stereotaxic needle-core biopsy and fine-needle aspiration cytologic evaluation of nonpalpable breast lesions. Radiology 1991; 181:633–634

25. Kopans DB. Fine-needle aspiration of clinically occult breast lesions. Radiology 1989; 170:313–314

26. Lofgren M, Andersson I, Lindholm K. Stereotactic fine-needle aspiration for cytologic diagnosis of nonpalpable breast lesions. AJR 1990; 154:1191–1195

27. Parker SH, Hopper KD, Yakes WF, Gibson MD, Ownbey JL, Carter TE. Image-directed percutaneous biopsies with a biopsy gun. Radiology 1989; 171:663–669

28. Parker SH, Lovin JD, Jobe WE, et al. Stereotactic breast biopsy with a biopsy gun. Radiology 1990; 176:741–747

29. Parker SH, Lovin JD, Jobe WE, Burke BJ, Hopper KD, Yakes WF. Nonpalpable breast lesions: stereotactic automated large-core biopsies. Radiology 1991; 180:403–407

Notes

Index

Where there are multiple page references, **boldface** indicates the main discussion of a topic.

Implant-displaced view, 274, 278
Implants. *See also* Saline-filled implants; Silicone-filled implants
  leakage, 281
  manual technique, 73
  rupture, 280–82
  subglandular, 269, 279
  subpectoral, 269, 274, 279
Incompletely evaluated calcifications
  differential diagnosis
    benign skin calcifications, 191–92
    calcifications suspicious for malignancy, 192
    probably benign calcifications, 191–92
    sedimented calcium in tiny benign cysts, 190–92
Inferior-approach needle placement, 322, 324
Inflammatory carcinoma, 305, 313
Inframammary fold, 3, 13, 37–38, 47–48, 54
Internal echo, 122–24
Internal necrosis, 139
Intracystic carcinoma, 96, 124, 287, 293–94
  differential diagnosis
    cyst, 115
Intracystic hemorrhage, 293–96
Intracystic papillary carcinoma, 122–23, 293
Intracystic papillary lesions, 293–96
Intralobular ducts, 5
Intramural cysts, 93
Invasive carcinoma, 106, 315–16, 350
Invasive ductal carcinoma, 306. *See also* Medullary carcinoma
  circumscribed carcinoma and, 96
  differential diagnosis
    complex cyst, 89
    ductal carcinoma *in situ*, 89, 239–40
    fibroadenoma, 89
    phyllodes tumor, 89
  intracystic papillary carcinoma and, 293
  ultrasonography, 122–23
  well-defined mass at mammography, 110–11
Invasive ductal carcinoma "not otherwise specified," 139
Invasive lobular carcinoma, 306, **315–16**
  differential diagnosis
    spiculated lesions, 134–35
Involuntary tremors, 57
Involuting fibroadenomas
  differential diagnosis
    cyst, 127
    hamartoma, 127–28
    lymph node, 127–28
    medullary carcinoma, 127

Isolated cluster of tiny calcifications
  additional mammographic projections, 193–95
  blurring of magnification mammograms, 198–99
  interpretation of test images, 189–92
  magnification technique, 194, **195–98**
  work-up steps, 192–93

K

Keloids, 217
kVp technique, 56–57, 63–68, 71, 78, 198–99, 278

L

Lactating accessory breast, 42
Lactation, 313
Large-gauge core biopsy, 350–51
Lateral shadowing, 120
Lateromedial needle approach, 322
Lateromedial view, 43, 45, 47, 207
LCIS. *See* Lobular carcinoma *in situ*
Lesions. *See also* Dermal calcifications; Malignant lesions; Masses; Nonpalpable lesions; Spiculated lesions
  anticipated location, 43–45, 47
  cystic, 287–89
  eczematoid, 224
  high-risk, 110
  imaging work-ups, 105–7
  raised skin lesions, 102–3
  specimen radiography, 330–34
  triangulation estimate using the oblique view, 3–15
  verrucous, 103
  visibility limited to one standard projection, 21–33
Linear-array transducers, 296
Linearly distributed calcifications, 151, 229
Lipofibroadenomas, 103
Lipoid cysts
  differential diagnosis
    ringlike calcifications, 264
Lipoma, 74
Liposarcoma, 147
Lobular carcinoma *in situ*, 110, 237, **240–41**, 262, 315
Lobular hyperplasia, 223, 226, 247
Lobular neoplasia, 110, 237, 240, 336
  differential diagnosis
    microcystic hyperplasia, 246
Lobulated cysts, 89–90
Local excision. *See* Lumpectomy
Localization needle systems, 327–30
Localized dermal calcifications. *See* Dermal calcifications
Low-amplitude echo, 26

Low-density radiopaque masses, 89
Low-level internal echoes, 120
Lumpectomy, 106–7, 154, 305
Lymph nodes, 108
    differential diagnosis
        involuting fibroadenoma, 127–28
        metastasis, 293
Lymphoma, 315
Lymphosarcoma, 147

M

Mach effect, 124
Macrolobulations, 108–9
Magnetic resonance imaging, 119, 277
Magnification techniques, 194, **195–98**. *See also* Spot-compression magnification view
    blurring of, 198–99
    cyst and solid mass similarity, 118
    evaluation of calcifications, 213–15
    specimen radiography, 331
    summation shadows, 28, 30
Malignancy
    clustered microcalcifications, 15
    correlation with calcifications in a solitary cluster, 232
    hamartomas and, 148
    likelihood in solitary cluster of microcalcifications, 250–51
    suspicious calcifications, 189, 191–92, 211–12
Malignant fibrous histiocytoma, 147
Malignant lesions, 85–86, 92. *See also* Ductal carcinoma *in situ*
    developing density, 159
    fibroglandular density obscuring small benign or malignant lesions, 177, 179–80, 182–84
    spot-compression magnification, 107–10
Mammographic positioning
    anticipated location of lesions, 43–45, 47
    axillary tail, 42–43
    blind areas, 47–48
    poorly marginated density, 37–39
Mammographic technique and image quality
    contrast and optical density, 63–68
    film processing, 71–77
    motion unsharpness, 56–58
    overview, 51–54, 56–60
    phototiming, 58–60, 71–77
    technical quality of test images, 51–54
Manual technique, 26, 64, 72, **73–74**, 278
Marker-guided view. *See* Metallic markers
mAs, 56–58, 63–68, 71, **78**

Masses, 42. *See also* Microlobulated masses; Solid masses
    with almost completely well-defined margins, 101–11
    anechoic, 120, 139, 287
    circumscribed, 257–62, 264
    fat-containing, 145, 147–48, 151, 154–55
    halo sign, 124
    hypoechoic, 122, 139, 148, 289, 313
    palpable mass obscured by dense fibroglandular tissue with mammographically visible mass in a different location, 177, 179–80, 182–84
    with partial halo sign and most margins obscured by isodense tissue, 115–20, 122–24
    suspicious for malignancy, 177, 179
    well-defined, noncalcified, smooth margins, 81–83
Mastectomy, 106, 154
Mastitis, 169, 305, **313**
Mediolateral needle approach, 322
Mediolateral oblique view. *See also* Augmented breast mammography
    anticipated location of identified lesions, 43–45, 47
    imaging sequence, 6–9, 12–13, 15
    isolated cluster of tiny calcifications, 189
    lesion seen on only one projection, 21, 23, 27–28
    mass with almost completely well-defined margins, 101
    milk of calcium in tiny benign cysts, 245, 247
    poorly marginated density in, 37–39
    preoperative needle localization, 32
    suboptimal inclusion of pectoral muscles, 51–53
    triangulation estimates of mammographic lesions, 3–4, 6–9, 10–12
Medullary carcinoma, 96, 110–11, 127, **139**
    differential diagnosis
        cyst, 115
        involuting fibroadenoma, 127
Meniscus calcifications, 247
Menopause
    postmenopausal women, 94, 169, 223, 305, 339
    premenopausal women, 168–69
Mesenchymal elements, 92
Metallic markers, **180, 182**, 184, 207, 217
Metastasis, 92, 315
Microcalcifications
    clustered, 3–7, 9–13, 15, 26
    ductal carcinoma *in situ*, 89
    ductal pattern, 225

T

U

V

W

X–Z